Methods in Immunology and Immunochemistry

VOLUME IV

Agglutination, Complement, Neutralization, and Inhibition

Methods in
IMMUNOLOGY
and IMMUNOCHEMISTRY

Edited by

CURTIS A. WILLIAMS

THE STATE UNIVERSITY OF NEW YORK
PURCHASE, NEW YORK

MERRILL W. CHASE

THE ROCKEFELLER UNIVERSITY
NEW YORK, NEW YORK

Volume IV

Agglutination, Complement, Neutralization, and Inhibition

1977

ACADEMIC PRESS   New York   San Francisco   London
A SUBSIDIARY OF HARCOURT BRACE JOVANOVICH, PUBLISHERS

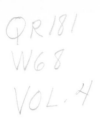

ACADEMIC PRESS, INC.
111 Fifth Avenue, New York, New York 10003

United Kingdom Edition published by
ACADEMIC PRESS, INC. (LONDON) LTD.
24/28 Oval Road, London NW1

Library of Congress Cataloging in Publication Data

Williams, Curtis Alvin,   Date
      Methods in immunology and immunochemistry.

      Includes bibliographies.
      CONTENTS.–v. 1.   Preparation of antigens and
antibodies.–v. 2.   Physical and chemical methods.
–v. 3.   Reactions of antibodies with soluble
antigens.–v. 4.   Agglutination, complement,
neutralization, and inhibition.
      1.   Immunology.   2.   Immunochemistry–Technique.
I.   Chase, Merrill W., joint author.   II.   Title.
QR181.W68   615$'$.37   67-22779
ISBN 0–12–754404–6

Topical Listing of Contents

Chapter 16. Agglutination and Flocculation

Slide Agglutination, 1; Tube Agglutination: Saline Agglutinins, 2; Quantitative Cell-Counting Method, 4; Tube Agglutination: Incomplete Antibodies and Cold Agglutinins, 9; Enzyme-Treated Erythrocytes, 14; Lectins, 19.

Direct Passive–Polysaccharide Adsorption on Untreated Erythrocytes, 26; Hemagglutination with Tannic Acid-Treated Erythrocytes, 30; Antigen–Erythrocyte Conjugates Prepared with Bisdiazobenzidine, 41; Preparation of Stable Formalinized Antigen–Erythrocyte Conjugates, 46.

Special Methods of Chemical Bonding for Preparing Antigen–Erythrocyte Conjugates, 47: Chromic Chloride, Carbodiimide Coupling, Difluorodinitrobenzene, 48; Specific Coupling to Erythrocyte Antigenic Sites, 48.

Antiglobulin Reactions with Erythrocytes, 49: Direct, Indirect Reactions, 50; Inhibition Tests, 52; Antiglobulin Consumption Test, 53; The Red Cell-Linked Antigen Test, 54.

Mixed Agglutination and Erythrocytes, 56; The Mixed Agglutination Reaction, 57; The Mixed Antiglobulin Reaction, 58; The Mixed Hemadsorption Test, 63.

Inhibition by Antibodies and Antibody-like Reagents: Semiquantitative Tube Tests, 67.

Quantitative Inhibition (Cell-Counting Method), 73.

Preparation of Bacteria as Antigens, 76; Special Antigens, 80; Antisera, 83; Agglutination Tests, 84: Tube Tests, 84; Cover Slip Tests, 86; Macroscopic Slide Tests, 87.

Enumeration of Bacterial Colonies in Liquid Media, 88; Antigens Inhibiting Agglutination, 89; Interpretation and Applications, 89.

JA 3 - '78

Appendix II

Contributors to Volume IV

Numbers in parentheses indicate the pages on which the authors' contributions begin.

E. R. ARQUILLA (41), Department of Pathology, College of Medicine, University of California, Irvine, California

RICHARD C. BLINKOFF (91),* The Rockefeller University, New York, New York

H. E. BOND (226),** National Cancer Institute, Bethesda, Maryland

WILLIAM C. BOYD (19),† Boston University School of Medicine, Boston, Massachusetts

J. BOZICEVICH (121),‡ Biomedics Research Laboratories, Inc., Division of Litton Industries, Kensington, Maryland

MERRILL W. CHASE (54, 61, 127, 136, 166, 180, 194, 198, 200, 226, 238, 241, 242, 250, 253, 254, 256, 258, 261, 266, 267, 269, 271, 275, 282, 285, 293, 296, 303, 407), The Rockefeller University, New York, New York

B. CINADER (313), Institute of Immunology, Departments of Medical Genetics, Medical Biophysics, and Clinical Biochemistry, Medical Sciences Building, University of Toronto, Ontario, Canada

HARVEY R. COLTEN (226), Department of Pediatrics, Harvard Medical School, Boston, Massachusetts

R. R. A. COOMBS (49, 54, 56), Department of Pathology, University of Cambridge, Cambridge, England

MARY B. GIBBS (1, 2, 4, 73), Department of Immunology, Walter Reed Army Institute of Research, Washington, D.C.

O. GÖTZE (219), Department of Molecular Immunology, Scripps Clinic and Research Foundation, La Jolla, California

* Present address: 830 Broadway, New York, New York.
** Present address: Electro-Nucleonics Laboratories, Inc., Bethesda, Maryland.
† Present address: 1241 Prospect Street, La Jolla, California.
‡ Present address: 6810 Hillmead Road, Bethesda, Maryland.

JOSEPH HAIMOVICH (386), Department of Chemical Immunology, The Weizmann Institute of Science, Rehovot, Israel

PETER M. HENSON (271), Department of Experimental Pathology, Scripps Clinic and Research Foundation, La Jolla, California

LOUIS G. HOFFMANN (127, 137, 167, 173, 225, 227, 228, 232), Department of Microbiology, College of Medicine, State University of Iowa, Iowa City, Iowa

ROLLIN D. HOTCHKISS (88), The Rockefeller University, New York, New York

M. A. JESAITIS (375), The Rockefeller University, New York, New York

MAURICE LANDY (26),* National Institute of Allergy and Infectious Diseases, Bethesda, Maryland

IRWIN H. LEPOW (180, 183, 186, 201, 242), Department of Medicine, University of Connecticut Health Center, Farmington, Connecticut

PHILIP LEVINE (9, 12), Immunohematology Division, Ortho Research Foundation, Raritan, New Jersey

STEPHEN D. LITWIN (115),† Department of the Army Headquarters, U.S. Army Medical Research Laboratory, Fort Knox, Kentucky

MANFRED M. MAYER (127, 137, 167, 173, 225, 227, 228, 229, 232, 235, 238, 241, 256, 261, 267), Department of Microbiology, The Johns Hopkins School of Medicine, Baltimore, Maryland

P. L. MOLLISON (49, 54), Wright-Fleming Institute of Microbiology, St. Mary's Hospital Medical School, London, England

HANS J. MÜLLER-EBERHARD (127, 176, 180, 190, 205, 209, 212, 217, 219, 220, 223, 250, 260, 263, 265, 269), Department of Molecular Immunology, Scripps Clinic and Research Foundation, La Jolla, California

ERWIN NETER (76, 89),‡ Departments of Pediatrics and Microbiology, State University of New York at Buffalo, Buffalo, New York

---

* Present Address: Schweizerisches Forschungs Institut, 7270 Davos, Switzerland.
† Present address: Division of Human Genetics, Cornell University Medical College, New York, New York.
‡ Present address: Department of Bacteriology, Children's Hospital, Buffalo, New York.

JACK PENSKY (242),* Department of Medicine, Case Western Reserve University, Cleveland, Ohio

M. RAYNAUD (277, 283, 288, 289, 292, 294, 301, 302, 310),† Institut Pasteur, Annexe de Garches, Garches, France

E. H. RELYVELD (277, 283, 288, 289, 292, 294, 301, 302, 310), Institut Pasteur, Annexe de Garches, Garches, France

MICHAEL SELA (386), Department of Chemical Immunology, The Weizmann Institute of Science, Rehovot, Israel

SIDNEY SHULMAN (94), Sperm Antibody Laboratory, Department of Microbiology, Departments of Urology and of Obstetrics and Gynecology, New York Medical College, New York, New York

GEORG F. SPRINGER (14, 67), Department of Microbiology, Northwestern University, Evanston Hospital, Evanston, Illinois

ABRAM B. STAVITSKY (30, 47), Department of Microbiology, Case Western Reserve University School of Medicine, Cleveland, Ohio

MARGARET TREACY (9, 12), Immunohematology Division, Ortho Research Foundation, Raritan, New Jersey

CURTIS A. WILLIAMS (127, 136, 166, 180, 194, 198, 200, 226, 238, 241, 242, 250, 253, 254, 256, 258, 261, 266, 267, 269, 271),‡ The Rockefeller University, New York, New York

N. D. ZINDER (375), The Rockefeller University, New York, New York

* Present address: Cleveland Veterans' Hospital, 10701 East Boulevard, Cleveland, Ohio 44106.
† Deceased.
‡ Present address: The State University of New York, Purchase, New York.

Preface

In planning an open-ended treatise on methodology in immunochemistry and immunology, we considered the needs not only of the specialist but of those whose primary concern in other areas of biology may suggest application of immunological tools. A rigid format was adopted for the first five volumes, a choice which has caused unexpected problems in publication. Volumes published to date have been very well received.

Volume I is concerned with typical preparative methods employed in handling antigens, antibodies, and laboratory animals. Volume II presents general chemical and physiochemical methods used in immunological research. Volume III deals with antigen-antibody and hapten-antibody reactions *in vitro*, in free solution, and in gels. Volume IV covers direct and indirect agglutination reactions, complement-fixation procedures, hemolytic intermediates, isolation of complement components, complement-related proteins, antisera to complement components, and neutralization reactions (toxins, enzymes, bacteria, bacteriophages). Volume V deals with antigen-antibody reactions *in vivo* : anaphylaxis, Arthus reactions, tolerance, immune suppression with chemical agents, radiation effects, phagocytosis and clearance, antibody synthesis *in vitro*, immunohistological methods, and applied electron microscopy.

Our aim has been to open our colleagues' notebooks to bring together detailed procedures that are hard to retrieve from the original literature and to provide indexes which can be used with confidence. Contributors were asked to include not only the details of procedures they had found most satisfactory in their own laboratory, but also critical remarks on common pitfalls and interpretation of results, references to alternative methods, and mention of applications to other problems. While not all topics are easily suited to this format, we feel that insofar as our general objectives are achieved, these volumes represent high potential energy.

Some important general topics as well as many specific methods are to be covered in future volumes including hypersensitivity, immunity to infection, transplantation, and immunogenetics.

We again express our appreciation to the advisory editors.

CURTIS A. WILLIAMS
MERRILL W. CHASE

Contents of Other Volumes

CHAPTER 16

Agglutination and Flocculation

A. Direct Hemagglutination

1. SLIDE AGGLUTINATION*

The slide agglutination technique provides a simple and rapid means of determining blood groups. The method is most frequently employed in ABO and Rh grouping. The procedure may be carried out on microscope slides, large glass plates, or white porcelain or plastic tiles. To avoid errors due to evaporation, antisera should be selected which produce agglutination within a few minutes. Whole blood or a 5% suspension of cells in saline may be used with antisera that give optimal results in saline. Saline-suspended red blood cells are not suitable for use with sera containing incomplete antibodies; whole blood must be used.

a. MATERIALS

Glass slides or plates with small circular wells about 1.5 cm in diameter made on the glass surface, either with a wax pencil or by dipping the rim of culture tubes into molten paraffin wax and pressing it onto the surface
Pasteur pipettes
Applicator sticks
Whole blood, either oxalated, heparinized, or citrated
Antiserum (known anti-A and anti-B sera or anti-Rh sera)
View box with transilluminated ground glass or flashed opal glass surface maintained at 37° to 47° by incandescent light bulbs inside the view box

b. PROCEDURE FOR ABO GROUPING

A drop of whole blood is placed in each of two circles on the slide with a Pasteur pipette. One drop of anti-A serum is added to the first circle and a drop of anti-B serum to the second circle. The drops are mixed with clean applicator sticks and spread out to fill the circles. The slide is tilted with a circular rolling motion and observed for agglutination. A circle containing a drop of the blood and a drop of normal human serum of of group AB serves as a control.

* Section 16.A.1 was contributed by Mary B. Gibbs.

Interpretation

Blood group	Anti-A serum	Anti-B serum
O	−	−
A	+	−
B	−	+
AB	+	+

c. PROCEDURE FOR Rh GROUPING

One drop of the Rh antiserum and a drop of whole blood are placed on a plain slide warmed to 37° to 45° on the view box. The drops are mixed and spread out to cover an oval area about $3\frac{1}{2} \times 1\frac{3}{4}$ cm. The box is rocked slowly from side to side and the slide is observed for agglutination up to 2 minutes. Each test has the following controls: (1) 2 to 3 drops of whole blood alone, (2) anti-Rh serum with known Rh-positive blood, and (3) anti-Rh serum with known Rh-negative blood.

Interpretation. Agglutination indicates that the red blood cells contain an Rh antigen corresponding to the Rh agglutinin in the serum used for the test.

Caution. Rouleaux formation may occur with evaporation and be mistaken for agglutination.

2. TEST TUBE AGGLUTINATION: SALINE AGGLUTININS*†

Blood group antibodies which agglutinate red blood cells suspended in saline are generally referred to as "saline agglutinins." Test-tube agglutinations are preferred for blood grouping with saline agglutinins which require more than a few minutes for agglutination, such as the determination of group A_2 cells, and when the chance for evaporation precludes the use of the slide technique. The method is especially useful in performing titrations when the relative activities of agglutinins of different sera are to be compared.

a. MATERIALS

Test tubes, 12×75 mm
Test tube racks
Pipettes, 1 and 0.1 ml
Isotonic saline solution (0.9% NaCl)
Centrifuge

---

* Section 16.A.2 was contributed by Mary B. Gibbs.

† See Section 16.A.4.a for agglutinins which require albumin or other macromolecules instead of saline.

b. Erythrocyte Suspensions

Freshly prepared 2% saline suspensions of washed, packed red blood cells are used in the test. Whole blood collected into sterile modified Alsever's solution (see Sections 16.B.2.a.iv and 17.B.1.b) or in acid citrate dextran as used in blood banks (see Section 16.A.5.c.i) and stored at +4° are suitable for use within 3 to 4 weeks.

c. Procedure for Blood Grouping

One-tenth milliliter of the antiserum and an equal volume of the cell suspension are delivered into a test tube. The contents are mixed and incubated at a temperature appropriate for the system, with occasional shaking (37° for 60 minutes with Rh agglutinins; 25° for 15 minutes with A and B agglutinins, 25° for 30 minutes before dismissing a diagnosis of group A₂). The reactions can be read in several ways: by hand loupe (5× to 6× magnification), or by removing a microdrop to a glass slide without cover slip and reading at 100× under the microscope,* or by centrifugation and resuspension. The latter method is given here. The tubes are centrifuged at 600 g for 1 minute. The cell pack is dislodged by gentle shaking over a mirror and observed for agglutination. Known positive and known negative sera, as well as cells suspended in buffered saline similarly are included with each test. For research purposes, microscopic observations on microdrops removed from a noncentrifuged reaction mixture with a 1 mm glass rod allow definitive end points.

d. Titration of Agglutinins

The following procedure used with A and B agglutinins can be applied to any saline agglutinating system with proper adjustment of the incubation time and temperature. The test is carried out in a series of 10 or more test tubes. Successively doubled dilutions are made in saline, and 0.1 ml of each dilution is delivered into each tube, the first tube containing neat serum or a 1:2 dilution. In each tube, 0.1 ml of the 2% suspension of red cells is then added. A control tube, preferably set up in duplicate, which contains 0.1 ml of saline and 0.1 ml of the cell suspension is included with each test. The contents of the tubes are mixed; the tubes are incubated at room temperature, agitated at 30 minutes, and read at 60 minutes. In the centrifuge method, the tubes are centrifuged at 600 g for 1 minute and the degree of agglutination is determined by shaking the tubes gently to dislodge the packed cells. The degree of ag-

---

* The test may be miniaturized by using small tubes (as 50 × 60 mm) and adding single drops of saline, known agglutinin, and erythrocyte suspension. The drop of saline prevents rouleaux formation.

glutination is arbitrarily graded from $++++$ to 0. The titer of the anti-serum is the highest dilution of serum given visible agglutination.

The method gives reproducible results when the same cell suspension is used. The results of titrations performed on different days may differ by a factor of 2 or more because of day-to-day variations in test conditions. For maximum accuracy, in comparing the activities of agglutinins, a standard reference serum should be tested simultaneously with each group of titrations of unknown antisera. The ratio of the titer of the reference serum to the titer of an unknown antiserum is reproducible under any test conditions. The method described here serves for most purposes. For fine quantitation and determination of "HD_{50}," that is, the amount of antibody needed to agglutinate 50% of the erythrocytes, Section 16.A.3 is applicable.

3. QUANTITATIVE CELL-COUNTING METHOD*

The cell-counting assay method of Wilkie and Becker[1] makes possible the quantitative estimation of hemagglutinin activity and describes the course of the reaction as a curve which relates agglutination response to concentration of hemagglutinins.

a. PRINCIPLE

When varying quantities of a given agglutinin are allowed to react with a given volume of red blood cells to the equilibrium state, the relation between the proportion of cells agglutinated and the logarithm of the amount of agglutinin used is sigmoidal within the region of incomplete or partial agglutination. The sigmoid curve is transformed to a straight line by converting the original function, proportions of cells agglutinated, to probability units or probits[2] which are plotted on semilog paper as described below. The 50% hemagglutinating unit of agglutinin, designated HD_{50}, is interpolated from a log probit plot of experimental results or, for a more accurate estimate, can be computed from the linear equation. The HD_{50} is defined as the amount of undiluted serum per milliliter of dilution (ml/ml) required to agglutinate 50% of the test cell suspension. The method is applicable to any hemagglutinating system in which the agglutination response is a sigmoidal function of the agglutinin concentration in the region of partial agglutination.

The procedure to be described is used in our laboratory with the iso-hemagglutinins of the ABO system. The modifications of Silber et al.[3] must

---

* Section 16.A.3 was contributed by Mary B. Gibbs.

[1] M. H. Wilkie and E. L. Becker, *J. Immunol.* **74**, 192 (1955).
[2] C. I. Bliss, *Science* **79**, 38 (1934).
[3] R. Silber, M. B. Gibbs, E. F. Jahn, and J. H. Akeroyd, *Blood* **17**, 282 (1961).

be used with Rh agglutinins: with anti-Rh "saline agglutinins," incubation at 37° is practiced for 2 to 4 hours before the cell suspensions are placed on the rotator (at 37°) for 30 minutes; with incomplete-Rh agglutinins, erythrocytes are first trypsinized under special conditions.

b. MATERIALS AND SPECIAL EQUIPMENT

Buffered saline at pH 7.3,* sterilized by filtration through Millipore or other membranes of ca. 0.22 μm pore size (Vol. I, Chap. 2.C.5) and stored at room temperature, is used for diluting serum and suspending red cells. All procedures with the Coulter counter are carried out in a saline–albumin solution (0.5 ml of 25% human serum albumin per 100 ml of hypertonic buffered saline to provide 1.25 mg of albumin per milliliter).

Red cells are obtained from blood collected into one volume of sterile modified Alsever's solution (Sections 16.B.2.a.iv and 16.A.2.a) and stored at 4°. Cell suspensions, prepared from washed cells, are made up to a concentration of 24 to 26 × 10^6 per milliliter of 0.5% cell suspension in plastic Erlenmeyer flasks and used within 4 hours of preparation. Reproducible assays depend to a large extent on the standardization of cell concentrations. Accurate standardizations can be made rapidly with the Coulter electronic cell counter with use of a 100-μm aperture.

Antiserum samples are represented by venous blood incubated at 37° for 1 hour and left overnight "on the clot" at 4°. The serum is removed and inactivated at 56° for 45 minutes. Sera are then allowed to stand for 72 hours at 4° (since freshly inactivated sera have seemed to show lesser titers) before storage in small samples at −20°. Prior to use, sera are thawed rapidly at 37° and allowed to reach room temperature.

Special test tubes, 12 × 40 mm are required. They are available commercially (Bellco 14-1710 SPL). Highly flexible rubber stoppers, size 00, café-au-lait, are recommended for these tubes. These stoppers fit the tubes snugly without trapping cells and will not "pop-off" during rotation.

Dacie-type bench rotators, 10 rpm, are used for agitation of test mixtures in the special tubes.† Commercial rotators are available which can be adapted to hold the 12 × 40 mm tubes. A Kahn shaker can be used with larger test volumes in plastic flasks.

---

* We employ a hypertonic PBS at pH 7.3, with 0.067 M phosphate and 0.8% NaCl: Dissolve per liter 8 gm of NaCl, 1.35 gm of KH$_2$PO$_4$, and 8.112 gm of Na$_2$HPO$_4$ (exsiccated). The buffer component corresponds to buffer 28 (Vol. II, Appendix II) at pH 7.5. Hypertonicity is necessary to preserve the cells during the long period on the Dacie-type rotator.

† A tilted plate, with attached clips to hold tubes, rotates slowly. The device is similar to the Multi-Purpose Rotator of Scientific Industries Inc., Queens Village, New York, with speeds from 6 to 60 rpm.

Pipettes, Mohr type, Class A (Kimax 37025) 1-ml and 2-ml sizes are recommended for delivery of serum dilutions and cell suspensions to the test tubes. Pipetting errors are negligible with these pipettes.

c. Preliminary Test

In the cell-counting procedure, a 2-fold titration of the antiserum is designed to give at least four points in the region of partial agglutination (between 12% and 95%), which will bracket the 50% agglutination end point. For selection of the antiserum concentrations to be employed, it is best to perform a preliminary qualitative test tube titration with a 2% cell suspension. (Section 16.5.A.2.d) to obtain a crude estimate of the serum dilution which will give 50% agglutination with 0.5% erythrocyte suspension. In general, the 50% end point for 0.5% cell suspension occurs about two tubes beyond the "one-plus" end point of the qualitative titration with use of 2% cell suspension. The dilutions of antiserum to be employed fall within a 4-fold range above and below this serum dilution.

d. Procedure

Each quantitative titration consists of four 2-fold serum dilutions which are chosen on the basis of the preliminary test. Serum dilutions are prepared individually in class A volumetric flasks, and 0.5-ml portions of each dilution are delivered into each of two tubes from a 1-ml Mohr pipette. Saline controls receive 0.5 ml of the buffered saline. Five-tenths milliliter of the standardized cell suspension is added to each test and each control tube (a 2-ml Mohr pipette is used to deliver into each set of four tubes). A fresh pipette is used for every four deliveries. The tubes are closed with rubber stoppers and placed on the rotator. Dependent upon the rapidity of the aggregation and disaggregation reactions of the iso-agglutinin being tested, test mixtures may remain on the rotator (aggregation method of equilibration), or they may be rotated for 45 minutes to assure optimal sensitization, then centrifuged at 600 g for 1 minute, and finally replaced on the rotator (disaggregation method of equilibration). The former method is used with antisera from individuals immunized with blood group substance; the latter is employed with sera containing only naturally occurring isoagglutinins. The time required for equilibrium reactions with either type of antiserum by the appropriate method is highly variable (1 to 5 hours). Our routine practice is to use a 5-hour period of rotation with all anti-A and anti-B equilibrated by the indicated methods. When a shorter rotation period is desired, or when agglutinins of blood group systems other than ABO are to be tested, the rates of aggregation and disaggregation must be determined for each antiserum as described by Wilkie and Becker.[1] A reaction rate study is also indicated when the assay curve is curvilinear.

i. Cell Counting

After equilibration, the extent of agglutination in each tube is measured by determining the number of unagglutinated (free) cells, either by hemacytometer or by the Model B Coulter electronic counter as described below.[4]

(a) *Hemacytometer*. Spencer Bright-Line hemacytometers and optical glass cover slips are cleaned in flowing warm tap water and rinsed with distilled water and two changes of ethanol (these hemacytometers have the "improved "Neubauer" ruling). The chambers of the hemacytometers and the cover slips are polished with lens paper. Both chambers of the hemacytometer are charged by holding a filled capillary tube (0.15 to 0.2 mm, OD) at a 45° angle to the cover slip. The free cells in the four corner squares and the central square of the red cell counting area are counted in the usual manner. When the free cell count for this area ($\frac{1}{5}$ mm^2) is less than 100 cells, cells lying in the entire red blood cell counting area (1 mm^2) are counted. This procedure is repeated on each tube, two counts being made on each tube (four counts per dilution of antiserum or saline control).

Calculations: Average the four counts for a given dilution of serum or for the saline control and multiply by 50 for $\frac{1}{5}$ mm^2 area counts or by 10 for 1 mm^2 area counts to obtain free cells/mm^3. Divide the value obtained with each cell–serum mixture by that of the saline controls (total cell count) and multiply by 100 to get the percentage of free cells: 100 − % free cells = % agglutinated cells.

(b) *Electronic counter*.[4] Equilibrated test mixtures or saline controls are diluted for counting by transferring 0.1 ml of test mixture to 20 ml (or 25 ml) buffered saline–albumin diluent. The sample is gently inverted three times and three successive instrument counts are made of each diluted sample, using a 70-μm aperture. Saline controls are counted with the upper threshold set at infinity (∞). The upper threshold setting for counting free cells in agglutinated samples must be determined for each erythrocyte population since distributions of cell sizes differ. With the proper gain adjustments and upper thresholds, it is possible with the instrument to obtain free-cell counts which are identical with hemacytometer counts. Information on gain adjustments and selection of upper thresholds can be obtained from the manufacturer.*

---

[4] M. B. Gibbs, J. C. Dreyfus, and L. A. Aguilu, *J. Immunol.* **94,** 62 (1965).
* Coulter Electronic Sales Co., 520 West 20th Street, Hialeah, Florida.

Calculations: Average of 6 counts for duplicate tubes + (coincidence − background) × dilution (201 or 251) × 2 = free cells per milliliter of reaction mixture or saline controls. The percentage of agglutinated cells is obtained in the manner used with the hemacytometer count. Instructions for determination of coincidence and background is found in the manufacturer's literature.

ii. Treatment of Data

The percentages of agglutination can be plotted on the ordinate of probability-log paper (Keuffel & Esser 359-22 or 359-22G) against the concentrations of antiserum on the abscissa. An alternative method is to plot the probit corresponding to the percentages of agglutination against the logarithms of the serum concentrations on semilog paper. Tables of probits are found in most texts of statistical tables. The HD_{50} unit of agglutinin activity is found by interpolation on the linear regression line at the ordinate of 50% agglutination (or probit 5.0). A simple formula for computing the HD_{50} is:

$$Y - \bar{Y} = b(X - \bar{X})$$

where $Y = 5.0$ (probit for 50% agglutination); $\bar{Y}$ = mean of the four experimentally determined probits; b = slope of the regression; X = the log of the HD_{50} value to be determined; and $\bar{X}$ = mean logarithm of the four serum concentrations used. The slope can be determined by the method of least squares using the logarithms of the antiserum concentration as the X values and the probits as the Y values.

In our hands, an HD_{50} is reproduced on the same day in independent assays with an error of 5.7% (one standard error) which represents the total error resulting from making the test preparations and estimating the free cells either by hemacytometer or instrument. Instrument estimates have a slightly smaller error but less than one would expect, because of the error in preparation of dilutions for counting. By using accurately standardized suspensions of cells of equal storage age, controlled incubation temperatures, and reagents at room temperature at the time of serum dilution, the standard error of the HD_{50} for ten assays of an antiserum performed on different days was 11.2%. The error increased to 42% when no effort was made to control the test conditions. Since adherence to rigid standard conditions or to universally uniform experimental conditions is not practical, it is advisable to express the results of an assay as the potency of an antiserum relative to the potency of a standard reference serum which is tested simultaneously under the same test conditions. The average standard error of the relative potency ratio (standard HD_{50}/unknown HD_{50}) is 5.8% (2.6% to 9.8%). A potency ratio is, of course, invalid if the assay curves of the standard and unknown sera are not parallel.

iii. Limitations

The only limitation to the method with reversible antigen–antibody systems and hemacytometer counting is the weak binding capacity of some agglutinins. The agglutinates formed by centrifugation of cells that are sensitized with these agglutinins will dissociate completely in the lower region of agglutination. Instrument counting is limited to use with agglutinins that form agglutinates bound sufficiently firmly so as not to dissociate within 3 minutes after dilution of the sample for counting.

4. TUBE AGGLUTINATION: INCOMPLETE ANTIBODIES AND COLD AGGLUTININS

a. Test Tube Agglutination: Incomplete Antibodies*†

Hemagglutinins are classified arbitrarily as "warm" or "cold" antibodies, the former reacting optimally at 37° and the latter reacting optimally at temperatures below 37°. Incomplete antibodies may be defined as immunoglobulins (IgG or IgA) capable of combining specifically with blood group antigens on red cells but incapable of agglutinating erythrocytes suspended in simple salt solutions. Several synonyms for incomplete antibodies are in use, such as: albumin agglutinins, blocking antibodies and hyperimmune antibodies.

Almost all incomplete antibodies, especially those of the Rh-Hr system, have been shown to be 7 S γ-globulins in contrast to complete antibodies (saline agglutinins) which are almost exclusively 19 S γ-globulins.[1]

Incomplete antibodies of various blood group specificities are responsible for all cases of hemolytic disease of the newborn and for the vast majority of intragroup transfusion reactions and decreased survival of transfused cells. They may also be present on the surface of red cells of patients suffering from "warm" acquired hemolytic anemia as is demonstrable in eluates.‡ These autoantibodies frequently have Rh specificity.

Incomplete antibodies may be detected by the following methods:

i. Agglutination in Macromolecular Media

It has been shown that the addition of certain macromolecules will decrease the force of repulsion between red cells, allowing them to

---

* Section 16.A.4.a was contributed by Philip Levine and Margaret Treacy.

† Agglutination of "saline" antibodies is discussed in Section 16.A.2.

[1] H. H. Fudenberg, H.G. Kunkel, and E. C. Franklin, *Acta Haematol.* **10,** 522 (1959).

‡ Methods for isolation of antibodies from blood cells or stromata are described in Vol. I, Chap. 3.B.2.

approach each other more closely, a condition necessary for agglutination.[2] Bovine albumin at concentrations varying from 20 to 30% is most widely used at present. Antibodies of the Rh-Hr system are effectively demonstrated by this procedure. Although tests conducted in albumin media usually will not detect certain antibodies—for example anti-K and anti-Fy[a],[*] which require the antihuman globulin test (see below)—the albumin tests do offer the advantage of identifying the occasional anti-c (hr′), which can be missed if only the antihuman globulin test were to be used. Red cells that fail to show agglutination in macromolecular media can be washed subsequently and tested by the antihuman globulin procedure (Section 16.B.5).

Procedure with Albumin-Saline (modified after Diamond and Denton[3]). Place two drops of the serum to be tested in a small (10 × 75 mm) test tube. Add 1 drop of a 5% suspension in saline of washed red cells of known antigenic composition. Add 2 drops of bovine albumin (20 to 30%). Incubate the tube at 37° for at least 15 minutes. Centrifuge at 3400 rpm for 15 seconds or 1000 rpm for 1 minute. Read for agglutination with the aid of a hand lens.

ii. Detection of Incomplete Antibodies by Agglutination of Enzyme-Treated Erythrocytes

This procedure is discussed in Section 16.A.5. Automated systems for typing large numbers of individuals often involve brief exposure of the erythrocytes to dilute bromelin, in connection with substances such as polyvinylpyrrolidone to induce rouleaux formation during part of the operating cycle.[4] M-antigen and Fy[a]-antigen are destroyed by proteases, and such tests must be made without enzyme exposure.[5]

iii. Anti-human Globulin Test (Synonym: Coombs Test)

Antibodies specific for certain systems, for example, Kell, Duffy, Kidd, and Lewis (Table I) may fail to agglutinate erythrocytes even in the

[2] W. Pollack, H. J. Hager, R. Reckel, D. Toren, and H. O. Singher, *Transfusion* **5**, 158 (1965).
[*] Intensive study of human erythrocytes has led to recognition of many different "systems" and varieties within each system. This multiplicity is well portrayed in Table I (reproduced by permission of authors and publisher from R. R. Race and R. Sanger, "Blood Groups in Man," 6th ed. Table I. Blackwell, Oxford, 1975). Detailed discussion of the systems is given in this volume and in P. L. Mollison, "Blood Transfusion in Clinical Medicine," 5th ed., Blackwell, Oxford, 1972.
[3] L. K. Diamond and R. L. Denton, *J. Lab. Clin. Med.* **30**, 821 (1945).
[4] R. E. Rosenfield, I. O. Szymanski, and S. Kochwa, *Cold Spring Harbor Symp. Quant. Biol.* **29**, 427 (1964).
[5] R. E. Rosenfield, personal communication (1968).

TABLE I[a]

BLOOD GROUP ANTIGENS IN MAN

System	Antigens detected by	
	Positive reaction with specific antibody	Positive reaction with one antibody, negative with another
A_1A_2BO	A_1, B H	A_2, A_3, A_x and other A and B variants
MNSs	M, N, S, s, U, M^g, M$_1$, M', Tm, Sj, Hu, He, Mi^a, Vw(Gr), Mur, Hil, Hut, M^v, Vr, Ri^a, St^a, Mt^a, Cl^a, Ny^a, Sul, Far	M_2, N_2, M^c, M^a, N^a, M^r, M^z, S_2
P	P_1, P^k, Luke	P_2
Rh	D, C, c, C^w, C^x, E, e, e^s (VS), E^w, G, ce(f), ce^s(V), Ce, CE, cE, D^w, E^T, Go^a, hr^s, hr^H, hr^B, $\bar{R}^N$, Rh33, Rh35, Be^a, LW	D^u, C^u, E^u, and many other variant forms of D, C and e
Lutheran	Lu^a, Lu^b, Lu^{a}Lu^b (Lu3), Lu6, Lu9, Lu4, Lu5, Lu7, Lu8, Lu10–17	
Kell	K, k, Kp^a, Kp^b, Ku, Js^a, Js^b, Ul^a, Wk^a, K11, KL, K12–17	
Lewis	Le^a, Le^b, Le^c, Le$^\alpha$, Le^x	
Duffy	Fy^a, Fy^b, Fy3, Fy4	
Kidd	Jk^a, Jk^b, Jk^{a}Jk^b (Jk3)	
Diego	Di^a, Di^b	
Yt	Yt^a, Yt^b	
Auberger	Au^a	
Dombrock	Do^a, Do^b	
Colton	Co^a, Co^b, Co^{a}Co^b	
Sid	Sd^a	
Scianna	Sc1, Sc2 (Bu^a)	
Very frequent antigens	Vel, Ge, Lan, Gy^a, At^a, En^a, Wr^b, Jr^a, Kn^a, El, Dp, Gn^a, Jo^a (and other examples)	
Very infrequent antigens	An^a, By, Bi, Bp^a, Bx^a, Chr^a, Evans, Good, Gf, Heibel, Hey, Hov, Ht^a, Je^a, Jn^a, Levay, Ls^a, Mo^a, Or, Pt^a, Rl^a, Rd, Re^a, Sw^a, To^a, Tr^a, Ts, Wb, Wr^a, Wu, Zd (and others)	
Other antigens	I, i, Bg (HL-A), Chido, Cs^a, Yk^a	
Xg	Xg^a	

[a] Reproduced by permission from R. R. Race and R. Sanger, "Blood Groups in Man," 6th ed., Table I. Blackwell, Oxford, 1975, with slight emendation.

presence of albumin or other macromolecules (see i). Such antibodies after fixation to the red cell surface may be detected by the Coombs test, employing a reagent antiserum made to human serum globulin (see Section 16.B.5). Red cells which have absorbed many of the antibodies occurring in the IgG fraction of serum, for example, anti-Rh, $-$K, $-$Fy^a, $-$S, and the warm antibody of acquired hemolytic anemia can be directly agglutinated by antiserum to human immunoglobulins. On the other hand, red cells sensitized with antibodies of the complement fixing variety, for example, anti-Le^a, $-P_1$, $-Tj^a$, $-Jk^a$, and $-Jk^b$,* immune anti-A and anti-B, and the cold antibody of acquired hemolytic anemia may not be agglutinated directly by the same antiserum; however, these sensitized cells will be agglutinated by an antiserum which recognizes those components of complement that have become fixed to the red cells along with the antibody (Section 16.B.5.a; see subsection e.*iii* for preparation of antiserum to complement components). Antibodies of the complement-fixing variety are potentially hemolytic.

It has been shown that the sensitization of red cells by human serum in the presence of bovine albumin enhances agglutination by an anti-human globulin reagent, presumably by allowing greater antibody uptake.[6] To be effective, the anti-human globulin procedure must employ a reagent which has been standardized carefully with respect to its content of antibodies to the immunoglobulins and to some of the components of complement.

Procedure Modified after Coombs and Associates.[7] To 2 drops of the serum to be tested, add 1 drop of a 5% suspension in bovine albumin of washed red cells of known antigenic composition. Incubate in a water bath at 37° for 15 minutes; wash 3 or 4 times with large volumes of saline; decant the last wash completely. Add 2 drops of anti-human globulin serum and mix. Centrifuge at 3400 rpm for 15 seconds or 1000 rpm for 1 minute. Gently resuspend the sedimented red cells and read for agglutination with the aid of a hand lens.

It must be emphasized that maximal sensitivity of methods for the detection of incomplete antibodies will be obtained only if due regard is given to such variables as red cell concentration, period of incubation, temperature, presence of serum complement, proper washing prior to the addition of the anti-human globulin serum, and the degree of gravitational force applied by centrifugation.

Anti-human globulin tests are discussed in detail in Section 16.B.5.

b. TEST TUBE AGGLUTINATION: COLD AGGLUTININS*

All normal human sera contain cold—complete or incomplete—antibodies which are active at 4°. In some sera, potent cold antibodies have a thermal range extending to 37° although their reactivity is seldom as strong as at room temperature or at 4°. Cold agglutinins may or may not behave as autoantibodies. Coombs recommends (Section 16.B.5.a) collecting venous blood in a warm syringe and keeping the blood at 37°

---

* Section 16.A.4.b was contributed by Philip Levine and Margaret Treacy.

[6] M. Stroup and M. MacIlroy, *Transfusion* **5**, 184 (1965).

[7] R. R. A. Coombs, A. E. Mourant, and R. R. Race, *Lancet* **2**, 15 (1945).

until the erythrocytes are separated and washed three times with warm saline. This is a useful procedure for selected cases, such as autoimmune hemolytic anemia of the cold variety.

Most cold antibodies are saline agglutinins; they have been shown to be 19 S IgM.[1] Specifically, they may be anti-A, anti-B, anti-A₁, anti-H, anti-I, anti-P + P₁ [also designated anti-Tj^a], anti-P₁, anti-Le^a, anti-Le^b, and anti-M and rarely may have other specificities (Section 16.A.4.a, Table I).*

While specific cold antibodies as a rule do not cause frank hemolytic transfusion reactions in ABO compatible recipients, they may reduce the survival time of donor red cells, particularly if one is dealing with antibodies active just below 37° or with patients subjected to hypothermia. Such antibodies can play no role in hemolytic disease of the newborn.

Apparently nonspecific cold agglutinins are found frequently in the sera of normal healthy individuals. Cold agglutinins with much stronger activity can be demonstrated in the sera of patients suffering from acquired hemolytic anemia of the cold variety. Actually their specificity has now been established as anti-I and/or anti-IH.[2] These agglutinins react with the vast majority of red cells including the patient's cells when tested at 4°. Their specificity is revealed if I negative red cells (cord cells or the very rare adult I negative cells) are included in the panel of test cells. The serology of Ii is extremely complex. The studies of Feizi et al.[3] indicate that Ii specificity is concealed in the internal structure of H, A, Le^a, and Le^b substances and antibodies such as anti-IA, -IB, -ILe^{bH}- and -IP₁ have been described. Some variations in the temperature behavior of anti-I with antigen on the intact red cell and antigen obtained by solubilization of the red cell membrane have recently been reported,[4] but these findings have been challenged.[5]

Cold antibodies usually fix complement and may occur in the incomplete form, the most striking example being anti-H, so frequently found adsorbed to the red cells of normal individuals (donor blood) kept at 4°. In performing compatibility tests, this finding could be a source of concern to those unaware of the fact that the antibody in these cases is derived not from the patient's serum but from the donor's serum and thus is behaving as an autoantibody. Serum removed from clots formed at

[1] H. H. Fudenberg, H. G. Kunkel, and E. C. Franklin, *Acta Haematol.* **10**, 522, (1959).
[2] A. S. Wiener, L. J. Unger, L. Cohen, and J. Feldman, *Ann. Intern. Med.* **44**, 221 (1956).
[3] T. Feizi, E. A. Kabat, G. Vicari, B. Anderson, and W. L. Marsh, *J. Exp. Med.* **133**, 39 (1971).
[4] W. F. Rosse and P. K. Lauf, *Blood* **36**, 777 (1970).
[5] A. Cooper, personal communication (1975).
* The ABO, P, MN, and Lewis systems are discussed in detail by R. R. Race and R. Sanger, "Blood Groups in Man," 6th ed. Blackwell, Oxford, 1975.

room temperature will retain cold agglutinins, whereas serum removed from chilled clots may show reduced amounts of cold agglutinins owing to absorption onto the patient's (or donor's) red cells. Erythrocytes which have become coated with cold antibody may give false positive reactions when tested for ABO, Rh, or other antigens.

We have found the following method useful for handling cold auto-agglutinins with the specificity of anti-I and anti-IH.

Procedure (modified after Taylor)[6]

1. At the bedside draw a fresh specimen of blood from the patient and place half in a tube containing oxalate and the remainder in a dry tube. Immediately transfer the tube containing the oxalated blood to a beaker of warm (37°) water.

2. Allow the second tube to clot at 4°, and then separate the serum as quickly as possible to maintain the low temperature.

3. Wash cells from the oxalated blood three times with warm (37°) saline and use for grouping and typing.

4. To determine whether the cold agglutinin has been completely absorbed from the blood clotted at 4°, test this treated serum at 4° against a saline suspension of the patient's washed oxalated red cells. If the cold agglutinin is still present in the serum, absorb the serum further by adding packed, washed red cells obtained from the oxalated specimen. Allow the suspension to stand in an ice bath for 0.5 hour, separate the serum quickly, and repeat the test for complete absorption. This procedure may be repeated to remove any residual cold autoantibody.

[6] J. F. Taylor, *Am. J. Med. Technol.* **21**, 193 (1955).

5. ENZYME-TREATED ERYTHROCYTES*

Enzyme treatment of erythrocytes is discussed here for two wholly practical purposes. One is to facilitate the detection of so-called blocking or "incomplete" antibodies (γ_G-globulins). The other is to prepare erythrocytes as tools to test sera containing a multitude of antibodies. The objective here is to render the serum either (a) functionally monospecific by removing interfering antigens from the erythrocyte surface, or (b) truly monospecific by absorption of the serum with enzyme-treated red cells. The discussion is restricted to treatment with proteases and to describing facilitation of detection of antigen–agglutinin interactions. Enzyme treatment of erythrocyte virus receptors, and also hemolysis caused directly by enzymes,[1] are not within the scope of this outline.

* Section 16.A.5 was contributed by Georg F. Springer.

[1] G. F. Springer, *Bacteriol. Rev.* **27**, 191 (1963).

a. Background and Basis of Technique

Since antibodies react specifically with chemical surface structures, they are not only sensitive indicators for the serologist, but also analytical tools for the chemist.[1] Although some basic knowledge of the action of enzymes on erythrocytes existed for many years,[2] it was not until the discovery of the Rh system that their practical importance was realized for diagnostic purposes. Pickles[3] was the first to show that "incomplete" antibodies were able to specifically agglutinate enzyme-treated erythrocytes in an aqueous physiological electrolyte medium. This phenomenon implicated a structural feature of the erythrocyte surface as determining the inability of some antibodies to cause agglutination. The two most obvious explanations for increased agglutinability of enzyme-treated erythrocytes are: (1) removal of blocking structures from the erythrocyte surface,[1] and (2) change in the electrostatic bonding forces on the erythrocyte surface with a subsequent decrease in hydration, which would lead to a decrease in intererythrocyte repulsion.[1,4]

Pickles' discovery changed the "univalent" concept of incomplete antibodies, since in both instances so-called "blocking" or "incomplete" antibodies would be at least bivalent but the action of one of the combining sites would be hindered unless the erythrocytes were enzymatically treated; such treatment is believed to give the second combining site on the antibody an improved possibility to unite with a complementary antigen structure of another cell. This interpretation finds some support in the observation that following high speed centrifugation red cells not pretreated with enzymes may be agglutinated by these antibodies.[5] However, these findings do not explain how a viscous hydrophilic environment per se (Section 16.A.4.b.ii), even if not charged significantly, such as a dextran solution, may enable blocking antibodies to agglutinate erythrocytes. Rise in the dielectric constant has been implicated in the latter instance as reducing repulsive forces and facilitating agglutination.[4]

b. Application

Enzyme-treated erythrocytes are especially useful in blood banking and in the serological diagnosis of infectious mononucleosis.[6-14, cf.15, 16] En-

[2] V. Friedenreich, *Acta Pathol. Microbiol. Scand.* **5**, 59 (1928).

[3] M. Pickles, *Nature (London)* **158**, 880 (1946).

[4] W. Pollack, H. J. Hager, R. Reckel, D. A. Toren, and H. O. Singher, *Transfusion* **5**, 158 (1965).

[5] L. Hirszfeld and S. Dubiski, *Schweiz. Z. Pathol. Bacteriol.* **17**, 73 (1954).

[6] W. J. Kuhns and A. Bailey, *Amer. J. Clin. Pathol.* **20**, 1067 (1950).

[7] W. E. Wheeler, A. L. Luhby, and L. Scholl, *J. Immunol.* **65**, 39–46 (1950).

[8] J. A. Morton and M. Pickles, *J. Clin. Pathol.* **4**, 189 (1951).

zyme treatment can be automated and an autoanalyzing system be used.[17] Enzymes are used to accomplish the following: (1) saline agglutination by "incomplete" antibodies; (2) removal of interfering erythrocyte antigens to produce a monospecific reaction with a serum although it contains several antibodies; (3) enhancement in titer or strength of a reaction; (4) uncovering "hidden" receptors; (5) preparing erythrocytes for subsequent procedures such as absorption of serum antibodies; (6) hemolysis of enzyme-treated erythrocytes by specific antibody reaction; (7) increase of the sensitivity of anti-human globulin test.

c. Agglutination Tests with Enzyme-Treated Erythrocytes

i. Test Tube Procedure after Morton and Pickles

We have worked predominantly with plant proteases.[14, 18] The following procedures patterned after Morton and Pickles[8] proved useful.

(a) *Solutions and Glassware.* Phosphate-buffered saline (PBS) at pH 7.2 is used as diluent in all tests.* Serological pipettes (0.1 ml) and test tubes of 7.5 by 0.9 cm size are used for the titrations.

(b) *Enzyme Preparations.* Crude or crystalline proteases may be employed (bromelin, ficin, papain, trypsin). The crude preparations are satisfactory for the present purpose. The manufacturer's directions should be followed if crystalline enzymes are used. With crude plant enzyme preparations, the procedure is as follows: One gram of crude enzyme is ground in a mortar with slow addition of 10 ml of 0.05 N HCl (reagent grade) and the mixture is left to steep overnight at 4°. It is then clarified by filtration or centrifugation at 13,000 g for 20 minutes. This stock solution is stable for at least 4 weeks at 4° and for approximately 3 months in the deep freeze (distributed in a series of small tubes). As working solution one part of stock solution is mixed with 49 parts of PBS; it should be kept at 4° and used within 24 hours.

---

[9] R. E. Rosenfield and P. Vogel, *Trans. N. Y. Acad. Sci.* [2] **13**, 213 (1951).

[10] A. S. Wiener and L. Katz, *J. Immunol.* **66**, 51 (1951).

[11] F. Stratton and P. Renton, "Practical Blood Grouping." Blackwell, Oxford, 1958.

[12] B. Pirofsky and M. E. Mangum, *Proc. Soc. Exp. Biol. Med.* **101**, 49 (1959).

[13] M. Brigid, *Transfusion* **1**, 321–330 (1961).

[14] G. F. Springer and H. J. Callahan, *J. Lab. Clin. Med.* **65**, 617 (1965).

[15] K. Boorman and B. Dodd, "An Introduction to Blood Group Serology." Little, Brown, Boston, Massachusetts, 1961.

[16] R. R. Race and R. Sanger, "Blood Groups in Man," 5th ed. Blackwell, Oxford, 1968.

[17] F. H. Allen, Jr., R. E. Rosenfield, and M. E. Adebahr, *Vox Sanguinis* **8**, 698 (1963).

[18] G. F. Springer and M. J. Rapaport, *Proc. Soc. Exp. Biol. Med.* **96**, 103 (1957).

* Phosphate-buffered saline formulas are given in Vol. II, Appendix II, buffer No. 35. The author uses 0.025 M phosphate at pH 7.2, containing per liter 0.68 gm of $NaH_2PO_4 \cdot H_2O$, 5.34 gm of $Na_2HPO_4 \cdot 7H_2O$, and 8.5 gm of NaCl.

(c) *Erythrocytes and Their Preparation.* Blood is collected in citrate–dextrose solution* and stored at 4°. It is to be used within 2 weeks after the bleeding. Immediately before use the erythrocytes are washed 3 times with 10 to 20 volumes of buffered saline. One volume of packed red cells is mixed with 5 volumes of the enzyme solution and incubated for 30 minutes in a water bath at 37° with occasional shaking. The proportion of enzyme solution to erythrocytes can be varied within limits. The treated cells are then centrifuged, washed 3 times with 10 volumes of buffered saline, stored at 4°, and used as a 3 to 5% suspension within 2 days.

(d) *Absorption of Antisera with Enzyme-Treated Erythrocytes.* Absorption of antisera is frequently necessary since enzyme treatment may uncover panagglutinable structures (T-like antigens) on the erythrocyte surface (cf. 1). Serum samples are divided into 2 portions. One part is absorbed with an equal volume of packed enzyme-treated red cells either at room temperature (22° to 25°) for 1 hour, or at 22° to 25° for 30 minutes, and at 4° for 30 minutes with frequent agitation. After centrifugation, the absorbed serum is titrated in parallel with the unabsorbed lot to check the efficiency of the absorption.

(e) *Titration.* Buffered saline, 0.1 ml, is added to each tube except the first of each row. Then serum titrations with 0.1 ml in 2-fold dilution steps are carried out from 22° to 25°. For greater accuracy and reproducibility a different pipette is to be used for each transfer. Subsequently 0.1 ml of the erythrocyte suspension is added to each tube. The tubes are shaken, incubated at room temperature, and read after 60 to 90 minutes with a hand lens or microscopically by placing small droplets on slides. As standard and positive control, include dilutions of a known serum containing the antibody in question. Enzyme-treated erythrocytes added to buffered saline serve as negative control. Panagglutinins can usually be removed by absorption of the serum with the donor's own enzyme-treated red cells [see paragraph (d) above].

ii. *The Papain Procedure of Stratton and Renton*[11]

Stratton and Renton performed enzyme tests on slides rather than in tubes: Drops of a 5% cell suspension, pretreated with cysteine-activated (see below) papain for 10 minutes at 37°, are mixed on a slide with each

* Although 1 to 1.2 volumes of buffered Alsever's solution per volume of blood are often used (Sections 16.A.2, 16.B.2, 16.B.3, 16.A.2.a), the writer prefers the "ACD" formulation of acid–citrate–dextrose known as NIH formula B. This is widely used in blood blanks to reduce the sodium content: 25 ml is added for each 100 ml of whole blood in blood bank practice; the writer customarily uses one-third the volume of whole blood: Na_3 citrate·$2H_2O$, 13.2 gm; citric acid H_2O, 4.8 gm; dextrose, 14.7 gm; make up to 1 liter with distilled water.

of several normal sera diluted 1:2, to ensure that the cells are not agglutinable "spontaneously." If this test is negative, the red cells are examined further for sensitivity,, using a standard incomplete anti-Rh antibody in a dilution that gives a strongly positive agglutination when equal volumes of antibody and cell suspension are mixed on a slide and rocked for 6 minutes at room temperature. Negative control tests are put up on each occasion consisting of papainized cells and normal serum diluted 1:2. Agglutination is first read by inspection: Tubes that appear negative are examined under the low power of the microscope.

Variations in these methods usually consist of alterations in hydrogen ion concentration (to approach the pH optimum of the enzyme used) or simplifications that save a procedural step; in the latter case accuracy may be sacrificed.

iii. The Papain Method of Löw[19]

(a) Preparation of Enzyme Solution. (1) Grind 2 gm of papain in a mortar with 100 ml of 0.066 M phosphate buffer, pH 5.4;* (2) filter and add 10 ml of 0.5 M cysteine (0.79 gm of L-cysteine·HCl in 10 ml of distilled water); neutralize with an equal volume of 0.5 M NaOH; (3) dilute to 200 ml with 0.025 M PBS at pH 7.2; (4) incubate 60 minutes at 37°; (5) store in small tubes in the deep freeze.

(b) Test Procedure. (1) Add 3 volumes of enzyme solution to 1 volume of serum under test. (For weakly reacting sera, use an equal volume of enzyme solution and serum.) (2) Add an equal volume of 3% cells in saline to above mixture. (3) Mix and incubate 60 to 90 minutes at 37°. (4) Observe for macroscopic agglutination without centrifugation.

Although most of the proteases commonly used have the same effect, some variations have been described previously.[1, 10, 11]

d. INTERPRETATION OF RESULTS

Enzyme treatment has the general advantage of securing strong and rapid agglutination reactions. In addition, some effects on erythrocytes can be obtained only by enzymes. "Unexplained" positive reactions, however, must be guarded against.

General precautions to be taken in all enzymatic and serological experiments have been adequately described elsewhere (cf. Stratton and

---

[19] B. Löw, Vox Sanguinis **5**, 94 (1955).

* KH$_2$PO$_4$-Na$_2$HPO$_4$ buffer (0.067 M) is given in Vol. II, Appendix II, buffer 28. The author prepares 1 liter of solution A (9.08 gm of KH$_2$PO$_4$) and 50 ml of solution B (0.594 gm of Na$_2$HPO$_4$·2H$_2$O or 0.894 gm of NaHPO$_4$·7H$_2$O) and mixes 964 ml of A with 36 ml of solution B.

Renton[11]). However, particular attention must be given to false positive and to false negative results.

False positive results may be due to (1) "spontaneous" agglutination of enzyme-treated cells; (2) infected serum, rouleaux-forming properties of serum and autoantibodies; (3) red cells contaminated with microbes; or (4) failure in the slide test to dilute the patient's serum at least 1:2.

False negative results may be due to (1) inadequate treatment of the red cells; or (2) destruction of antibody by enzyme, occurring in the Löw modification 3 to 4 hours after addition of the enzyme.

6. LECTINS*

Phytohemagglutinins have been known for a long time; different seed extracts had been noted to agglutinate erythrocytes of various species somewhat selectively.[1] *Phaseolus vulgaris* (the black bean) yields such an extract formerly known as "Phasin"; it is the usual source of commercial phytohemagglutinin used to stimulate mitosis of lymphocytes *in vitro*. Specific agglutination of human blood groups by extracts of the seeds of certain plants was reported independently in 1947 and 1948 by Boyd[2, 3] and Renkonen,[4, 5] and these phytohemagglutinins were later termed lectins by Boyd.[6] In some cases lectins also precipitate specifically with the appropriate soluble blood group antigens. General reviews have been published by Krüpe,[7] Mäkelä,[8] Bird,[9] Boyd,[10] and Tobiška,[11] Sharon and Lis,[12, 13] and by multiple authors in a special Conference.[14] It is found that lectins bind electively with particular polysaccharides on cell surfaces and will sometimes precipitate polysaccharides and glycoproteins.[12, 14]

* Section 16.A.6 was contributed by William C. Boyd.

[1] K. Landsteiner, "The Specificity of Serological Reactions," 2nd ed. Harvard Univ Press, Cambridge, Massachusetts, 1945 (reprinted by Dover, New York, 1962).

[2] W. C. Boyd, "Fundamentals of Immunology," 2nd ed. Wiley (Interscience), New York, 1947.

[3] W. C. Boyd and R. M. Reguera, *J. Immunol.* **62**, 333 (1949).

[4] K. O. Renkonen, *Ann. Med. Exp. Biol. Fenn.* **26**, 66 (1948).

[5] K. O. Renkonen, *Ann. Med. Exptl. Biol. Fenn.* **28**, 45 (1950).

[6] W. C. Boyd and E. Shapleigh, *J. Lab. Clin. Med.* **44**, 235 (1954).

[7] M. Krüpe, "Blutgruppen-spezifische pflanzliche Eiweisskörper." Enke, Stuttgart, 1956.

[8] O. Mäkelä, *Ann. Med. Exp. Biol. Fenn.* **35**, Suppl. 11 (1957).

[9] G. W. G. Bird, *Brit. Med. J.* **1**, 165 (1959).

[10] W. C. Boyd, *Vox Sanguinis* **8**, 1 (1963).

[11] J. Tobiška, "Die Phytohämagglutinine." Akademie-Verlag, Berlin, 1964.

[12] N. Sharon and H. Lis, *Science* **177**, 949 (1972).

[13] H. Lis and N. Sharon, *Annu. Rev. Biochem.* **42**, 541 (1973).

[14] E. Cohen, ed., Biomedical Perspectives of Agglutinins of Invertebrate and Plant Origin, *Ann. N. Y. Acad. Sci.* **234**, 1–412 (1974).

Many plants, such as the castor bean, *Ricinus communis*, yield extracts that agglutinate blood of all blood groups, and are thus called nonspecific for human erythrocytes. Many more plants contain no detectable hemagglutinins in their seeds. Some other species contain substances which agglutinate human erythrocytes with demonstrable selectivity (Table II). Some seeds, perhaps most, contain proteins that combine firmly but nonspecifically with erythrocytes of any blood group, without agglutinating them or producing any visible change in their behavior. The coating of lectin can be detected by certain procedures.[15] The plant hemagglutinins are plant globulins, though they contain some carbohydrate, as do most proteins.

In 1965, lectin activity was found in extracts of snails (Boyd and Brown[16] with *Otala lactea*, Prokop *et al.*[17] with *Helix*), after which time considerable research has been done with invertebrate species. The word lectin (from the Latin *legere*, meaning to choose or pick out) originally applied to *plant* agglutinins. It has since been broadened to include all proteins (other than antibodies) which possess the ability to react with specific receptors—apparently all carbohydrates—on the surfaces of erythrocytes or other cells.[14, 18] Thus concanavalin A, which agglutinates human erythrocytes of all blood groups by reason of its sugar specificity, is a lectin, as is the castor bean agglutinin which is specifically inhibited by certain sugars[19] and is distinct from ricin, the castor bean toxin.[12] In fact the question has been raised whether there can be any large molecule–large molecule interactions which are nonspecific.[20]

Lectins have been used to (a) determine the subgroups of blood groups A and AB,[6] (b) diagnose "secretors,"[21, 22] (c) make routine ABO blood grouping,[23] (d) determine MN blood grouping,[24] (e) separate mixtures of erythrocytes of different groups,[25] (f) initiate mitogenesis,[12] (g) differentiate malignant from normal cells.[12] Other applications bearing on an understanding of specific agglutination and precipitation have included: (h) determining the number of specific combining sites on a single

[15] G. W. G. Bird, *Brit. Med. Bull.* **15**, 165 (1959).
[16] W. C. Boyd and and R. Brown, *Nature (London)* **208**, 593 (1965).
[17] O. Prokop, A. Rackwitz, and D. Schlesinger, *J. Forensic Med.* **12**, 108 (1965).
[18] W. C. Boyd, *Ann. N. Y. Acad. Sci.* **234**, 53 (1974).
[19] W. C. Boyd and E. Waszczenko-Zacharczenko, *Transfusion* **1**, 223 (1961).
[20] W. C. Boyd, *Experientia* **30**, 1473 (1974).
[21] W. C. Boyd and E. Shapleigh, *Blood* **9**, 1195 (1954).
[22] P. Speiser, K. Baumgarten, and O. Kaserer, *Z. Immunitaetsforsch.* **111**, 168 (1954).
[23] M. Saint-Paul, *Transfusion* **4**, 3 (1961).
[24] W. C. Boyd, *Vox Sanguinis* **8**, 1 (1963).
[25] K. C. Atwood and S. L. Scheinberg, *J. Cell. Comp. Physiol.* **52**, Suppl. 1, 97 (1958).

erythrocyte,[26] (i) changing, by chemical alteration, the specificity of lectins (and potentially of antibodies),[27-30] (j) testing the lattice theory of immune reactions. (The observations of Springer and Desai[31] that the anti-H(O) lectin of the eel precipitates specifically with certain molecularly dispersed monosaccharides seems to have demolished the once prevailing lattice theory.[32])

In place of physical chemical methods[32] modeled on cold-alcohol protein fractionations developed by Cohn et al.,[33] chromatography and affinity chromatography have resulted in preparations that are highly purified. Using such methods, Hammarström and Kabat[34] purified and characterized the anti-A lectin from the snail *Helix pomatia*, and Etzler and Kabat[35] purified the anti-A from *Dolichos biflorus*. Many lectins have now been separated or purified.[12, 14] Some of these, such as the lectin of *Limulus polyphemus* (the horseshoe crab)[36-38] and concanavalin A,[39] have been investigated extensively; but failure to differentiate between human blood groups makes them of less concern in this presentation. The lectin of *Dolichos biflorus* is specific for terminal α-linked N-acetylgalactosamine, that of *Sophora japonica* is predominantly specific for α-galactose, while that of *Lotus tetragonolobus* has L-fucose specificity.[40]

Lectin solutions are prepared by extraction of the appropriate part of the plant with physiological saline (extensive trials with hypo- and hypertonic solutions of NaCl and other salts have not revealed any superior method of extraction). Seeds should be ground fine before extraction. For small amounts a mortar and pestle suffice; larger amounts can be ground in a suitable mill (an electric coffee mill serves well). The extraction may

[26] W. C. Boyd, H. M. Bhatia, M. A. Diamond, and S. Matsubara, *J. Immunol.* **89**, 463 (1962).
[27] S. Matsubara and W. C. Boyd, *J. Immunol.* **91**, 641 (1963).
[28] S. Matsubara and W. C. Boyd, *J. Immunol.* **96**, 25 (1966).
[29] S. Matsubara and W. C. Boyd, *J. Immunol.* **96**, 829 (1966).
[30] S. Matsubara and W. C. Boyd, *Immunology* **25**, 909 (1973).
[31] G. F. Springer and P. R. Desai, *Biochemistry* **10**, 3749 (1971).
[32] W. C. Boyd, *Experientia* **29**, 1565 (1973).
[33] E. J. Cohn, J. L. Oncley, L. E. Strong, W. L. Hughes, Jr., and S. H. Armstrong, Jr., *J. Clin. Invest.* **23**, 417 (1944).
[34] S. Hammerström and E. A. Kabat, *Biochemistry* **8**, 2696 (1969).
[35] M. E. Etzler and E. A. Kabat, *Biochemistry* **9**, 869 (1970).
[36] J. J. Marchalonis and G. M. Edelman, *J. Mol. Biol.* **32**, 453 (1968).
[37] C. L. Finstad, G. W. Litman, J. Finstad, and R. A. Good, *J. Immunol.* **108**, 1704 (1972).
[38] C. L. Finstad, R. A. Good, and G. W. Litman, *Ann. N. Y. Acad. Sci.* **234**, 170 (1974).
[39] G. N. Reeke, Jr., J. W. Becker, B. A. Cunningham, G. R. Gunther, J. L. Wang, and G. M. Edelman, *Ann. N. Y. Acad. Sci.* **234**, 369 (1974).
[40] G. W. G. Bird, *Ann. N. Y. Acad. Sci.* **234**, 129 (1974).

TABLE II
SELECTIVITY OF VARIOUS LECTINS FOR HUMAN ERYTHROCYTES

Specificity	Source	Common name	Notes[a]
Anti-A	*Phaseolus limensis* *Phaseolus lunatus*	Lima beans Sieva (small pole lima beans)	At suitable dilutions, can discriminate between A_1 and A_2. Concentrated by alcohol at low temperature to be 36% precipitable by blood group A substance.[b] Has been crystallized but method is not published[c]
	Dolichos biflorus	Horse gram	[d, e]Virtually specific for A_1. Affinities for $A_1 : A_2$ cells = 500:1
	Vicia cracca	—	[f]A_1 reactivity very high; reacts only weakly on A_2 cells. Glycoprotein (30% carbohydrate) after some purification. Mobility between those of human β- and γ-globulins
	Vicia villosa	—	—
	Vicia peregrina	—	—
	Crotolaria aegyptica	—	—
	Crotolaria falcata	—	—
	Hyptos suaveolens	—	—
	Clitocyba nebularis	Mushroom	—
	Otala lactea	Snail (edible, imported from N. Africa)	[g]Expressed juice agglutinates A_1 to 1:8000, A_2 to 1:2000. Precipitates blood group A substance from hog gastric mucin[h]
	Helix pomatia	Edible Roman snail	[i,j]Affinity for A_2 exceeds that for A_1
Anti-B	*Sophora japonica*	Japanese pagoda tree	[k]Both anti-A and anti-B activities are present. Anti-A is suppressed by privine,[l] see text
	Bandeiraea simplicifolia	—	Not suitable for routine use[m]
	Marasmius oreades	Mushroom	Not suitable for routine use[n]
	Polyporus fomentarius	Tree fungus	Not suitable for routine use[o]

TABLE II (*Continued*)

Specificity	Source	Common name	Notes[a]
Anti-H*	*Ulex europaeus*	Furze, gorse, whin	[n]
	Cytisus sessifolis	—	[o]
	Laburnum alpinum	—	[o]
	Lotus tetragonolobus	—	[o]Inhibition studies by Morgan and Watkins[p]
	Tetragonolobus purpureus	—	—
	Ononis spinosa	Root	—
	Xylaria polymorpha	Mushroom	—
Anti-M	*Iberis amara*	Rocket candytuft	Certain varieties, only, exhibit the property
Anti-N	*Vicia graminea*	—	[q]
	Bauhinia purpurea	—	Certain species, only[r]
Anti-Gy	*Arachis hypogaea*	Peanuts	"Peanut factor" detecting a new blood property,[s] extracted in 5 volumes 10% saline and dialyzed to 0.15 M NaCl. Erythrocytes 1% in 30% bovine serum albumin
Anti-(B+H)†	*Euonymus europaeus*	—	—

* Agglutinates groups O, A_2, A_2B.

† Agglutinates groups B, AB, O, A_2, A_2B.

[a] The systematic botanical description of most of the listed plants is presented in L. H. Bailey, "Manual of Cultivated Plants," rev. ed., Macmillan, New York, 1949, and in A. Gray's "Manual of Botany, A Handbook of the Flowering Plants and Ferns of the Central and Northeastern United States and Adjacent Canada" (revised by M. L. Fernald), 8th centennial ed. American Book Company, New York, 1950.

[b] W. C. Boyd, E. Shapleigh, and M. McMaster, *Arch. Biochem. Biophys.* **55**, 226 (1955).

[c] S. Matsubara, cited by W. C. Boyd (1962).

[d] G. W. G. Bird, *J. Immunol.* **69**, 319 (1952).

[e] G. W. G. Bird, *Brit. Med. Bull.* **15**, 165 (1959).

[f] K. O. Renkonen, *Ann. Med. Exp. Biol. Fenn.* **28**, 45 (1950).

[g] H. M. Bhatia, W. C. Boyd, and R. Brown, *Transfusion* **7**, 53 (1967).

[h] W. C. Boyd, R. Brown, and L. G. Boyd, *J. Immunol.* **96**, 301 (1966).

[i] S. Hammarström and E. A. Kabat, *Biochemistry* **8**, 2696 (1969); S. Hammarström, *Ann. N. Y. Acad. Sci.* **234**, 183 (1974).

[j] I. Ishiyama, M. Mukaida, and A. Takatsu, *Ann. N. Y. Acad. Sci.* **234**, 75 (1974.)

[k] M. Krüpe and C. Braun, *Naturwissenschaften* **39**, 284 (1952).

[l] A Chattoraj and W. C. Boyd, *J. Immunol.* **96**, 898 (1966).

[m] W. C. Boyd, M. H. McMaster, and E. Waszczenko-Zacharczenko, *Nature (London)* **184**, 898 (1959).

[n] P. Cazal and M. Lalaurie, *Acta. Haematol.* **8**, 73 (1952).

[o] K. O. Renkonen, *Ann. Med. Exp. Biol. Fenn.* **26**, 66 (1948).

[p] W. T. J. Morgan and W. M. Watkins, *Brit. J. Exp. Pathol.* **34**, 94 (1953).

[q] F. Ottensooser and K. Silberschmidt, *Nature (London)* **172**, 914 (1953).

[r] W. C. Boyd, D. L. Everhart, and M. H. McMaster, *J. Immunol.* **81**, 414 (1958).

[s] W. C. Boyd, D. M. Green, D. M. Fujinaga, J. S. Drabik, and E. Waszczenko-Zacharczenko, *Vox Sang.* **4**, 456 (1959).

be carried out at +4° overnight with a weight of saline equal to 5 to 10 times the weight of the ground seed. Van Loghem[41] recommends for *Vicia graminea* 80 parts of saline, added in three portions, the supernatant suspension being poured off each time before fresh saline is added. Lectin preparations keep well in the frozen state. Most of them can be lyophilized.

The specificity of lectins is in some cases greater, in some cases less, than that of human and animal antibodies having similar specificities.

For agglutination, it is often necessary to have traces of calcium present. Surface pretreatment of human red cells with trypsin or ficin can be useful at times.[14] Lectins which have practical usefulness for human blood grouping are listed in Table II. Other lectins, not listed here, differentiate in part between special human bloods and so help in "dissecting" surface carbohydrate structures.[40] It is to be mentioned that *Vicia graminea* lectin served to demonstrate the presence of antigen N in chimpanzee blood.[42] The anti-H lectin of *Ulex europaeus* differentiates satisfactorily between salivas of secretors and nonsecretors of antigens H, A, and B.

a. ANTI-A LECTINS

Several good reagents are listed in Table II.

Lectin of sieva lima beans has been purified[43] by discarding the precipitate formed upon acidification to pH 4.5 with 1 N HCl, dialyzing against water to precipitate the active material, and extracting the precipitate twice in succession with 0.15 M NaCl. The solution is chilled and cold alcohol is added to 7%: discard this precipitate, increase the alcohol to 20% at −6°, and collect. Finally extract with 0.15 M NaCl. The purified lectin is specifically inhibited by N-acetyl-D-galactosamine.[44] Crude sieva extracts may have limiting dilution titers of 1:200 to 1:300, purified preparations may have anti-A titers of about 1:30,000.

The potent lectin present in the expressed juice of the snail *Otala lactea* appears to come only from the "albumin gland." Precipitin curves secured with blood group A substance from hog gastric mucin are shown in Figs. 1 and 2. A simple purification method for this agglutinin was described by Bhatia, Boyd, and Brown.[45] Some albumin gland extracts may have anti-A titers of 1:1,000,000.

[41] J. J. Van Loghem, communication to W. C. Boyd (1958).
[42] P. Levine, F. Ottensooser, M. J. Celano, and W. Pollitzer, *Amer. J. Phys. Anthropol.* **13**, 29 (1955).
[43] W. C. Boyd, E. Shapleigh, and M. McMaster, *Arch. Biochem. Biophys.* **55**, 226 (1955).
[44] S. Matsubara and W. C. Boyd, *J. Immunol.* **96**, 25 (1966).
[45] H. M. Bhatia, W. C. Boyd, and R. Brown, *Transfusion* **7**, 53 (1967).

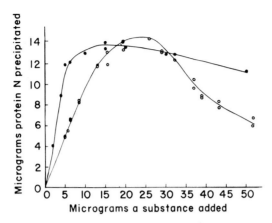

FIG. 1. Protein precipitated from sieva lectin solution by "A substance." The open circles show nitrogen precipitated from the lectin by hog A substance. For comparison, a precipitation curve given by mixing human anti-A serum and hog A substance is shown in filled circles. [Reproduced by permission from W. C. Boyd, E. Shapleigh, and M. McMaster, *Arch. Biochem. Biophys.* **55**, 226, Fig. 1 (1955).]

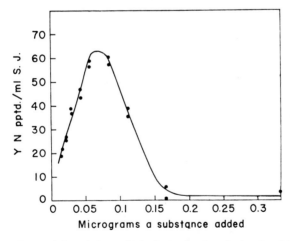

FIG. 2. Protein precipitated from *Otala lactea* lectin solution by "A substance." Blood group A substance was added in varying amounts to 1-ml portions of expressed tissue juices of the snail *Otala lactea*. [Reproduced by permission from W. C. Boyd, R. Brown, and L. G. Boyd, *J. Immunol.* **96**, 301, Fig. 2 (1966).]

b. ANTI-B REAGENT

The most effective anti-B lectin is prepared from *Sophora japonica*. The seed kernels are secured by flotation from the seed coats by placing the ground seeds in a mixture of 1 part of benzene and 2.8 parts of chloroform;[21] the seed kernels are freed of solvents, ground further, and extracted with 9 volumes of saline. This stock extract is kept frozen. Quantitative studies have been made,[46] using highly purified extract.[47] For use as an anti-B reagent, make a preliminary titration on B cells (*ca.* 1:10 to 1:20 dilution) and mix twice the concentration of the effective, desired dilution with an equal volume of 0.004 M privine hydrochloride (Ciba) and hold at 4° for 24 hours or at 37° for 1 hour before use.[48] This mixture is stable for 1 week. It is to be noted that 0.004 M privine hydrochloride does not inhibit human anti-B, rabbit anti-M (absorbed with N cells), rabbit anti-N, human anti-D, anti-C, anti-E, anti-c, anti-e, anti-H of *Ulex europaeus*, or anti-N of *Vicia graminea*.

The *Sophora japonica* lectin, normally reactive with both A- and B-cells (unless treated with privine) is not separable into two classes of molecules.[49]

c. ANTI-H LECTINS

Reagents for detecting H-substance are especially valuable in determining secretors of H-substance among individuals of group O, who display no obvious blood-group reactivity. Extracts of *Ulex europaeus* are recommended highly. The reaction between O cells and *Lotus tetragonolobus* lectin is inhibited by a variety of reagents,[49] namely, human and hog H-substances, L-fucose, α-methyl-L-fucopyranoside to very high degree, and well by β-methyl-L-fucopyranoside and 2-deoxy-L-fucose. Matsubara and Boyd[27–29] were able to alter the specificity of certain lectins by chemical modification.

[46] J. T. Miller and W. C. Boyd, *Vox Sanguinis* **13**, 209 (1967).
[47] J. T. Miller, W. C. Boyd, and M. A. Diamond, *Vox Sanguinis* **13**, 449 (1967).
[48] A. Chattoraj and W. C. Boyd, *J. Immunol.* **96**, 898 (1966).
[49] W. T. J. Morgan and W. M. Watkins, *Brit. J. Exptl. Pathol.* **34**, 94 (1953).

B. Indirect (Passive) Hemagglutination

1. DIRECT PASSIVE-POLYSACCHARIDE ADSORPTION ON UNTREATED ERYTHROCYTES*

The technique of passive hemagglutination, in which additional specificities are conferred on erythrocytes by the adsorption of foreign antigens was established as a principle in 1948.[1] It has come into widespread use as a standard procedure in immunology. It is generally recognized that protein antigens cannot be adsorbed directly onto normal erythro-

* Section 16.B.1 was contributed by Maurice Landy.

[1] E. V. Keogh, E. A. North, and M. F. Warburton, *Nature (London)* **161**, 687 (1948).

cytes and that the utility of the direct procedure involves antigens whose structure is predominantly or wholly polysaccharide. Capsular and somatic antigens from an extensive array of microbial species are readily adsorbed by normal erythrocytes, resulting in the acquisition by these cells of a new serological specificity characteristic of the microbial source.

a. COMPOSITION OF MICROBIAL POLYSACCHARIDES

The classification of microbial polysaccharides is undoubtedly complex, and there is a paucity of information as regards composition, structure, and the physicochemical attributes involved in their attachment to erythrocytes. For the most part, these complex polysaccharides of high molecular weight fall into two major categories: (1) the capsular uronic acid polymers such as the Vi antigen and certain pneumococcal type-specific polysaccharides which adsorb directly without prior treatment, and (b) the somatic–endotoxic complexes of gram-negative bacteria which contain considerable amounts of associated lipid and protein, and which generally fail to fix effectively unless they are first subjected to various modifying treatments, discussed below.[2] *

A more complex situation is presented in the case of fractions from *Mycobacterium tuberculosis*.[3] A heat-stable polysaccharide contained in Old Tuberculin was found to be absorbed on sheep erythrocytes, such cells then being agglutinable by rabbit antituberculosis sera and by sera from patients with mycobacterial infection ("Middlebrook-Dubos test").[4] † Seibert's "polysaccharide I" of mycobacterial origin[5] was found to give the test,[5a] and finer studies were made on the chemical properties, the material being called α-hemosensitin.[6, 7] A second polysaccharide, heat labile, was isolated from unheated culture filtrate as a product capable of sensitizing sheep erythrocytes; it differed from Seibert's Polysaccharide II[8] which was obtained from unheated filtrate but lacked this property. The second sensitizing material was termed β-hemosensitin.[3]

[2] D. A. Davis, M. J. Crumpton, I. A. Macpherson, and A. M. Hutchison, *Immunology* **1**, 157 (1958).

* Variations among the cell wall antigens extracted from gram-negative bacteria are described in Vol. I, Chap. 1, B.2.

[3] S. V. Boyden and E. Sorkin, *Bibl. Tuberc.* **7**, Part 10, 17 (1956).

[4] G. Middlebrook and R. J. Dubos, *J. Exp. Med.* **88**, 521 (1948).

† A factor in Old Tuberculin which showed cross-reactivity with staphylococci could be separated by drying and extracting with 90% phenol: The tuberculin-specific material was soluble, the staphylococcal material insoluble (G. M. Middlebrook, personal communication, 1968).

[5] F. B. Seibert and D. W. Watson, *J. Biol Chem.* **140**, 55 (1941).

[5a] G. Middlebrook, personal communication (1968).

[6] E. Sorkin and S. V. Boyden, *J. Immunol.* **75**, 22 (1955).

[7] E. Sorkin, S. V. Boyden, and J. M. Rhodes, *Helv. Chim. Acta* **39**, 1684 (1956).

[8] F. B. Seibert, *Amer. Rev. Tuberc.* **59**, 86 (1949).

A large and diffuse body of literature has developed on the spectrum of the microbial antigens taken up directly by erythrocytes. The ability to adsorb to erythrocytes appears to involve patches of the polysaccharide surfaces other than those bearing the specific antibody-receptor. Marked differences in the properties of antigens isolated from the same microbial sources by different procedures,[2] as well as wide variations in the coating of red cells, mammalian *vs* avian cells, performance of the test (macro *vs* micro, centrifuged or settling patterns, etc.) make it unprofitable to attempt to summarize, or even to assess the total experience to date. However, some generalizations can be offered and appear broadly applicable, independent of the source of the antigen, its particular mode of preparation, or details of the manner in which the test is performed.

b. Modification of Certain Polysaccharides for Adsorption of Erythrocytes

Some polysaccharides complexes, as mentioned above, are "activated" for maximal uptake by erythrocytes, as by exposure to heat (100° for 1 hour) or to dilute alkali or both, viz., 18 hours at 37° in the presence of 0.02 N NaOH. The nature of the alteration responsible for uptake of these antigens remains obscure.[9] For example, *Salmonella typhi* O antigens will coat erythrocytes when used in a concentration of 500 μg/ml, but after the heat or alkali treatment described the preparations can sensitize red cells in a concentration of only 3 to 6 μg/ml, and the capacity for agglutination is enhanced such that 16-fold less immune serum is needed than for cells coated with untreated O-antigen.

Another instance is provided by pneumococcal capsular polysaccharide type 6, which fixed to erythrocytes only after it had been oxidized with periodate.[9a]

c. Techniques

Since normal serum interferes markedly with the uptake of these antigens by erythrocytes, it is essential to wash the red cells thoroughly prior to exposure to antigen. The red cells take up only a very small proportion of the antigen which must be present to secure optimal coating. Again, because free antigen effectively blocks agglutination of coated cells by antibody, it is also necessary to wash the antigen-treated cells thoroughly prior to their use. The presence of electrolyte is known to be essential for fixation, and the rate of uptake of antigen is temperature-dependent, being very slow at 4° and rapid at 37°

[9] E. Neter, *Bacteriol. Rev.* **20**, 166 (1956).
[9a] P. A. Rebers, E. Hurwitz, M. Heidelberger, and S. Estrada-Parra, *J. Bacteriol.* **83**, 335 (1962).

Erythrocytes from a large number of mammalian species are suitable for this purpose, although not all are equally effective. Sheep erythrocytes have been employed most extensively and successfully, but it is often advantageous to utilize erythrocytes from the same species as the serum under test so as to obviate the necessity of absorbing out natural hemagglutinins.

Sensitization, coating, or specific modification of erythrocytes with these polysaccharide antigens is effected by simply exposing a suspension of the washed erythrocytes to a solution of the antigen in PBS at pH 7.2 for 1 to 2 hours at 37°. It has been found convenient to sensitize erythrocytes as a 10% suspension in physiological saline and then to wash and adjust the cells to a 1% suspension for use in agglutination tests. The concentration of antigen is critical in determining the reactivity of the coated erythrocytes with the specific antibody. It is necessary to ascertain for each product the optimum concentration for coating of red cells, since even different batches of antigen prepared in the same way frequently differ in this regard, a fact which emphasizes the essentiality of antigen titrations.

The red cell surface appears to possess various receptors for different polysaccharides. Thus when 1 ml of 10% sheep erythrocytes was exposed to 20 μg amounts of six polysaccharidic antigens of different specificity, either in turn or simultaneously (*Salmonella typhi* O-antigen, *Escherichia coli* Vi antigen, *Diplococcus pneumoniae* capsular polysaccharide Type III, *Pasteurella tularensis* antigen "Schu," *Pseudomonas aeruginosa* antigen "PC-9," *Serratia marcescens* antigen "P-15"), the coated cells reacted with each of the panel of antisera.[10] Even a great excess of a single polysaccharide did not prevent or greatly alter the subsequent uptake of other polysaccharide antigens. Consequently attachment is not likely to be a simple charge phenomenon. Once adsorbed to erythrocytes, the fixation of polysaccharide is remarkably firm; the stability of the coated cell is similar to that of the erythrocyte itself. However, significant dissociation of this antigen from red cells occurs on exposure to temperature of 52° to 62°. Since the polysaccharides themselves are heat stable, this elution from cells is probably a reflection of heat denaturation of key erythrocyte structures.

An appreciable amount of definitive work has been carried out with highly purified and well-characterized bacterial polysaccharides. However, it has frequently been practical and occasionally highly advantageous to employ incompletely defined bacterial fractions, simple extracts of bacterial cells or even crude culture filtrates. For example, in the case of the type-specific pneumococcus polysaccharides, most antigenic prepa-

[10] M. Landy, *Amer. J. Pub. Health* **44**, 1059 (1954).

rations fail, as commonly isolated, to absorb on red cells, yet culture filtrates of the same type pneumococci do confer on erythrocytes their type-specific antigenicity; hence, it seems reasonable to assume that purification and isolation procedures have significantly altered groupings that can interact with erythrocyte receptors. This issue merits further study.

d. Discussion

Although not generally appreciated, the coating of erythrocytes with high molecular weight microbial polysaccharides endows the red cell with the distinctive physicochemical attributes of these polymers as well as an additional serological specificity. An indication of the magnitude and consequences of some of these physical changes is provided by studies on capsular antigens such as Vi, pneumococcal "specific soluble substance" of type III (SSS III), and the products derived from *Klebsiella* strains. In these instances the erythrocytes were shown to assume the physico-chemical characteristics of these uronic acid polymers. Human erythrocytes acquired a pronounced negative charge and became so markedly "stabilized" as to be inagglutinable by potent blood grouping antisera directed against antigens indigenous to the red cell itself.[11]

In view of the known polydisperse character of many of these high molecular weight polysaccharides, it is entirely possible that only a certain proportion of the molecules, possibly of a critical size or charge, actually fix to cells. Little is known regarding the sites or receptors on erythrocytes which are involved in the fixation of polysaccharides.[12] The fact that lipid extracts from erythrocyte stromata, serum fractions rich in lipid, lecithin, and cephalin all inhibit the fixation of bacterial antigens on red cells has been interpreted by some as indicating that the lipoproteins on red cell stroma are the receptors for attachment of polysaccharide antigens.

[11] R. Ceppellini and M. Landy, *J. Exp. Med.* **117**, 321 (1963).
[12] S. Gard, *Acta Pathol. Microbiol. Scand.* **91**, 107 (1951).

2. HEMAGGLUTINATION WITH TANNIC ACID-TREATED (TANNED) ERYTHROCYTES*

Agglutination is a sensitive method for the detection of antibody since much less antibody is required to agglutinate particles containing antigenic patches on their surfaces than is needed to aggregate (precipitate) antigens in free solution. The finding by Boyden[1] that proteins can be

* Section 16.B.2 was contributed by Abram B. Stavitsky.

[1] S. V. Boyden, *J. Exp. Med.* **93**, 107 (1951).

absorbed on tannic acid-treated erythrocytes and that these cells can then be agglutinated by specific antiprotein sera extended the range of application of agglutination methods to the detection of antibodies to proteins and other substances such as haptens[2]—the latter via soluble hapten–protein conjugates which could be absorbed to tanned erythrocytes. (Haptenic groups also have been coupled directly to cell surfaces by various workers to study antihapten antibodies by agglutination and by complement-lysis, e.g., by direct diazotization of certain haptens[3–5] and by coupling with dinitrophenyl groupings.[6, 7])

The following account incorporates several emendations of methods originally recommended for tanned cell agglutination.[8, 9] Antigen can also be covalently coupled to erythrocytes by bisdiazotization (see Section 15.B.3); the former process will be described as *coating* the red cells, the latter as *coupling to* the red cells. The binding of antigen on tanned cells is somewhat reversible, yet it may be advantageous to employ this procedure rather than coupling protein to red cells. The protein-coated red cells are more stable than the protein-coupled red cells. More antigen often is required for coupling to cells than for coating tanned cells.

The hemagglutination method is a convenient procedure to detect and ascertain the concentration of γ_G and γ_M agglutinating antibodies to proteins, blood group substances, and haptens. It is particularly sensitive in detecting γ_M antibodies since small concentrations of these antibodies may yield significant titers, disproportionately high in comparison with hemagglutination by γ_G. Accordingly, a falsely low concentration of γ_G antibody may be inferred. Divalent antibodies are required for hemagglutination, hence so-called "incomplete" antibodies may not be detected. The hemagglutination reaction probably detects so-called "blocking" antibodies in sera of allergic patients. The reaction may detect also antigen–antibody complexes, which in some cases can be an advantage, in other cases a disadvantage.

According to the experience of this laboratory, the results of hemagglutination titrations on different antisera to a single well-defined protein often do not correlate with quantitative precipitin titrations. A recent study, however, indicates that hemagglutination titers may closely re-

[2] J. R. Battisto and M. W. Chase, *J. Exp. Med.* **118**, 1021 (1963).
[3] J. S. Ingraham, *J. Infec. Dis.* **91**, 268 (1952).
[4] A. M. Silverstein and F. Maltaner, *J. Immunol.* **69**, 197 (1952).
[5] J. S. Ingraham and H. O. Foley, *J. Infec. Dis.* **107**, 43 (1960).
[6] W. E. Bullock and F. S. Kantor, *J. Immunol.* **94**, 317 (1965).
[7] B. B. Levine and V. Levytska, *J. Immunol.* **98**, 648 (1967).
[8] A. B. Stavitsky, *J. Immunol.* **72**, 360 and 368 (1954).
[9] A. B. Stavitsky and E. Arquilla, *Int. Arch. Allergy Appl. Immunol.* **13**, 1 (1958).

flect the antibody nitrogen content of the serum as determined by quantitative precipitation.[10]

For most purposes, highly purified antigens should be chosen for coating tanned red cells or for immunization, since protein contaminants in antigen preparations may cause hemagglutination by small amounts of antibodies against the contaminants which may be present in the immune sera. This reaction is especially useful in the detection and estimation of antigens and antibodies in fractions of tissues, proteins, sera, or body fluids which are separated by chromatography, electrophoresis, ultracentrifugation, or other procedures.

The problem of desorption of antigen from tanned cells can be overcome by coupling antigen to erythrocytes with the bisdiazobenzidine reagent (Section 16.B.3). With this method, hemagglutination-inhibition can be used to quantitate antigen in a fluid, and antibody-coated erythrocytes can be agglutinated by homologous antigen.[11] Further, protein-sensitized cells can be used as an immunoabsorbent and the complex employed as an immunizing agent.

a. REAGENTS

i. Buffers for Tanned Cell Hemagglutination Procedures

Strongly buffered saline (0.075 M phosphate)* was introduced by Boyden[1]; solutions are used at pH values of 7.2, 6.4, and 5.6 and are prepared according to Table I.

TABLE I

PHOSPHATE BUFFERS (0.075 M) FOR TANNED CELL HEMAGGLUTINATION[a]

Desired pH	0.15 M NaH$_2$PO$_4$ anhydrous, 18.0 gm/liter; or monohydrate, 20.7 gm/liter	0.15 M KH$_2$PO$_4$, 20.4 gm/liter	0.15 M Na$_2$HPO$_4$ anhydrous, 21.3 gm/liter; or heptahydrate, 40.2 gm/liter; or dodecahydrate, 53.7 gm/liter	Sodium chloride
7.2	—	119.5 ml/liter	380 ml/liter	4.5 gm/liter
6.4	—	338.5 ml/liter	161 ml/liter	4.4 gm/liter
5.6[b]	467.5 ml/liter	—	32.5 ml/liter	4.4 gm/liter

[a] After preparation the pH should be tested and adjusted as necessary.

[b] This buffer, which is used only with formalinized cells, falls at the extreme acid side of phosphate buffers (Vol. II, Appendix II, buffers 27–35).

[10] W. J. Herbert, *Immunology* **13**, 453 (1967).
[11] F. Cua-Lim, M. Richter, and B. Rose, *J. Allergy* **34**, 142 (1963).
* Compare buffer 35 in Appendix II of Vol. II.

ii. Tannic Acid

Stock 1% solution is prepared by dissolving reagent grade tannic acid in saline and keeping it in a dark bottle at 4°. The stock solution is discarded after 1 month, or earlier if it becomes turbid or discolored. A dilution of 1 part of stock with 199 parts of saline (0.00005%) is prepared daily.

iii. Formaldehyde

Reagent grade formaldehyde (approximately 40%) is employed. A solution with a final concentration of 3% formaldehyde is prepared by dilution in pH 7.2 phosphate-buffered saline (Table I).

iv. Erythrocytes

Sheep blood freshly defibrinated or taken sterilely into Alsever's solution,* or into ACD solution (Section 16.A.5.c.i), and cells from other species, such as human cells of type O or rabbit erythrocytes, have been used successfully. Sheep erythrocytes are advantageously small (4.5 μm average diameter); the number per cubic millimeter of whole blood is 12×10^6, thus giving a Wintrobe hematocrit value of 29 to 35 (average, 32).[12] Blood cells are washed several times with 5 to 10 volumes of pH 7.2 phosphate-buffered saline before use. Blood is not used if appreciable hemolysis occurs during washing.

v. Preparation of Formalinized Erythrocytes (Method of Daniel et al.[13])†

Fresh, washed, and packed erythrocytes are mixed with 8 volumes of cold 3% formaldehyde (5°) and gently agitated or stirred at 4° for 24

---

* The original Alsever formulation [J. B. Alsever and R. B. Ainslie, *N.Y. State J. Med.* **41**, 126 (1941)] is modified by titrating to pH 6.1 with 10% citric acid, monohydrated, which requires about 5.5 ml per liter [S. C. Bukantz, C. R. Rein, and J. F. Kent, *J. Lab. Clin. Med.* **31**, 394 (1964)]. Preparation is described in Chap. 17.A.2.b. The solution can be autoclaved at 10 pounds pressure for 15 minutes or filtered sterilely. Add 1 volume of sterile whole blood to 1.2 volumes of sterile modified Alsever's solution and store at 4°. Allow 3 to 7 days for stabilization of the cells; the erythrocytes are overly fragile at first. As long as sterility is maintained, cells may be used for 5 or more weeks: They are discarded when the first washing fluid shows excess hemoglobin. Herbert advises adding an antibiotic such as Aureomycin at 5 mg per 100 ml [W. J. Herbert, *in* "Handbook of Experimental Immunology" (D. M. Weir, ed.), 2nd ed., p. 202. Davis, Philadelphia, Pennsylvania, 1973].

[12] O. W. Schelm, "Veterinary Hematology," 2nd rev. ed. Lea & Febiger, Philadelphia, Pennsylvania, 1967.

[13] T. M. Daniel, J. G. M. Weyand, Jr., and A. B. Stavitsky, *J. Immunol.* **99**, 741 (1963).

† Another procedure is given in Section 16.B.3.c.; see also L. Csizmas, *Proc. Soc. Exp. Biol. Med.* **103**, 157 (1960).

hours. Two volumes of cold 40% formaldehyde are added, and agitation is continued for another 24 hours. The cells are then filtered through 4 layers of gauze, washed 8 times with 8 to 10 volumes of saline, and resuspended in 6 to 8 volumes of saline. The cells may be stored at this point by refrigeration, or they may be agitated vigorously and frozen at −20° or lower, or lyophilized; they remain usable for many months. If preferred, these cells may be sensitized with antigen immediately.

vi. Diluents and Antisera

Antisera are diluted in 1% normal rabbit serum (1 ml per 100 ml of phosphate-buffered saline, pH 7.2) or in 0.2% solutions of gelatin, bovine γ-globulin, bovine serum albumin, or rabbit γ-globulin in the same buffer. The use of fetal calf serum and dextran as diluent proved highly favorable for titering anti-DNP sera since hemagglutination titers were increased 20- to 40-fold over titers of sera diluted in the phosphate buffer.[7] Diluents other than normal rabbit serum are more apt to cause spontaneous hemagglutination of red cells. Normal rabbit serum for preparing the diluent and diluents containing γ-globulin, as well as antisera to be tested, are heated at 56° for 30 minutes to inactivate hemolytic complement. These reagents are then absorbed with washed, packed erythrocytes of the desired species in order to remove normal hemagglutinating antibodies. (The absorption step can be omitted if the diluted antiserum or proteins are found in preliminary tests not to agglutinate the protein-coated cells.) After incubation for 10 minutes at room temperature with a volume of packed erythrocytes equal to the volume of undiluted serum or γ-globulin stock solution, the cells are sedimented by centrifugation and the serum or diluent is carefully separated. Occasionally, when the normal rabbit serum happens to exhibit a high agglutinating titer for the erythrocytes to be coated, more than one absorption with red cells is required before the absorbed serum, diluted to 1%, will lack all capacity to agglutinate the erythrocytes. After absorption the diluents are stored at −20°. They are diluted on the day of use with saline.

Askonas et al.[14] absorbed hemagglutinins from rabbit antiserum with packed sheep erythrocytes in the presence of 0.1% neutral sodium ethylenediamine tetraacetate to chelate Ca^{2+} and Mg^{2+} required for complement activity. Complement activity can also be inactivated with zymosan.[15] Alternative methods of removing complement activity are presented in Vol. III, Chap. 13.A.2.a.vi.

---

[14] B. A. Askonas, C. P. Farthing, and J. H. Humphrey, *Immunology* **3**, 336 (1960).
[15] K. P. Mathews, *J. Immunol.* **82**, 279 (1959).

b. SENSITIZATION OF ERYTHROCYTES

i. Sensitization of Fresh Erythrocytes after Treatment with Tannic Acid

Packed, washed sheep erythrocytes are resuspended in pH 7.2 phosphate-buffered saline to a final concentration of 2.5% by volume. The concentration of cells is determined by measuring hemoglobin released from an aliquot; 1.0 ml of the suspension is lysed by adding 5.0 ml of distilled water, the lysate is centrifuged clear, and hemoglobin is read spectrophotometrically. After this reading, correction of the volume of the "2.5%" suspension is made to a standard density according to the formula used by Kent et al.,[16] namely, $V_2 = (V_1 OD_1)/OD_2$, where V_2 is the adjusted volume to give OD_2, the optical density desired after the laking procedure; OD_1 is the optical density read upon laking an aliquot of the original volume V_1. This author adjusts to a reading of 0.400 in a Klett-Summerson colorimeter with a (green) No. 54 filter, using a 14-mm round cuvette; Kent et al.[16] adjusted to a reading of 0.500 in a Coleman, Jr., spectrophotometer at 580 nm, using a 2-ml volume in a 12-mm Kahn serological tube and a special cuvette holder; Battisto and Chase[2] used Coleman, 10 mm i.d. "perfect-round" cuvettes and adjusted to an absorbancy of 0.440 at 550 nm.*

One volume of this adjusted cell suspension is mixed with an equal volume of 1:20,000 (0.00005%) tannic acid and incubated at 37° for 15 minutes. The cells are spun out, washed with 1 volume of pH 7.2 phosphate-buffered saline, and resuspended in 5 volumes of pH 6.4 phosphate-buffered saline. One volume of the antigen solution of suitable concentration (see Table II) is then added to the cell suspension. The mixture is incubated for 30 minutes at room temperature. The cells are spun out and *the supernatant may be saved.*† After washing in 2 volumes of 1% normal rabbit serum in pH 7.2 buffered saline, the cells are suspended in 1 volume of 1% normal rabbit serum (the original "2.5%" concentration).‡ At 4° these preparations may remain stable and suitably sensitive for hemagglutination for 2 to 3 days.

---

[16] J. F. Kent, S. C. Bukantz, and C. R. Rein, *J. Immunol.* **53**, 27 (1946).

* The comparison was made on sheep cells which read 2% by hematocrit and 2.5% by pipetting "packed" cells; after laking with 5 volumes of water, the supernatant read 0.400 in the Klett-Summerson colorimeter under the stated conditions and 0.440 in the Coleman, Junior spectrophotometer at 550 nm.

† The supernatant antigen solution from the reaction mixture of tanned cells and antigen can be frozen at −20° and subsequently used to sensitive a similar volume of washed, packed, standardized tanned cells. Supernatants of some antigens have been used 4 times with no loss in sensitivity or specificity when tested with standard antisera, but bovine γ-globulin can be reused only once.

‡ Reproducibility of the end point of antibody titrations is dependent upon maintain-

Different preparations of the same antigen may vary in the effectiveness with which erythrocytes are sensitized. Divalent ions present in some preparations of diphtheria toxoid inhibit sensitization of the cell by these proteins. Electrodialysis of such preparations will render them satisfactory for sensitization of erythrocytes.

ii. Sensitization of Formalinized Erythrocytes[13]

Frozen formalinized cells are thawed and stirred vigorously to disperse, then washed 4 times with saline and resuspended in a convenient volume of saline. The cell volume of this suspension is determined in a hematocrit tube and diluted to a cell volume of 2.5%. These cells are mixed with an equal volume of 0.0005% tannic acid and incubated at 37° for 10 minutes. The suspension is centrifuged and the cells are washed in 1 volume of pH 7.2 phosphate-buffered saline. The cells are suspended in 5 volumes of saline buffered at the correct pH (Table II) and 1 volume of antigen at the concentration appropriate for formalinized cells (Table II). The mixture is kept at room temperature for 30 minutes and then centrifuged. After washing in 2 volumes of 0.005% normal rabbit serum in saline buffered at pH 7.2, the cells are finally suspended in 1 volume of 0.005% normal rabbit serum. Cells prepared according to this method are found to be stable at 4° and to withstand repeated freezing and thawing or lyophilization without loss of sensitivity or specificity, but at room temperature they will slowly lose activity, probably owing to desorption of antigen. Accordingly, it is important to keep these cells cold at all times. (Supernatants of reaction mixtures from these cells may be reused provided the formalinized cells are washed twice after tanning before addition of antigen.)

Ingraham [17, 18] found that formalinized cells will bind proteins or couple with diazotized haptens without previous tanning when mixtures are rotated slowly for several days, and he used such cells for the detection of antibodies to haptens and proteins.

---

ing the cell concentration constant from one day to another. Owing to slight but significant lysis of erythrocytes, averaging 12% loss, which was found to occur during the procedures of tanning, coating the cells with antigen, and subsequent washings, M. W. Chase (personal communication, 1968) found it necessary to restandardize the cell suspension. Accordingly, the cells were taken up in less than 1 volume of buffer containing normal rabbit serum, an aliquot was lysed as before with 5 volumes of distilled water, and hemoglobin was read after clarifying. Adjustment of cell density to give a reading of 0.470 at 550 nm in a Coleman, 10 mm i.d. "perfect round" cuvette was optimal in the hemagglutination test, when 0.05 ml of the corrected cell suspension was added to 0.5-ml portions of antibody dilutions.

[17] J. S. Ingraham, *Proc. Soc. Exp. Biol. Med.* **99**, 452 (1958).

[18] J. S. Ingraham, *in* "Immunological Methods" (J. F. Ackroyd, ed.), pp. 386–387. Blackwell, Oxford, 1964.

TABLE II

OPTIMAL CONDITIONS FOR SENSITIZATION OF TANNIC ACID-TREATED SHEEP
ERYTHROCYTES WITH VARIOUS PROTEINS[a]

Antigen[b]	Fresh cells, antigen conc./ml	pH	Formalinized cells, antigen conc./ml	pH
BGG	2.0 mg	6.4	0.1 mg	6.4
BSA	2.0 mg	6.4	0.1 mg	5.6
HSA	2.0 mg	6.4	0.05–0.01 mg	5.6
KLH	2.0 mg	6.4	1.0 mg[c]	5.6
D toxoid	130.0 Lf units	6.4	13.0 Lf units	6.4
EA	Not suitable[d]	—	0.5–1.0 mg[c]	5.6

[a] Data are based on the experience of this laboratory; modification may be necessary with different preparations of these antigens.

[b] BGG = bovine γ-globulin (Cohn fraction II); BSA = bovine serum albumin (fraction V); HSA = human serum albumin (fraction V); KLH = keyhole limpet hemocyanin; D toxoid = diphtheria toxoid (purogenated preparation of Lederle Laboratories); EA = egg albumin, 5× crystallized.

[c] Considerable variability in titers has been experienced with formalinized cells sensitized with these antigens.

[d] Not suitable since only low titers are obtained.

c. ASSAY METHODS

i. Titration of Antisera

Prior to assay, all sera are inactivated by heating at 56° to prevent hemolysis of the protein-coated red cells. When formalinized cells are employed, however, this inactivation can usually be omitted before undertaking absorption. Instead of the batch absorption, 0.1 ml of serum may be mixed with 0.9 ml of 0.00005% (1:200 of 1%) normal rabbit serum in pH 7.2 buffered saline and with 2 drops of packed, washed sheep erythrocytes. After centrifugation the diluted serum is used to prepare serial 2-fold dilutions in 10 × 100 mm round-bottomed tubes with final volumes of 0.5 ml. The pH 7.2 buffered saline diluent to be used with formalinized–sensitized cells contains 0.5% serum, not 1% serum as is used with fresh sensitized cells. A suspension of uniformly dispersed, sensitized erythrocytes (0.05 ml volume) is added to each tube, and the tubes are shaken vigorously to suspend the cells evenly. The following controls are required:

1. Tests with dilutions of a known positive serum; these tubes indicate the end point of the tests with the batch of antigen-coated tanned cells used on the day of the test.

2. Tests with dilutions of a normal serum (a *complete* dilution series parallel to all tubes of series (1) above is not needed); these tubes show

that antigen-coated tanned cells are not agglutinated nonspecifically. It is to be recalled that traces of detergents or dichromate in the tubes can lead to false patterns in the settling cells.

3. Serum diluent, 0.5 ml, plus sensitized cells; this tube should yield a completely negative reaction, indicating that "normal" antibodies for sheep red cells have been fully absorbed from the inactivated and absorbed serum used as diluent.

4. A series of dilutions of antiserum plus 0.1 to 0.2 mg of homologous antigen per tube, followed by the addition of sensitized cells; the homologous antigen at this concentration should inhibit hemagglutination more or less completely. This test proves that agglutination of the coated cells depends upon reaction of antibody with specific antigen.

5. A series of dilutions of antiserum plus 0.1 to 0.2 mg of heterologous antigen per tube, followed by addition of sensitized cells; the heterologous antigen should not inhibit hemagglutination at all.

Alternative methods to those given above have been suggested to miniaturize the test, especially where reagents (such as serum of individual mice) must be conserved.[19] Dilutions of antiserum can be made within Lucite wells using calibrated capillary pipettes or spiral loops of the Takătsy-type or the slotted ball of the "Microtiter-type"* to hold 0.025 ml or 0.05 ml. Tests can be conducted in hemispherical depressions in clear plastic trays fitted with flat plastic lids to avoid evaporation.† Patterns of the sedimented erythrocytes can be examined easily under the low power of a binocular dissecting microscope.

The cells in the tubes are allowed to settle at room temperature or in the cold for 3 to 15 hours and the cell settling patterns are observed. If antigen is slowly being desorbed from the cells, the titer may decrease with time. Figure 1 illustrates typical patterns. The last 2-plus patterns in the series provides the most clear-cut and reproducible end point, although undoubtedly specific hemagglutination occurs in some tubes which display a "one-plus" pattern. Small negative prozones are occasionally observed. More precise quantitation of end points may be achieved by reading the end point photometrically[18] or by counting cells electronically and measuring size distribution changes in an antigen-coated cell population by varying concentrations of antibody.[20]

Studies with rabbit antisera taken during the early part of the primary

---

[19] J. L. Sever, *J. Immunol.* **88**, 320 (1962).

* Available as "Microtiter," Cooke Engineering Company, Alexandria, Virginia.

† Available from Linbro Chemical Co., Inc., New Haven, Connecticut, as No. 96U-CV, using only the hemispherical base of the wells, or—if applicable to a given problem—the tiny (0.2 ml) wells of model MCR-96 or S-MCR 96.

[20] H. F. Mengoli, J. C. Pruitt, and H. M. Carpenter, *Lab. Invest.* **12**, 365 (1963).

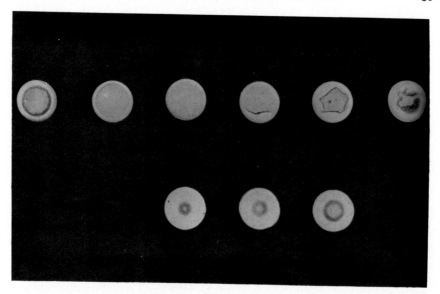

FIG. 1. Appearance of hemagglutination patterns as observed by mirror in the base of tubes having perfect, hemispherical bottoms; the tubes are not shaken. Top row, left to right: $++++$, $+++$, $++$, $+$, $\pm$, 0 reactions. The designations are as follows: $++++$, compact, granular agglutinate; $+++$, smooth mat on bottom of tube with folded edges; $++$, smooth mat, edges somewhat ragged; $+$, narrow ring of red around edge of smooth mat; $\pm$, lesser area covered by erythrocyte sediment than in $+$ reactions, but heavier peripheral ring than in negative tubes; 0, discrete button of erythrocytes in bottom of tube. Bottom row, left: type of pattern seen with early antibody-containing sera, predominantly IgM globulin. Bottom row, right: negative ($-$) pattern. (Note that tubes which contain a button of glass in the bottom will show "doughnut-like" clear centers where the cells, sliding down the walls of the tube, fail to join as a uniform layer.)

response to protein antigens[21] showed the presence of predominantly γ_M hemagglutinating antibodies. These sera often produced hemagglutination patterns different from those observed with hyperimmune sera. Figure 1, bottom row, illustrates this type of pattern. It is now known that these early sera also contain γ_G antibodies.[22] The hemagglutination patterns may, therefore, result from the interaction of both γ_M and γ_G antibodies with the sensitized erythrocytes.

ii. Estimation of Small Amounts of Antigen by Inhibition Tests

Several series of dilutions of antiserum are made. In one series, 0.05 or 0.1 ml of a suitable concentration of the unknown protein is added to

[21] A. B. Stavitsky, in "Immunological Methods" (J. F. Ackroyd, ed.), pp. 363–396. Blackwell, Oxford, 1964.
[22] M. Wei and A. B. Stavitsky, *Immunology* **12**, 431 (1967).

each tube. The same volume of saline is added to each tube of a second control series. The same volume of various known concentrations of the standard antigen are added to tubes of additional series. All tubes are incubated overnight at room temperature. A suspension of sensitized cells (0.05 ml volumes) is then added to all tubes and the control tubes, and the amount of protein in the unknown is estimated by comparison of its inhibition titer with that of the standard antigen. Alternatively, serial dilutions are made of the unknown and standard proteins in dilute, inactivated, and absorbed normal rabbit serum. To each tube, 0.1 ml or 0.05 ml of a suitable dilution of the antiserum in 1:100 normal rabbit serum are added, likewise to a control tube which does not contain antigen. After overnight incubation at room temperature, 0.05 ml of sensitized cells is added to each tube, and the amount of protein in the unknown is estimated by comparison of its inhibition titer with that of the standard.

An extension of the inhibition test is the determination of pregnancy by examining urine for human chorionic gonadotropin (HCG). Formalinized tanned sheep cells coated with HCG and specific antiserum are commercially available.* Tests employ small amounts of filtered urine, added as inhibitor. Latex particles also have been used (Section 16.E.1.c).

d. General Factors That Affect Hemagglutination

To sensitize cells for maximal sensitivity, specificity, and stability, the antigen must be used in an optimal concentration and at an optimal hydrogen ion concentration (Table II). With certain soluble kidney antigens coated on fresh, tanned erythrocytes, a pH of 7.0 may be preferable to pH 6.4; and with certain preparations of diphtheria toxoid, the highest titers are observed when sensitization of fresh, tanned cells is performed at pH 5.0.[23] There is a linear relationship (logarithmic scale) between number of cells and titer, such that the agglutinin titer is doubled when the number of cells added is halved. Accordingly, it is essential to standardize the density of the final erythrocyte suspension. The sensitivity of the inhibition reaction in detecting certain antigens may increase progressively as the time for combination of antigen and antibody is lengthened before the sensitized erythrocytes are added. The incubation temperature has no marked effect on the reaction of γ_G rabbit antibody with protein-sensitized cells, but γ_M rabbit antibody yields highest titers at about 4°. Formalinized cells and formalinized–sensitized cells tend to

---

* Typical sets of reagents are provided by several laboratories, such as Wampole Laboratories, Stamford, Connecticut ("UCG-test"), and Organon's "Prognosticon."
[23] M. Reynaud, personal communication (1961).

aggregate spontaneously and must be mixed or shaken vigorously before use.

It is reported that higher hemagglutination titers are found with an antiserum to native bovine serum albumin when the tanned erythrocytes are coated with partially denatured BSA, the cells coated with the denatured protein apparently detecting additional antibodies. Wolberg et al.[24] concluded that antibodies to hidden determinants of bovine albumin were usually produced during immunization but that such antibodies do not react with cells coated with the native protein. T2 phage-coated red cells do not detect phage antibodies unless the phage are first solubilized with detergent.[25] The resultant hemagglutination reaction appears to be as sensitive as the conventional neutralization test (Section 18.C). The tanned cells can be coated with various fractions of the solubilized phage for assay of antibodies directed against distinct antigens of the phage.

[24] G. Wolberg, C. T. Liu, and F. L. Adler, J. Immunol. **105**, 797 (1970).
[25] W. S. Walker, C. T. Liu, and F. L. Adler, J. Immunol. **103**, 907 (1969).

3. ANTIGEN–RED CELL CONJUGATES PREPARED WITH BISDIAZOBENZIDINE*

The use of antigen–red cell conjugates prepared with bisdiazobenzidine has several advantages, and one major disadvantage. The disadvantage is the fragility of the cells. The advantages are that (1) there is essentially no desorption of antigen from the conjugate; (2) the end points of hemagglutination are more sharply read than with tanned cells (Section 16.B.2); and (3) the preparation can be used, in the presence of complement, for a precise measure of relative antibody concentration.

a. REAGENTS

i. Preparation of Bisdiazobenzidine (BDB)

Benzidine (0.92 gm) is dissolved at room temperature in a solution containing 200 ml of H_2O and 6 ml of 6 N HCl. It is then cooled in an alcohol Dry-ice bath until ice crystals are floating free. At this time, about 6 ml of freshly prepared 10% $NaNO_2$ are added with continuous stirring. Ice should always be present in the reaction mixture in order to maintain the temperature constant. The solution may turn a transient reddish brown, yet, with continuous stirring the color of the solution will become a pale lemon yellow. The stirring is continued until the solution gives a negative reaction for nitrite on starch iodide paper. About 6.5 ml of sodium nitrite can be added to this mixture. The last 0.5 ml is added

---

* Section 16.B.3 was contributed by E. R. Arquilla.

slowly. BDB has been standardized empirically by adding 7 ml of 0.11 M phosphate buffer (pH 7.4) to 0.5 ml of BDB (1:15 BDB). A deep reddish brown color develops immediately, and the solution becomes turbid within 90 $\pm$ 5 seconds. When the solution does not turn deep reddish brown immediately, the time before turbidity appears is also prolonged. A few crystals of benzidine can then be added and the solution retested. If the turbidity develops rapidly (in less than 80 seconds), small amounts (0.05 to 0.1 ml) of 10% sodium nitrite are added to the solution. When the desired preparation is obtained, the stock BDB is divided into 0.5 ml aliquots and stored at $-80°$. Under these conditions BDB remains active for at least 9 months.

ii. Antigens

Since antigen solutions used to prepare erythrocyte conjugates with BDB must not contain any material capable of reacting with this reagent, antigens are therefore dissolved in phosphate-buffered saline.

iii. Erythrocytes

Fresh, defibrinated sheep blood or sheep blood in Alsever's solution (Sections 16.B.2.a.iv or 17.A.2.a), human type O cells, and cells from other species such as rabbit, have been used successfully. Blood cells are washed several times with 5 to 10 volumes of pH 7.4 phosphate-buffered saline before use. Blood is not used if appreciable hemolysis occurs during washing.

iv. Solutions

Buffered saline consists of 0.15 M NaCl in 0.01 M phosphate buffer, pH 7.4 (Vol. II, Appendix II, buffer 33B diluted 1:4 and 8.5 gm of NaCl added).

Barbital (Veronal)–Buffered Saline (VBS). This diluent is used for titrating complement and for making immune hemolysis titrations at pH 7.4 with $MgCl_2$ and $CaCl_2$ (Vol. II, Appendix II, buffer 6B).

VPS–Albumin. For hemagglutination titrations, barbital-buffered saline containing 0.15% BSA (1.5 gm/liter) is prepared. Prior to use, the diluent is held at 80° for 1 hour and then cooled at once to 0° in a water bath. Much of the nonspecific agglutination observed at high dilution of antiserum is eliminated by using this diluent.

v. Sheep Cell Stromata

Stromata needed to absorb complement are prepared according to the method of Eylar et al.[1] Sheep red cells (100 ml of packed cells or less) in

[1] E. H. Eylar, M. A. Madoff, O. V. Brody, and J. L. Oncley, *J. Biol. Chem.* **237**, 1992 (1962).

Alsever's solution are washed with saline until the supernatant is clear. The cells are suspended in a small volume of saline (500 ml) and hemolysed by adding 12 volumes of water. The pH is adjusted with 0.1 N HCl to between 5 and 6, where a heavy floc forms. The supernatant is decanted, water is again added to a final volume of 6 liters, and the pH is readjusted to between 5 and 6. This procedure is repeated until the supernatant is clear. The precipitate is washed with distilled water, taken up in a small volume of distilled H_2O, and lyophilized. Stromata are used on a dry-weight basis for absorption of serum.

vi. Complement

Absorbed complement (C'_{abs}) is used for the hemolytic titration of insulin antibodies. Pools of fresh guinea pig sera are absorbed with 10 mg/ml of sheep red cell stroma at room temperature (25°) for 10 minutes during gentle agitation, and then are centrifuged at approximately 2000 g for 15 minutes at 4°.

vii. Titration of Complement

Titers of C'_{abs} are determined by 50% hemolytic end points (Section 17.A.4.b). A unit of complement is defined as the smallest amount of C'_{abs} which will cause lysis of 50% of the sensitized cells (1 ml of a 1.25% suspension) in a final volume of 1.5 ml after 30 minutes at 37°.

b. PREPARATION OF ANTIGEN CONJUGATES WITH FRESH ERYTHROCYTES

i. Estimation of the BDB:Antigen Ratio Necessary for Optimal Conjugation of Antigen to Red Cells

The ratio of BDB to antigen required for optimal sensitization of red cells varies with the particular antigen, but this ratio is nearly constant with different batches of BDB. If excess of antigen is used, homologous antisera give only low specific agglutination of the cells. If too little antigen is used, nonspecific agglutination and obvious hemolysis will occur. A rough approximation of the amount of antigen is obtained by adding varying amounts of antigen to a given amount of washed red cells and BDB. Usually 0.1 ml of packed washed red cells are suspended to constant volume with variable amounts of antigen (0.5 to 3 mg). The red cells are evenly suspended by gentle agitation, and 0.4 ml of BDB (diluted 1:15 with 0.11 M phosphate buffer, pH 7.4) is added. These suspensions are shaken gently for 10 minutes at room temperature, washed twice with approximately 5 volumes of barbital-buffered saline–albumin, and then suspended in 5 ml of this diluent. The amount of antigen needed for optimal sensitization of red cells is approximated in the preparations where no spontaneous agglutination of red cells by BDB is noted. Next, several batches of sensitized cells are prepared with the concentration of antigen varied over a much narrower range (e.g., 2.0 to 2.5 mg). These antigen–red cell conjugates are then tested comparatively against some antiserum accepted as a "standard."

The criteria for an optimal ratio of antigen to BDB are: (1) agglutination of the conjugated cells by the least amount of the standard antisera; (2) a ready discrimination between agglutinated and nonagglutinated antigen–red cell conjugates, by finding a clearly defined end point; (3) maximal inhibition of agglutination of the conjugated erythrocytes when the standard antiserum is preincubated with soluble antigen; and (4) nonspecific agglutination of antigen–red cell conjugates is not found.

ii. Antigen Conjugates Made with Fresh Erythrocytes

(a) *Stability of the Conjugated Erythrocytes.* The antigen-conjugated red cells can be maintained at 3° to 4° for 4 to 5 hours and still be used for hemagglutination or immune hemolysis. The hemagglutination end points should be read 2 to 3 hours after the antigen-conjugated red cells have been added to the antiserum. After the addition of the erythrocyte–antigen conjugate to antiserum, some lysis will be noted, at approximately 6 hours of incubation at room temperature, and at approximately 12 hours when a temperature of 3° to 4° is employed.

(b) *The Detection of Antibodies by Hemagglutination.* Two series of successively doubled dilutions of each test antiserum are prepared in 10 × 75 mm test tubes, using VBS–albumin as the diluent in a final volume of 0.5 ml. To the inhibition series, 10 μg of antigen in 0.1 ml is added to each tube, and 0.1 ml of saline is added to each tube of the controls. After mixing, 0.05 ml of a suspension of antigen–red cell conjugate is added to all tubes, making a final volume of 0.65 ml. Nonspecific agglutination owing to the possible presence of heterophile antibodies is sought by preparing control tubes containing 0.05 ml of a 2% suspension of washed, unsensitized erythrocytes and 0.6 ml of the lowest dilution (highest concentration) of antiserum used. All tubes are shaken to disperse the cells evenly and the tubes are then allowed to stand for 3 to 4 hours, without disturbing the cells as they settle.

Agglutination is determined by the pattern given by the sensitized erythrocytes in the bottom of the tube. In the absence of agglutination, a discrete button of red cells is observed. A slight degree of agglutination produces a halo surrounding a central pink film. Positive agglutination results in an evenly distributed sheet of erythrocytes. When agglutination is maximal, this sheet is wrinkled and folded since the agglutinated cells slide down the side walls and become compressed. The test tubes used (10 × 75 mm) must be uniform and free of distorted hemispherical bottoms. Arbitrary criteria for the presence of antibodies are established as follows: (1) antigen–red cell conjugates are agglutinated by the test antiserum; (2) agglutination is inhibited when the test antiserum has been preincubated with antigen; (3) the test antiserum does not agglutinate nonsensitized erythrocytes.

The titer of an antiserum is designated as the highest dilution in which there is definite evidence that agglutination has taken place. Attempts to quantitate degrees of hemagglutination are subjective in nature and are unnecessary if the technique of passive immune hemolysis, which gives precise measurements of antibody activity, is used subsequently.

iii. The Technique of Passive Immune Hemolysis for Titrating Antisera

As in agglutination titration, serial dilutions of antisera are prepared and cooled to 0° in an ice bath. To each tube is added an excess of C'_{abs} (20–50 hemolytic units). Finally the antigen–red cell conjugate is added; usually about four times as many cells are employed in the immune hemolysis reaction as are used for hemagglutination. After the cells are suspended uniformly by gentle shaking, all samples are incubated in the 37° water bath for 30 minutes. The nonhemolysed cells are then separated by centrifugation at approximately 2000 g for 5 minutes at 3°. After the supernatant solutions are decanted, 2 ml of water is added to each erythrocyte sediment to effect hemolysis. Hemolysis in each sample is then measured by extinction at 580 nm with a spectrophotometer. This method is valid and reliable, when standardized antisera and large pools of standardized C'_{abs} are available. The reagents (C'_{abs}, BDB, insulin, or cells) must be tested again when any of them is changed. Specific inhibition of immune hemolysis should be demonstrated by adding a known amount of antigen (10 μg in 0.05 ml) to samples of diluted antisera prior to the addition of C'_{abs} and red cell–antigen conjugates.

Antibody measurement by the technique of immune hemolysis can be made very precisely by estimating the area under the curve which is obtained when hemoglobin released *by immune hemolysis* is plotted against the logarithm of the reciprocal of the dilution of the test antisera. The area under the curve can be measured by cutting out and weighing the respective segment of the graph (Table III).[2] The reproducibility and precision of the method are shown in Table III. In this table, the hemolytic titration curves obtained from 5 aliquots of the same insulin antiserum,

[2] E. R. Arquilla and J. Finn, *J. Exp. Med.* **118**, 55–71 (1963).

TABLE III
PRECISION OF IMMUNE HEMOLYTIC TITRATION OF ANTISERUM

Aliquots	Antiserum dilution				Area of curve[a] (mg of paper)	Percent of mean area
	1/20	1/80	1/320	1/1280		
1	0.495[b]	0.340	0.125	0.065	1273	102.0
2	0.480	0.330	0.115	0.070	1220	97.8
3	0.500	0.340	0.115	0.070	1250	100.2
4	0.485	0.330	0.125	0.070	1251	100.3
5	0.500	0.330	0.115	0.075	1241	99.5

[a] Area of the hemolytic titration curve determined by weighing the appropriate portion of the graph paper to the nearest milligram. Mean curve area, 1247 mg. Calculated standard deviation, $\pm 1.5\%$ from mean.

[b] Absorbancy of hemoglobin released from erythrocytes in the hemolytic test, found by determining total hemoglobin in the erythrocyte volume added to each tube, subtracting the hemoglobin in each residual cell sediment after water lysis of both and reading absorbancy at 580 nm.

tested simultaneously, showed a standard deviation of 1.5% when the mean area of the hemolytic titration curves was taken as 100%.

c. PREPARATION OF STABLE FORMALINIZED ERYTHROCYTE– ANTIGEN CONJUGATES

Formalinized red blood cells* have been used previously in hemagglutination reactions for assay of human chorionic gonadotropin.[3] Red blood cells stored in Alsever's solution for 2 to 14 days are washed 3 to 4 times in 8 to 10 volumes of saline and diluted in saline as an 8% suspension (8 ml of packed cells plus 92 ml of saline). Formalin solution (3%) is prepared by adding 50 ml of USP formalin (37%) to 567 ml of saline and adding 0.1 N NaOH to an apparent pH of 7.1. One volume of the freshly prepared (8%) suspension of washed red blood cells is mixed with one volume of 3% formaldehyde and incubated at 37° for 18 to 24 hours. The cell suspension is shaken occasionally during incubation. The red cells are then washed 4 times in 8 to 10 volumes of distilled water and stored at +4° as a 10% suspension in distilled water. It is convenient to store cells in a 10% solution to avoid pipetting packed cells, a procedure which is not precise. The 10% suspension of formalinized red cells is determined by cell volume (hematocrit), using aliquots of the stock cell suspension. Stock formalinized red cells, stored as long as one year at 3° to 4°, have shown no significant alteration in their properties.

* Another technique is given in Section 16.B.2.b.ii.

[3] L. Wide, *Acta Endocrinol.* **41**, Suppl. 70 (1962).

i. Conjugation of Antigen to Formalin-Treated Red Cells

Determining the proper ratio of BDB to antigen for optimal sensitization of formalin-treated red cells is similar in principle to its determination when conjugates of antigen–BDB and fresh red cells are used. Three times as much BDB is needed for optimal sensitization of formalinized red cells as for fresh red cells. Consequently, the stock BDB is diluted with 0.11 M PO$_4$ buffer at pH 7.4 to 1:5 rather than to 1:15. Conjugation of antigen to formalinized red cells is otherwise carried out as for conjugates made with fresh cells.

ii. Storage of Antigen–Formalinized Erythrocyte Conjugates

Conjugates of antigen with formalinized red cells can be stored as a 10% suspension for many weeks; such preparations can be used after one washing with 8 to 10 volumes of diluent, followed by dilution to the desired suspension. As a rule, the suspension of antigen–formalinized red cells to be used in antiserum titration can be somewhat more dilute (ca. 1.5%) than conjugates of antigen with fresh red cells (2%).

Lyophilization of antigen–formalinized red cell conjugates, already diluted to the final desired concentration (1.5%) with diluent VBS–albumin, is conveniently carried out using small aliquots (2 to 3 ml). After lyophilization, the tubes are sealed and stored in a desiccator at room temperature. Prior to use, the cake within a vial is resuspended with as much distilled water as was present in the sample before lyophilization (i.e., 2 to 3 ml). After thorough mixing, this preparation can be used directly.

When antigen–formalinized red cell conjugates are to be lyophilized in large batches, the hardened red cells are suspended in a minimal volume of distilled water, to which 0.5 gm of sucrose is added for each 0.5 ml of packed red cells; a homogeneous dark brown powder is obtained. This material should be sealed securely and stored in a dry environment. Prior to use it is washed twice with distilled water (50 ml per 0.5 ml of packed red cells) and suspended in VBS–albumin.

4. ANTIGEN-RED CELL CONJUGATES PREPARED BY SPECIAL METHODS OF CHEMICAL BONDING*

Several methods have been introduced, other than coupling by bisdiazobenzidine (Section 16.B.3), to circumvent the tendency of tanned cells to adsorb proteins nonspecifically from the serum being titrated, or the possibility of desorption of antigen from the conjugate.

* Section 16.B.4 was contributed by Abram B. Stavitsky.

a. CHROMIC CHLORIDE

Metallic cations can be used to attach proteins to red cells.[1] The most useful of these is chromium, and tests based on chromic chloride coupling have been used to measure antibodies to several proteins, including ovalbumin and bovine γ-globulin.[1-3] Since these conjugates do not adsorb protein from the immune serum, they can be used in experiments with antiglobulin reagents (Coombs test).[2] An excess of rabbit complement will lyse the protein–erythrocyte complex,[3] a feature of passive lysis to be emphasized because tanned cells can be lysed by complement alone in the absence of antibody.

Theoretically, nonagglutinating concentrations of antibody can be coupled to cells by the CrCl$_3$ method and the immunoglobulin class of the antibody can be determined by use of hemagglutinating concentrations of specific anti-class sera.

b. CARBODIIMIDE COUPLING

The water-soluble 1-ethyl-3(3-dimethylaminopropyl) carbodiimide (ECDI) can be employed to couple proteins to red blood cells for hemagglutination tests.[4-6] The coupling steps are shown in Vol. I, Chap. 1.E.6.

c. 1,3-DIFLUORO-4,6-DINITROBENZENE (DFDNB) COUPLING

This reagent can be used to couple proteins to human red cells.[7] This method has also been employed to couple human chorionic gonadotropin to formalinized cells.[8]

d. SPECIFIC COUPLING TO ANTIGENIC SITES OF ERYTHROCYTES

Coombs *et al.* have developed alternative methods for coating red cells with antigen.[9, 10] The erythrocytes are coated by attaching agents that bind strongly with the cells, do not damage them, and do not agglutinate them at the concentrations used. The "antigens" consist of immunoglobu-

[1] J. H. Jandl and R. L. Simmons, *Brit. J. Haematol.* 3, 19 (1957).

[2] H. H. Fudenberg, G. Drews, and A. Nisonoff, *J. Exp. Med.* 119, 151 (1964).

[3] P. J. Perucca, W. P. Faulk, and H. H. Fudenberg, *J. Immunol.* 102, 812 (1969)

[4] L. Gyenes and A. H. Sehon, *Immunochemistry* 1, 43 (1964).

[5] H. M. Johnson, K. Brenner, and H. E. Hall, *J. Immunol.* 97, 701 (1966).

[6] H. M. Johnson, B. G. Smith, and H. E. Hall, *Int. Arch. Allergy Appl. Immunol.* 33, 511 (1968).

[7] N. R. Ling, *Immunology* 4, 49 (1961).

[8] A. J. Fulthorpe, I. M. Roitt, D. Doniach, and K. Couchman, *Brit. Med. J.* 1, 1049 (1963).

[9] R. R. A. Coombs, A. N. Howard, and L. S. Mynors, *Brit. J. Exp. Pathol.* 34, 525 (1953).

[10] R. R. A. Coombs and M. L. Fiset, *Brit. J. Exp. Pathol.* 35, 472 (1954).

lins, lectins, and bacterial lipopolysaccharides. Examples are Rh antibody coated on Rh positive cells,[9] photooxidized anti-Forssman antibody and erythrocytes carrying the Forssman antigen[11] (sheep and other red cells),[10] certain lectins that combine with red cells of many species but have only weak agglutinating properties (Section 16.A.6),[12] and bacterial lipopolysaccharides (Section 16.B.1).[12]

[11] K. Landsteiner, "The Specificity of Serological Reactions," rev. ed., p. 96ff. Harvard Univ. Press, Cambridge, Massachusetts, 1945; and Dover, New York, 1962.

[12] C. J. Sanderson, *Immunology* **18**, 353 (1970).

5. ANTIGLOBULIN REACTIONS WITH ERYTHROCYTES*†

The antiglobulin reaction may be used to demonstrate the presence of antibody on the cell surface in cases where the antibody on its own fails to produce agglutination. The reaction came into general use after it had been shown to be a very suitable method of revealing the presence of "incomplete" Rh antibodies,[1] although the principle of the reaction had been described a good deal earlier.[2]‡ The greatest application so far has been with respect to red cell antigen–antibody systems and particularly to the detection of human blood group antibodies, but the reaction is also applicable to other cell systems, for example, those of bacteria.§

The antiglobulin reaction may also be used as a final stage in certain passive hemagglutination methods, especially where polysaccharide antigens are concerned but also with protein antigens so long as the coupling of the protein to the red cells is effected without changing the nonspecific adsorptive properties of the cell membrane.

Tissue cells may also be subjected to examination by this method, but here modifications such as the mixed antiglobulin reaction (Section 16.B.6.c) may be more appropriate. As the reaction is based essentially on the detection of globulin at the cell surface, precautions are needed to guard against the complication of nonspecific absorption of globulin.

Various elaborations of the antiglobulin reaction have been introduced. For example, by labeling the antiglobulin serum with fluorescein it is possible to localize immunoglobulins in tissues under investigation (Section

* Sections 16.B.5.a–d were contributed by R. R. A. Coombs and P. L. Mollison.

† Testing for erythrocyte-bound antibody by adding antiglobulin antibody is popularly known as the "Coombs test." [Ed.]

[1] R. R. A. Coombs, A. E. Mourant, and R. R. Race, *Brit. J. Exp. Pathol.* **26**, 255 (1945).

[2] C. Moreschi, *Zentralbl. Bakteriol., Parasitenk,* **46**, 49 and 456 (1908).

‡ Procedure as submitted in 1964 supplemented by Editor.

§ Thus nonagglutinating antibody has been demonstrated in chronic brucellosis by absorption to brucella organisms followed by application of the Coombs test. R. R. A. Coombs, *Amer. J. Clin. Pathol.* **53**, 131 (1970). [Ed.]

17.F.4 and Vol. V, Chap. 27.B). Other elaborations are discussed below and in Section 16.B.6.

Many types of antiglobulin reagent can be prepared: Thus, sera can be made that are specific for the individual immunoglobulins or complement components. [Among these are antisera against IgG, IgM, IgA, IgE, or particular portions of immunoglobulins (γ-, μ-, α-, ϵ-heavy chains or κ or λ light chains, or Fab or Fc pieces) or for complement components C1q, C3, C4, and others. Production of some of these sera is discussed in Sections 16.B.5.f, 17.F.3.b, and 17.F.4.a.—Ed.]

a. THE DIRECT ANTIGLOBULIN TEST

This procedure is used to demonstrate that red cells, taken directly from the circulation, are already sensitized with antibody, with complement components, or with both of these. Positive results are observed in subjects with autoallergic (autoimmune) hemolytic anemia, in infants with hemolytic disease of the newborn, and occasionally as a transient phenomenon in subjects who have been transfused with incompatible red cells.

For most purposes the antiglobulin reagent need contain only anti-γ_G and antibodies to complement components. It is unlikely that any single dilution of the antiglobulin reagent will react optimally with red cells weakly sensitized with Ig and anti-complement globulins respectively. It will, therefore, be necessary to use each antiglobulin serum at two dilutions, or to blend two different antiglobulin sera, so that the final reagent, when suitably diluted, reacts optimally with antibody-coated and complement-coated cells, respectively.

If reasonably potent antiglobulin sera are used so that the optimal dilution is 1 in 50 or more it will probably be unnecessary to absorb the antiglobulin serum, but control tests must always be made with unsensitized red cells of different ABO groups. If necessary, the antiglobulin serum must be absorbed with thoroughly washed red cells.

A special instance of the direct antiglobulin test is given in Section 16.B.5.e.

Procedure

A few drops of blood may be taken from a skin prick directly into 2 to 3 ml of saline, or venous blood may be mixed with an anticoagulant. Red cells are washed three times, each time in approximately 50 volumes of saline and then resuspended to 10% for white porcelain tile or slide tests or 2% for tube tests. In each case 1 drop of suspension is added to 1 drop of suitably diluted antiglobulin serum.

In testing red cells from patients with potent cold autoantibodies the red cells must be kept at 37° until they have been washed. The best method is to take venous blood with a warm syringe, to transfer the blood to a screw-capped container, and to drop this into water at 37° to 40° in a thermos flask. The flask is then transported to the laboratory, and the red cells are washed three times in warm saline, preferably using a heated centrifuge.

b. The Indirect Antiglobulin Test

This procedure is used when sera are to be examined for "incomplete" antibodies. In some cases only undiluted serum is tested, as when the test is being used as part of the cross-matching procedure prior to blood transfusion. In other cases, in which a quantitative estimate of the amount of antibody present is required, serial dilutions of the serum are prepared and each is tested separately.

i. Procedure

Four volumes of serum or of diluted serum are mixed with 1 volume of a 20% suspension of red cells. This gives a ratio of serum to red cells of 20:1; for greater sensitivity this ratio may be increased to 100:1 by using a 4% suspension of red cells. The mixture of serum and cells is incubated at 37° for 1 to 2 hours, and the cells are then washed three times and tested as in the direct test.

ii. Use of Antiglobulin Sera of Different Specificities

Most "incomplete" antibodies are composed of γ_G-globulin and may be detected by using an anti-γ_G-globulin serum. Many γ_G-globulin antibodies bind complement, and it may then be easier to detect complement components on the sensitized red cells than to detect the antibody directly. Accordingly, the sensitized red cells, as in the direct test, should be tested with antiserum to complement components, as well as with anti-Ig. A few incomplete antibodies are IgM, but since, as far as present experience goes, these all bind complement, they may also be detected by using an antiserum to complement components.[3]

Some antibody-containing sera are anticomplementary, particularly if they have been stored, and it may then be easier to detect them by a two-stage test; that is to say, they can be detected by incubating the red cells first with the antibody-containing serum and second with fresh serum as a source of complement. The first stage is carried out as in the test described above (Section B.5.b.i) except the antibody-containing serum is first treated with EDTA (final concentration, 4 mg per milliliter of serum). After incubation at 37° for 1.5 hours the cells are washed three

[3] M. J. Polley, P. L. Mollison, and J. F. Soothill, *Brit. J. Haematol.* **8,** 149 (1962).

times and are then incubated with 2 volumes of fresh serum at 37° before being washed again and tested with antiglobulin serum.[4]

c. Inhibition of Antiglobulin Serum as a Method of Estimating Certain Serum Proteins

i. Principle

Inhibition of antiglobulin serum can be used as a method of obtaining quantitative estimates of any of the proteins involved in the antiglobulin reaction. For example, inhibition of the reaction between anti-IgG and red cells sensitized with a IgG-antibody such as incomplete anti-Rh can be used to estimate the amount of IgG present. In practice, antisera against the various separated immunoglobulins are found to behave as almost specific reagents, although one might expect that the L chains common to all immunoglobulins would cause cross-reactions such as the known partial precipitation of IgG by anti-IgM.* In inhibition reactions, however, slight cross-reactions may be observed; for example, IgM may inhibit slightly the reaction between anti-IgG and Rh-sensitized red cells.[3]

ii. Procedure for Estimating the Concentration of IgG

The procedure is to prepare, first, red cells weakly sensitized with anti-Rh(D) and, second, suitable dilutions of antiglobulin serum. Serial dilutions are now prepared of the IgG solution to be assayed and, as standards, serial dilutions are needed either of a purified preparation of IgG or of a serum of known IgG concentration. The "unknown" and "known" dilutions are added, respectively, to a series of tubes each containing a volume of diluted antiglobulin serum and are then mixed before the sensitized red cells are added. The amount of IgG in the "unknown" serum is determined by comparison. For example, if a 1:1000 dilution of the "unknown" serum produces the same degree of inhibition as a 1:5000 dilution of a 1% solution of IgG, the "unknown" solution contains 0.2% of IgG. It should be noted that assays of IgG by the immunological method give higher results than those obtained by electrophoresis because IgG is electrophoretically heterogeneous and the immunological method detects comparatively rapidly migrating IgG which is not included in the electrophoretic analysis.

The immunological method can also be used to estimate IgM globulin

---

[4] M. J. Polley and P. L. Mollison, *Transfusion* **1**, 9 (1961).

* Anti-IgM does not agglutinate red cells sensitized with incomplete anti-Rh (IgG), presumably because the predominant antibody in the anti-IgM serum is against the heavy chain (μ chain in this case) and the concentration of anti-L (light) chain is low. Similarly, anti-IgG does not agglutinate erythrocytes sensitized with incomplete anti-Le^a (IgM).

by inhibition of the reaction between anti-IgM and Le(a+) red cells sensitized with EDTA-treated anti-Le^a, and to estimate the concentrations of IgA and of complement components C3 and C4 using suitably sensitized red cells.

iii. Application in Forensic Work

The reaction between anti-human globulin serum and red cells sensitized with human antibody will be inhibited by diluted human serum, but not by diluted animal serum. Thus, in order to discover whether a particular blood stain is of human or animal origin the dried blood is extracted in saline and dilutions of this are added to diluted anti-human globulin serum and the mixtures are then tested with Rh-sensitized red cells. The method is capable of detecting less than 1 μg/ml of human γ-globulin.

d. ANTIGLOBULIN CONSUMPTION TEST

In certain circumstances agglutination may provide an unreliable means of detecting the reaction between antiglobulin serum and antibody-coated cells. For example, in testing platelets or white cells suspected of being sensitized with antibody, interpretation of the results is made difficult by the fact that these cells tend to clump spontaneously. Here, the antiglobulin consumption test is valuable. The principle of the test is to discover whether antiglobulin is "consumed" when it is incubated with cells suspected of being sensitized with antibody. Equally, as in the method described below, the test can be used to detect antibodies against normal cells by incubating the cells with serum suspected to contain antibody.

A discussion of the scope of the antiglobulin consumption test may be found in reviews by Moulinier,[5] Steffen,[6] and Gell and Coombs.[7] Dausset and Columbiani provide technical details.[8] The procedure has detected antibody in the serum of patients with idiopathic thrombocytopenia.[7]

Procedure

The following method can be used to detect antibodies against white cells and platelets. Suspensions of the cells are treated with the serum under investigation and, in parallel, with normal serum as a control. After incubation, the cells are washed thoroughly (at least 8 times). Two sets of serial dilutions of antiglobulin serum are prepared, one set then being incubated with the test cells, the other with the control cells. After

[5] J. Moulinier, Rev. Fr. Etud. Clin. Biol. 1, 355 (1956).
[6] C. Steffen, Rev. Fr. Etud. Clin. Biol. 5, 831 (1960).
[7] "Clinical Aspects of Immunology" (P. G. H. Gell and R. R. A. Coombs, eds.), 2nd. ed. Davis, Philadelphia, Pennsylvania, 1968.
[8] J. Dausset and J. Columbiani, in "Immunological Methods" (J. F. Ackroyd, ed.), p. 575. Blackwell, Oxford, 1964.

incubation, the supernatant of each tube is tested with Rh-sensitized cells. Consumption of antiglobulin by the test cells is taken as evidence of sensitization with antibody.

e. THE RED CELL-LINKED ANTIGEN TEST*

As the result of long-extended investigations, Steele and Coombs[9] were able to prepare erythrocytes linked serologically with antigens and so to search for anti-protein antibodies of the "incomplete" variety. Crude globulins [50% $(NH_4)_2SO_4$ precipitate] of rabbit anti-sheep erythrocytes, mixed with soluble antigens (e.g., BSA, casein, milk lactoglobulin), were photooxidized in the presence of 0.1% Rose Bengal against northern light with shaking. During the photooxidation (1) the agglutinating capacity of the antibody was lost and (2) the added soluble protein became bound to the oxidized globulin. The final reagent would attach to human red cells of group O (incubation in the dark). The presence of bound antibody was shown by the antiglobulin reaction and attachment of the protein antigen in agglutination tests with specific antiserum.

When milk proteins were bound to human erythrocytes in this manner,[10] it was possible to detect IgG and IgA antibodies in serum of infants by testing the washed cell suspensions with anti-IgG, and anti-IgA and anti-IgM.[11] Prior to use of the final antiglobulin test, it is useful to sediment the erythrocytes and suspend in a solution of Vi polysaccharide at 2.5 μg/ml to stabilize the cell suspension.[12]

In a special case, castor bean allergen was linked to human O erythrocytes, which were then exposed to the sera of patients allergic to castor bean. The presence of IgE antibody on the coated cells was detected by adding specific anti-IgE.[13] [Detection of specific allergic IgE is now sought by use of the *radioallergosorbent test* (RAST).]

* Section 16.B.5.e was contributed by Merrill W. Chase.

[9] A. S. V. Steele and R. R. A. Coombs, *Int. Arch. Allergy Appl. Immunol.* **25**, 11 (1964).

[10] A. Hunter and R. R. A. Coombs, *Int. Arch. Allergy Appl. Immunol.* **36**, 354 (1969).

[11] R. R. A. Coombs, W. E. Jonas, P. J. Lachmann, and A. Feinstein, *Int. Arch. Allergy Appl. Immunol.* **27**, 321 (1965).

[12] R. R. A. Coombs, W. E. Jonas, and P. J. Lachmann, *Immunology* **10**, 493 (1966).

[13] R. R. A. Coombs, A. Hunter, W. E. Jonas *et al.*, *Lancet* **1**, 1115 (1968).

f. PRODUCTION OF ANTIGLOBULIN SERA*†

i. *Production of Anti-IgG*

Human IgG can be obtained by first dialyzing human serum against 0.0175 M phosphate buffer, pH 6.5, and then fractionating the serum

* Section 16.B.5.f was contributed by R. R. A Coombs and P. L. Mollison.

† Compare also P. L. Mollison, "Blood Transfusion in Clinical Medicine," 5th ed. Davis, Philadelphia, Pennsylvania, 1972.

on a DEAE-cellulose column, using the same buffer as eluant*; after a second passage through the column, highly purified IgG is obtained. For the primary stimulation of an animal a solution of IgG is mixed with an equal volume of Freund's adjuvant and injected into four sites (two shoulders and two thighs); a suitable dose for a rabbit is 8 mg of IgG (total). Secondary stimulation can be carried out 4 weeks later by injecting a similar amount of γ-globulin precipitated by alum†; again, the injections are given into four sites. The animals may be bled 2 weeks later. (Details in this section are from a special MRC Report.[14])

If rabbits are used, it is convenient to select those whose serum has only weak natural agglutinins for human group A red cells; otherwise it may be found necessary to absorb the antisera. Similarly, if sheep are used, R-positive animals[15] should be selected.

ii. Production of Anti-IgM

IgM myeloma protein from human patients has been used with success. It is not possible to obtain a preparation which is entirely free of IgG, and the resulting antiserum will therefore have to be absorbed with IgG if a specific reagent is required.

iii. Production of Antibodies to Complement Components

If animals are injected with whole human serum, anti-C3- and anti-C4-globulin are usually produced in addition to anti-Ig and other antibodies. Sera which are almost specific for human complement may be produced by injecting an antigen–antibody–complement complex in which the antigen and antibody are of nonhuman origin. For example, the precipitate formed by mixing ovalbumin with rabbit antiovalbumin may be mixed with fresh human serum and injected into a rabbit. The resulting antiserum should contain mainly anti-human C3-globulin but may also contain antibodies against other human proteins, such as IgG-globulin.

Almost pure reagents may be produced in the following way: Red cells of the animal (e.g., rabbit) in which the reagent is to be produced are exposed to agglutinin prepared in an animal such as the horse, and these cells are used to attach human complement. Thus, rabbit red cells may be treated with hydrazine-treated horse serum. The hydrazine inactivates C4 so that only horse antibody (and horse C1) become attached to the rabbit red cells. The cells are now washed and suspended in zymosan-

---

* See Vol. I, Chap. 3.A.3.
† Absorption of proteins to nascent alumina is described in Vol. I, Chap. 2.A.2.b.ii. See also H. Proom, *J. Pathol. Bacteriol.* **55**, 419 (1943). Alumina cream can be used also (Vol. I, Chap. 2.A.2.b).
[14] Medical Research Council (Great Britain), *Immunology* **10**, 271 (1966).
[15] A. N. Sorensen, J. Rendel, and W. H. Stone, *J. Immunol.* **73**, 407 (1954).

treated fresh human serum; the zymosan inactivates part of the C3 complex but leaves C5 in addition to C1, C4, and C2. Treatment of the sensitized rabbit cells with the zymosan-treated serum thus results in red cells carrying horse antibody and horse C1 with human C4 and C5. If these cells are injected into the rabbit, the predominant antibodies formed against human serum components will be anti-C3 and anti-C4. (This method is based on that of Polley et al.[16])

Other methods appear in Sections 17.F.2 (anti-guinea pig C2), 17.F.3.b and 17.F.4.a (anti-rabbit C3 and anti-human complement components) [Ed].

[16] M. J. Polley, E. M. Rochna, and P. L. Mollison, Vox Sang. **9,** 91 (1964).

6. MIXED AGGLUTINATION AND ERYTHROCYTES* †

a. INTRODUCTION

Mixed agglutination is the formation of aggregates of two different cell types (or particles) by antibody reacting with similar antigenic determinants on both cells.

The mixed agglutination reaction concerns the examination of one of the cell types for a specific antigen using the second cell type (or particle), carrying the known antigen, as the indicator suspension. Coombs et al.[1] developed this technique as an investigative tool to examine isolated skin epidermal cells for the A and B blood group antigens; it has been employed also for detecting minor populations in erythrocyte mixtures, that is, below 2% of the cells.[2]

The mixed antiglobulin reaction, which is an elaboration of the mixed agglutination technique, was developed as a means of showing combination of antibody.[3, 4] In this procedure, aggregates composed of two different cell types (or particles) will form in the presence of antiglobulin providing *both* cell types bear attached globulin. One of the cell types is first coated with globulin to serve as the indicator cell.

Both reactions were introduced originally for tests on cells which were unsuited for ordinary agglutination tests: mixed agglutination was used to display antigenic determinants which were available also on indicator cells, and mixed antiglobulin to reveal antibody sensitization.

* Sections 16.B.6.a–c were contributed by R. R. A Coombs.

† Procedure as submitted in 1964 supplemented by Editor.
[1] R. R. A. Coombs, D. Bedford, and L. M. Rouillard, *Lancet* **1,** 461 (1956).
[2] A. R. Jones and S. Silver, *Blood* **13,** 763 (1958).
[3] R. R. A. Coombs, J. Marks, and D. Bedford, *Brit. J. Haematol.* **2,** 84 (1956).
[4] D. G. Chalmers, R. R. A. Coombs, B. W. Gurner, and J. Dausset, *Brit. J. Haematol.* **5,** 225 (1959).

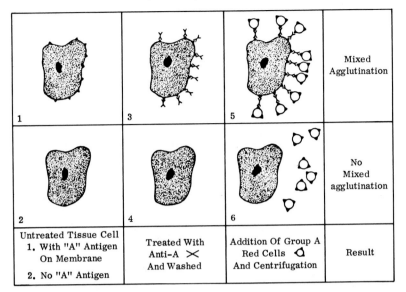

1	3	5	Mixed Agglutination
2	4	6	No Mixed agglutination
Untreated Tissue Cell 1. With "A" Antigen On Membrane 2. No "A" Antigen	Treated With Anti-A ✕ And Washed	Addition Of Group A Red Cells ◁ And Centrifugation	Result

FIG. 2. Diagrammatic illustration of the mixed agglutination reaction, showing the presence of the A isoantigen on tissue cells. Reproduced by permission of author and publisher from "Immunological Methods" (J. F. Ackroyd, ed.), p. 444. Blackwell, Oxford, 1964.

The development of these two investigative reactions came as a natural development of the earlier academic experiments on mixed aggregation,[5, 6] performed in critical examination of the "lattice" hypothesis of agglutination.

With the recent formation of synthetic "hybrid" dual-specificity antibodies, true mixed agglutination can be achieved even between cells possessing different antigenic determinants which share no common determinant,[7, 8] yet this is a very special circumstance. However, the possibility that antibodies with dual specificity occur naturally cannot be ruled out.[9]

b. THE MIXED AGGLUTINATION REACTION

There is no set way of performing the mixed agglutination reaction. The subject is reviewed in detail by Coombs and Franks.[9a] Each situation may demand its own special treatment.

In one form of the test (Fig. 2) the tissue cells in suspensions are incu-

[5] W. W. C. Topley, J. Wilson, and J. T. Duncan, *Brit. J. Exp. Pathol.* **16**, 116 (1935).

[6] A. S. Wiener and M. Herman, *J. Immunol.* **36**, 255 (1939).

[7] H. Jacot-Guillarmod and H. Isliker, *Vox Sang.* **7**, 675 (1962).

[8] H. H. Fudenberg, G. Drews, and A. Nisonoff, *J. Exp. Med.* **119**, 151 (1964).

[9] B. E. Dodd, *Brit. J. Exp. Pathol.* **33**, 1 (1952).

[9a] R. R. A. Coombs and D. Franks, *Progr. Allergy* **13**, 174 (1969).

bated with antiserum heated at 56° for half an hour (this is important if complement-dependent reactions are to be avoided) and then washed free of uncombined antibody. The indicator cell suspension is added, and the tubes are lightly centrifuged to bring the two cell types into intimate contact. If mixed agglutinates are seen on microscopic examination of the deposited cells, the test is positive (Figs. 2(5) and 3a and b).

Various modifications and elaborations are possible; red cells may be used as the indicator cells or soluble antigen absorbed on latex may be used to form the indicator particles[10]; the tissue cells under test may be examined in suspension or may be examined as monolayers growing on glass.[11]

To date, the reaction has found its main application in demonstrating the presence of blood group isoantigens, or heterophile antigens, or species-specific antigens on tissue cells growing in culture. This has provided a valuable method for checking the identity of cell cultures.[12] The antigens on spermatozoa may be studied by this reaction.[13] The method has also found forensic application in grouping very small blood stains[14] and in identifying fragments of skin[15] and other applications.[15a]

c. The Mixed Antiglobulin Reaction

This reaction involves two principles—those of mixed agglutination and of the antiglobulin reaction. It offers a method of revealing antibody combination or globulin-coating of cells or of particles which may be unsuited for ordinary antiglobulin agglutination tests.[9a]

After the mixture of indicator cells and serum is incubated, the cells are washed well to remove all globulin other than that attached as specific antibody. In the original tests for platelet antibodies,[1] indicator cells were prepared either by sensitizing sheep red cells with photooxidized rabbit anti-Forssman antibody which did not agglutinate the sheep red cells, or by treating human red cells with incomplete anti-D Rh antibody. This supplied indicator red cells bearing, respectively, attached rabbit or human globulin. After serum-treated test cell suspension and the indicator red cell suspension have been mixed together with antiglobulin serum, a positive reaction is indicated by the occurrence of mixed aggregation.

[10] A. Hagiwara, *Exp. Cell Res.* **28,** 615 (1962).

[11] C. Högman, *Vox Sang.* **4,** 12 (1959).

[12] R. R. A. Coombs, *Nat. Cancer Inst. Monogr.* **7,** 91 (1962).

[13] R. G. Edwards, L. C. Ferguson, and R. R. A. Coombs, *J. Reprod. Fert.* **7,** 153 (1964).

[14] R. R. A. Coombs and B. E. Dodd, *Med. Sci. Law* **1,** 359 (1961).

[15] L. M. Swinburne, *Med. Sci. Law* **3,** 3 (1962).

[15a] B. Dodd, *in* "Clinical Aspects of Immunology" (P. G. H. Gell and R. R. A. Coombs, eds.), 2nd ed., p. 250. F. A. Davis, Philadelphia, Pennsylvania, 1968.

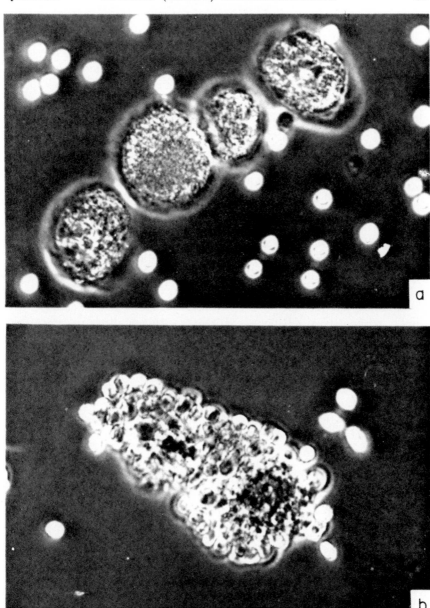

FIGS. 3a and b. Negative and positive mixed agglutination reaction between tissue cells and indicator red cells. Reproduced by permission from R. R. A. Coombs, *Nat. Cancer Inst. Monogr.* **7,** 100, Plate 6 (1962).

In a negative reaction, the cells of the indicator suspension are agglutinated by the antiglobulin serum but no mixed aggregates are formed.

In the light of present knowledge on the antigenic specificity of human immunoglobulins, in order to ensure detection of all human antibodies indicator cell suspensions should be available carrying globulin of specificity IgM (and possibly IgA) besides that of IgG, which would be the specificity supplied by human red cells sensitized with human incomplete anti-D antibody. Again, if the antibody reaction under investigation takes place optimally only in the presence of complement (like certain of the human blood group antibodies), then indicator cells carrying anti-C3 and anti-C4 should be used, and also anti-β-globulin antiserum. In such a test the phenomenon of immune adherence* may be superimposed.[16]

The mixed antiglobulin reaction was used originally in the examination of human sera for antibodies against human platelets and leukocytes. These antibodies were also shown to react with HeLa cells.[4] Like direct mixed agglutination, this reaction also has found forensic application for the recognition of human blood stains.[9a,17]

Fagraeus and Espmark[18] reported on what is essentially a mixed antiglobulin reaction (although in their report it is called "mixed haemadsorption") to show viral antibody combining with measles virus infecting monkey kidney cells in monolayer culture. Not only does this study open up a wide field, but it suggests improvements in the indicator suspension by having the antiglobulin molecules already attached to the cells of the indicator suspension. Barron et al.[19] used this procedure with success to measure antibody to the measles virus in human sera.

The potentialities of the method have received preliminary exploration in a study of species-specific antigens on the membrane of tissue cells growing as monolayers.[20, 21] Tönder et al.[22] have further extended the

---

* "Immune adherence" is the attachment to human or monkey erythrocytes of antigens complexed with specific antibody and serum complement. Trypanosomes, bacteria, rickettsiae, vaccinia virus, and even inert materials, such as starch and zymosan, are found to attach to red cells. Adhesion to platelets has been observed also. The effect can be quantitated by microscopic observation, as by determining the percentage of erythrocytes having particles adherent to them. In an appropriate system, the phenomenon allows titration of very small amounts of antibody or of complement.[16]

[16] J. L. Turk, in "Immunological Methods" (J. F. Ackroyd, ed.), p. 405. Blackwell, Oxford, 1964.

[17] W. McN. Styles, B. E. Dodd, and R. R. A. Coombs, Med. Sci. Law 3, 257 (1963).

[18] A. Fagraeus and Å. Espmark, Nature (London) 190, 370 (1961).

[19] A. L. Barron, F. Milgrom, D. T. Karzon, and E. Witebsky, J. Immunol. 90, 908 (1963).

[20] Å. Espmark and A. Fagraeus, Acta Pathol. Microbiol. Scand. Suppl. 154, 258 (1962).

[21] F. Milgrom, K. Kano, A. L. Barron, and E. Witebsky, J. Immunol. 92, 8 (1964).

[22] O. Tönder, F. Milgrom, and E. Witebsky, J. Exp. Med. 119, 265 (1964).

principle to demonstrate antibody combining with intracellular antigens in fixed tissue sections. Likewise Abeyounis *et al.*[23] have adapted the method to show H-2 antibodies in homografted mice reacting with cell monolayer cultures. Another development (see discussion in Espmark and Fagraeus[20]) adapts the principle to the demonstration of antibody combining with soluble antigens such as PPD (Purified Protein Derivative of tuberculin) or thyroglobulin fixed to glass.

d. PRACTICAL DEVELOPMENTS*

Following the early days of the Mixed Agglutination Reaction and the Mixed Antiglobulin Reaction, there have been extensive developments, summarized through 1969 in a thorough review by Coombs and Franks[9a] entitled, "Immunological Reactions Involving Two Cell Types."

Progress in understanding of the structure of immunoglobulins and their antigenic structure has enlarged the scope of the antiglobulin reaction, as noted in Section 16.B.5. Specific reagents now exist for the heavy chains and the light chains individually, for allotypes and even idiotypic determinants. The particular antibody which coats sensitized cells can be characterized in many particulars, also many of the complement components may be measured with antibodies against the purified components.

One particular line of study opened when lymphocytes were recognized as differing functionally—B cells and T cells; and Ig receptors were found on B cells. Since these "patches" appeared to be formed of chain sequences of immunoglobulins, the mixed antiglobulin reaction was appropriate to study lymphoid cells.

As an example, rabbit lymphocytes were shown to possess determinants of γ-, μ-, Fab-, and allotypic A4 and A6 specificities.[24] The antisera to rabbit immunoglobulin structures were raised in sheep or goats; frozen washed rabbit lymphocytes were thawed, exposed to a reagent, and washed. The indicator cells were sheep red cells coated with anti-Forssman antibody of IgG or IgM specificities or with Fab fragments of this antibody prepared by pepsin and mercaptoethanol treatment. Observation slides and cover slips were siliconized, and slides were further prepared with evaporated droplets of toluidine blue (0.5% in methanol). The dye was dissolved in a trace of cell diluent (0.2% bovine albumin in buffered

---

* Sections 16.B.6.d and e were submitted by Merrill W. Chase.

[23] C. J. Abeyounis, F. Milgrom, and E. Witebsky, *Nature (London)* **203**, 313 (1964).

[24] R. R. A. Coombs, B. W. Gurner, C. A. Janeway, A. B. Wilson, P. G. Gell, and A. S. Kelus, *Immunology* **18**, 417 (1970).

saline), and prepared lymphocytes and indicator cells were added to the dye. The preparations were sealed and total lymphocytes and rosetted lymphocytes counted, easily visible because dyed. Individual rabbits varied in numbers of IgG-reacting lymphocytes (26 to 61%). The findings on a typical rabbit showed 35% bearing IgG-determinants, 18% IgM- and 54% Fab-, although the ratio of IgG:IgM was often reversed on other animals. Lymphocytes of typed rabbits showed light-chain A4 and A6 determinants varying between 11 and 37%.

In contrast to the rabbit, the frequency of Ig determinants on human peripheral lymphocytes was much lower: 0.3% for γFc-, less than 1% for αFc-, up to 5% for light-chain determinants.[25] Also in studies with the mouse, the frequency of γFc determinants was 1 to 2% and of μFc < 1%.[26] Only certain antiserum specimens were able to detect Ig determinants. With favorable sera, 15-25% of mouse lymphocytes would react, apparently because of determinants related to the Fab- fragment.

The mixed antiglobulin reaction was also used to study immunoglobulin determinants in chicken lymphocytes because of bursal control of the B-cell population in the avian species.[27] By the use of specific Fab-, γ- and μ-reagents prepared from (a) chicken anti-sheep red cell antibodies and (b) rabbit and anti-chicken globulins, it was shown that normal chickens had 2.5 to 15.8% of Fab sites on peripheral lymphocytes (γ-determinants ran around 1% and μ-determinants $\sim$5.3%). Bursectomy, however, prevented the appearance of lymphocytes with Ig determinants, in accord with fluorescent antibody studies of Kincade et al.[28] and Rabellino and Grey.[29] Thymectomy increased 3-fold the number of circulating lymphocytes bearing Fab sites.

A special instance of rosette formation in a mixed agglutination reaction (opsonic adherence) was found to be restricted to use of *fresh* human lymphocytes.[30] Separated lymphocytes were added directly to ox erythrocytes coated with rabbit anti-ox red cell sera. Positive rosetting occurred with 24 to 59% of lymphocytes of normal individuals and 41 to 87% of cells in chronic lymphocytic leukemia. This is the first indication that use of frozen cells may not always be adequate for study.

[25] R. R. A. Coombs, A. Feinstein, and A. B. Wilson, *Lancet* **2**, 1157 (1969).
[26] R. R. A. Coombs, B. W. Gurner, I. McConnell, and A. Munro, *Int. Arch. Allergy Appl. Immunol.* **39**, 280 (1970).
[27] R. M. Aitken, W. H. Penhale, and R. R. A. Coombs, *Int. Arch. Allergy Appl. Immunol.* **43**, 469 (1972).
[28] P. W. Kincade, A. R. Lawton, and M. D. Cooper, *J. Immunol.* **106**, 1421 (1971).
[29] E. Rabellino and H. M. Grey, *J. Immunol.* **106**, 1418 (1971).
[30] T. Hallberg, B. W. Gurner, and R. R. A. Coombs, *Int. Arch. Allergy Appl. Immunol.* **44**, 500 (1973).

e. The Mixed Hemadsorption Test

The special case of mixed antiglobulin reaction which is carried out with "target preparations" fixed to glass rather than with suspensions of "target cells" has been denoted *mixed hemadsorption* and outlined in Section 16.B.6.c. Numerous applications have been made already, with use of multiple types of indicator cells (Table IV). Each investigator will need to adapt such techniques to his own purposes. Critical controls must be introduced, and the proper concentration of reagents must be worked out carefully. Workers will of necessity be guided in their approaches by consulting the original literature, yet it appears useful to list some of the systems in which *mixed hemadsorption* has solved problems. The original studies[18] showed that measles virus present in infected monolayer cultures of monkey kidney cells could bind antiviral antibodies, this event being detected upon addition of prepared indicator cells (Table IV, row F).

Table IV lists methods for examining tissue antigens as cultured cells or sections (rows A–C, I, J), cell cultures for cell contaminants (row H), virus-infected tissues (rows D–F), and soluble materials fixed on glass (rows K–M). The *antiserum* can be known or suspected. Indicator cells or reagents range from simple (rows B, Dii) to typical and standard (as in row A) up to specialized preparations as in rows E, Fii, and Ii.

By means of a technique based on that introduced by DeSomer and Prinzie,[31] antibodies that act on the test object can be titrated. Fagraeus and Espmark overlay the monolayer cultures with a 3-mm layer of 0.75% agar and distribute over the surface 8 to 12 filter paper discs 5 or 12 mm in diameter which have been wetted with successive 4-fold or 10-fold dilutions of the antiserum. Antibody diffuses through the agar overlay laterally for 2 to 3 days, after which time the agar layer and the paper discs are poured out easily. Indicator cells (10 ml of 0.2 to 0.5% suspension per 200 cm² surface) are then added. After a reaction period of 30 to 60 minutes, nonattaching cells are floated off and readings of "hemadsorption" are made. Positive reactions show well-demarcated red areas where erythrocytes have become attached: The diameters are characteristically greater than the area of the filter paper discs owing to diffusion of antibody through the agar and are related directly to the antibody present originally in the individual discs.[20, 32] Iron staining of the erythrocytes can improve photographic recordings.[33]

[31] P. DeSomer and A. Prinzie, *Virology* **4**, 387 (1957).
[32] J. Å. Espmark and A. Fagraeus, *J. Immunol.* **94**, 530 (1965).
[33] A. Fagraeus, J. Å. Espmark, and J. Jonsson, *Immunology* **9**, 161 (1965).

TABLE IV

Typical "Hemadsorption" Mixed Antiglobulin Tests

Test object	Antiserum	Indicator cells or test	Reference
A. Bovine adrenal medulla monolayers, etc.	Rabbit anti-bovine organ, etc.	Sheep RBC minimally sensitized with inactivated rabbit antibody, then agglutinated with goat anti-rabbit serum	a
B. Human embryonic tissue monolayers (kidney, heart, lung, skin, liver, spleen) of various A-B-O-Rh groups, grown with human AB serum	Human isoagglutinins (anti-A_1 or anti-B) or anti-Rh_0 (anti-D)	Human RBC A_1, B, or O, or trypsinized or papainized O-Rh_0 and O-Rh-negative	b
C. Human HeLa monolayers	Rabbit anti-HeLa cells	As in row A or F(i) or H(i)	c
D. Human HeLa monolayers infected with vaccinia virus	Rabbit anti-vaccinia serum (or antiserum prepared in rats, guinea pigs, mice calves, roosters, monkeys, humans)	i. As in row A or F(i) or H(i) ii. Fluorescent sheep anti-rabbit globulin	c
E. Human amnion cells infected with measles virus	Human measles-convalescent or immune sera, or random sera for diagnosis	Tanned human group O cells coated with human Cohn Fr. II, then agglutinated with rabbit anti-human globulin	d
F. Monkey kidney tissue monolayer infected with vaccinia virus (or measles or canine distemper viruses)	(1) Rabbit anti-vaccinia serum (or rabbit anti-measles or anti-distemper virus) or	(i) Sheep RBC sensitized with rabbit anti-sheep RBC and coated with horse anti-rabbit serum	c

(2) Rat anti-vaccinia serum	(ii) Tanned sheep RBC with adsorbed rat γ-globulin and coated with rabbit anti-rat serum	f
G. Mouse "L-cell" fibroblast monolayers (C3H strain origin)	Mouse serum, C57BL line bearing or rejecting C3H skin	Human group O RBC sensitized by mouse anti-human RBC, and coated with rabbit anti-mouse serum
H. Tests for species contamination of cultured cell lines	(1) Rabbit antisera to kidney cells of human or monkey or calf or HeLa human cells*	(i) Sheep RBC minimally sensitized with inactivated rabbit antibody, then coated with sheep anti-rabbit γ-globulin	g
	or	
	(2) Rat antisera to above panel of cells*	(ii) Sheep RBC sensitized with rat anti-sheep RBC, coated with rabbit anti-rat γ-globulin
	or	
	(3) Cynomolgus monkey antisera to kidney cells of human or *Cercopithecus* monkey or HeLa human cells*	(iii) Sheep RBC sensitized with human anti-sheep RBC, coated with rabbit anti-human γ-globulin
I. Appropriate test objects	Human antibodies	(i) Tanned sheep RBC with absorbed staphylococcus toxoid, treated with human anti-staphylococcus serum globulin; coated with rabbit anti-human serum	c,h
		(ii) Tanned sheep RBC with absorbed human γ-globulin; then coated with rabbit anti-human globulin	c
		(iii) Sheep cells sensitized with human mononucleosis heterophile serum, then coated with rabbit anti-human globulin	c

(continued)

TABLE I (*Continued*)

Test object	Antiserum	Indicator cells or test	Reference
J. Bovine tissue and brain sections fixed on glass slides	Rabbit anti-bovine organ sera	As in row A above	i
K. Human thyroglobulin fixed to glass (1 μg/cm^2)	Human anti-thyroid serum, followed by rabbit anti-human γ-globulin	Sheep RBC sensitized with human anti-sheep RBC	c
L. Human thyroglobulin fixed to glass (1 μg/cm^2)	Human anti-thyroid IgG *or* anti-thyroid IgM, used separately	(i) Sheep RBC sensitized with human anti-sheep RBC (IgM); outer coating of rabbit anti-cynomolgus globulin, forming specific anti-IgM reagent (ii) Sheep RBC sensitized with cynomolgus anti-sheep RBC; outer coating of rabbit anti-human γ-globulins, forming anti-(IgG and anti-IgM) reagent	c,j
M. Nucleoprotein fixed to glass	Human serum with anti-DNA factor	Appropriate indicator cells bearing anti-human globulin	h

* Sera inactivated and absorbed with sheep RBC or human Ab − Rh(+)RBC.

[a] F. Milgrom, K. Kano, A. L. Barron, and E. Witebsky, *J. Immunol.* **92**, 8 (1964).

[b] C. Högman, *Vox Sang.* **4**, 12 and 319 (1959).

[c] A. Fagraeus, J. Å. Espmark, and J. Jonsson, *Immunology* **9**, 161 (1965).

[d] A. L. Barron, F. Milgrom, D. T. Karzon, and E. Witebsky, *J. Immunol.* **90**, 908 (1963).

[e] A. Fagraeus and Å. Espmark, *Nature (London)* **190**, 370 (1961).

[f] C. J. Abeyounis, F. Milgrom, and E. Witebsky, *Nature (London)* **203**, 313 (1964).

[g] J. Å. Espmark and A. Fagraeus, *J. Immunol.* **94**, 530 (1965).

[h] J. Å. Espmark and A. Fagraeus, *Acta Pathol. Microbiol. Scand.* Suppl. 154, 258 (1962).

[i] O. Tönder, F. Milgrom, and E. Witebsky, *J. Exp. Med.* **119**, 265 (1964).

[j] J. Jonsson, Å. Espmark, and A. Fagraeus, *Int. Arch. Allergy Appl. Immunol.* **29**, 329 (1966).

C. Inhibition of Hemagglutination

1. INHIBITION OF HEMAGGLUTINATION BY ANTIBODIES AND ANTIBODY-LIKE REAGENTS IN SEMIQUANTITATIVE TUBE TESTS*†

Inhibition of antigen–antibody reactions was first used by Landsteiner[1] in order to assess the specificity and activity of substances not precipitable by antibodies. The reaction is an indirect way of demonstrating and measuring antigens and haptens or antibodies. (See Vol. III, Chap. 13.B.1.) Its principle is based on the competition for antibody combining sites between a fixed antigen (here the erythrocyte serves as antigen carrier) and soluble antigen or hapten.‡ The inhibiting compound has a structure identical or closely similar to the specific determinant on the agglutinogen, here the red cell, and therefore interacts with the corresponding agglutinin. The extent of inhibition is related not only to the amount of inhibitor, but also its affinity for the antibody combining sites.[2]

The *procedure* necessitates only a small expenditure of reagents, which often are scarce in structural studies. The *sensitivity* is one of the highest among serological methods and readily detects 1 μg or even less of antigen per milliliter. The *specificity* of hemagglutination inhibition reactions is of the same order as that of precipitin and agglutination reactions. In addition, the hemagglutination inhibition method can be used for systems where soluble antigens have not been obtained or where only nonprecipitating antibodies including so-called blocking antibodies are available.

The *limitations* of hemagglutination inhibition tests lie in their lack of precision. By its very nature the procedure has an inherent error of at least $\pm 50\%$; furthermore, the reactions may become unspecific beyond

---

* Section 16.C.1 was contributed by Georg F. Springer.

† This section is restricted to specific inhibition of antibodies and of agents with serological properties similar to those of antibodies. It is not concerned with inhibition of hemagglutination resulting from "blocking" antibodies (prozone phenomenon), or with the destructive effects of biochemical, chemical, or physical agents on antibodies or with inhibition of agglutination by microbial agents.

[1] K. Landsteiner, *Biochem. Z.* **104**, 280 (1920).

‡ Such inhibition is seen by comparing reactions between antigen and antibody run in the presence and in the absence of inhibitor or by measuring the amount of nitrogen in the respective precipitates when full equilibrium has been reached (Vol. III, Chap. 13.B). It is measurable in some cases also by equilibrium dialysis across a semipermeable membrane (Vol. III, Chap. 15.A and 15.B).

[2] E. A. Kabat, *in* "Experimental Immunochemistry" (E. A. Kabat and M. M. Mayer, eds.), 2nd ed., pp. 241–267. Thomas, Springfield, Illinois, 1961.

a certain maximal concentration of inhibitor or below a minimal concentration of agglutinin. Therefore, these tests should be complemented wherever possible with quantitative precipitin or precipitation inhibition techniques in order to quantitate the results and to avoid overinterpretation; qualitative disparity in inhibiting power of certain substances may occur in these various systems.[3]

The method has proved to be of value in the elucidation of the determinant structures of blood-group antigens[2, 4–6] and in addition in the characterization of structures with which erythrocytes may become sensitized,[7] including microbial antigens.[8] It has been used successfully in genetic investigations of human serum groups,[9] in the diagnosis of diseases such as rheumatoid arthritis,[10] and in investigation of nonimmunological protein–carbohydrate interactions.[11]

A *modification of the original principle* employs antibodies to *viral hemagglutinins*. The potency of such antisera can be measured by determining the minimum amount of serum capable of completely inhibiting hemagglutination by viruses under standard conditions. This procedure is widely used in assaying antisera to influenza and other viruses.[12, 13]

Certain *protein extracts* from lower animals and plants (Section 16.A.6), although not antibodies, also agglutinate erythrocytes, occasionally in a highly specific way; these reactions may also be inhibited by the addition of antigens and haptens. For conducting hemagglutination–inhibition tests, standardization of all reagents is of prime importance as will be discussed in some detail.

a. HEMAGGLUTININS AND THEIR PREPARATION

Serum containing the desired agglutinins, or the isolated serum- or plant-agglutinins are employed; between 2 and 20 units of "anti-reagent" are used. One unit is defined as the amount of agglutinin present at the

[3] G. F. Springer and P. Williamson, *Vox Sang.* **8**, 177 (1963).

[4] E. A. Kabat, "Blood Group Substances." Academic Press, New York, 1956.

[5] M. Heidelberger, *Fortschr. Chem. Org. Naturst.* **18**, 503 (1960).

[6] W. T. J. Morgan, *Proc. Roy. Soc. Ser. B* **151**, 308 (1960).

[7] G. F. Springer, *in* "The Amino Sugars" (R. W. Jeanloz and E. A. Balazs, eds.), Vol. 2B, pp. 267–336. Academic Press, New York, 1966.

[8] G. F. Springer, P. Williamson, and W. C. Brandes, *J. Exp. Med.* **113**, 1077 (1961).

[9] R. Grubb and A. B. Laurell, *Acta Pathol. Microbiol. Scand.* **39**, 390 (1956).

[10] M. Ziff, P. Brown, J. Lospalluto, J. Badin, and C. McEwen, *Amer. J. Med.* **20**, 500 (1956).

[11] G. F. Springer, P. R. Desai, and B. Kolecki, *Biochemistry* **3**, 1076 (1964).

[12] G. K. Hirst, *J. Exp. Med.* **75**, 49 (1942).

[13] Committee on Standard Serological Procedures in Influenza Studies, *J. Immunol.* **65**, 347 (1950).

titration end point of a given quantity of antiserum, i.e., the minimum amount of a hemagglutinin causing agglutination of a standardized suspension of washed erythrocytes.

If the hemagglutinin solution is a serum, it should be inactivated at 56° before use for the shortest effective period (usually 15 to 20 minutes). It may be kept in lots of 1 to 5 ml at −20° or sterilized, e.g., with 0.25% phenol and 1:20,000 thimerosal or 0.1% sodium azide (all final concentrations), and stored at 3 to 6°. It should be clarified by centrifugation at ca. 1700 at 4° overnight. The reagent should contain no anti-erythrocyte antibodies except those reacting with the structure under investigation. The reagent can be rendered specific by absorption or adsorption and elution.[4, 14, 15]

b. Erythrocytes and Their Preparation

In the author's laboratory, blood is collected and stored aseptically for no more than 2 weeks at 3° to 6° in one-third volume of acid–citrate–dextrose (ACD) solution NIH formula B (Section 16.A.5.c). Immediately before use the erythrocytes are washed 3 times with 10 to 20 volumes of "buffered saline." Erythrocytes are used as 0.5, 1.0, or 2.0% suspensions.

c. Solutions

The diluent and the erythrocyte suspending solution in all tests is 0.85% aqueous NaCl, containing 0.025 M phosphate buffer, pH 7.3 ("buffered saline"—Section 16.A.5.c).

d. Glassware

Tubes of various sizes can be employed. The 8-mm by 75-mm size has been found most useful. Commonly used tubes of larger capacity have a size of 12 × 75 mm or 13 × 100 mm. Graduated, calibrated pipettes of 0.1-, 0.2-, or 1.0-ml capacity are used, depending on the volume of reagents.

e. Inhibitors

The test material should be standardized in terms of weight or moles of substance. This is usually done by preparing stock solutions, in buffered saline, which contains 5 to 10 mg of inhibitor per milliliter. Before weighing it is desirable to dry the substances to constant weight in a desiccator

[14] F. Stratton and P. H. Renton, "Practical Blood Grouping." Blackwell, Oxford, 1958.
[15] G. F. Springer and R. E. Horton, *J. Gen. Physiol.* **47**, 1229 (1964).

in vacuo over a drying agent at room temperature. Care must be taken to assure maximal solution of the substances and to maintain a pH between 6.8 and 7.6. With some fluids, e.g., saliva, it may not be feasible to determine the weight of material to be added to each tube, and the results may then be expressed in terms of dilution of the original volume of the inhibitory solution.

f. Test Procedure

A number of techniques are in use.[4, 11, 16] The *test* is conveniently *performed* as follows: To all except the first tube, 0.1 ml of buffered saline is added. After the addition of 0.1 ml of inhibitor each to the first and second tube, 2-fold serial dilutions of 0.1 ml are made beginning with the second tube. A different 0.1-ml serological pipette is used for each transfer. The last transfer should be kept in case no end point is reached. Solutions of different inhibitor concentrations may be made instead and successively diluted—not necessarily—twofold. To the titrated solutions 4 to 8 units of hemagglutinin are added, and the samples are shaken and incubated for 1 to 2 hours at room temperature (22° to 26°). Erythrocytes, 0.1 ml, carrying the antigen corresponding to the antireagent are then added to each tube and the test mixtures again are shaken and examined after an additional 1 to 2 hours' incubation at room temperature. The incubations may also be carried out at other temperatures, varying from 4° to 37° depending on the agglutinin under investigation. For a given test all incubations should be at the same temperature.

Each titration series includes *controls* consisting of (a) a serum standard, diluted to 4 to 8 minimum hemagglutinating doses and then titrated in 2-fold geometrical dilutions to which 0.1 ml of buffered saline is added instead of inhibitor followed by 0.1 ml of erythrocyte suspensions, as well as (b) one tube containing an erythrocyte suspension in buffered saline. It is also desirable to include (c) a standard inhibitor. If possible, materials should be retested at least twice. Samples to be compared must be run in parallel in the same tests. Active substances should also be tested in two unrelated hemagglutination inhibition systems, in order to assess specificity in inhibition.

The *end point* of inhibition lies between the last tube showing complete inhibition and the first tube indicating slight agglutination. Either of these tubes might be taken as the end point, but this interpretation must be kept uniform throughout. The test is most reliably read under the low

---

[16] A. S. Wiener, "Blood Groups and Transfusion," 3rd ed. Hafner, New York, 1962 (reprint).

power of a microscope at the same temperature at which the inhibition was carried out. Specificity and reproducibility are wanting at concentrations of more than 5 mg of inhibitor per milliliter or less than 2 to 4 units of hemagglutinin. Therefore, samples that do not inhibit at concentrations of 5 mg/ml should be considered inactive.

Activities are best *expressed* on a weight or molar basis and may be conveniently stated in terms of dilution of the inhibiting material before addition of serum and erythrocyte suspension. Final concentrations of inhibitor are then obtained by dividing the given values by 3.

g. MODIFICATIONS OF THE PROCEDURE

The volume of all reagents may be increased 2- to 4-fold, if macroscopic interpretations are desired. Also, the volume of all solutions may be decreased to 0.02 ml; calibrated 0.1-ml pipettes are then used. Although it is tedious to make dilutions in such small volumes, it does not, in the hands of experienced individuals, decrease the accuracy of the procedure.

A procedure has been described[17, 18] which employs standardized loops with which similarly small amounts of each reagent are used (0.025 ml) and in which up to 8 titrations can be carried out simultaneously on plastic trays. We have not found this method to be as reproducible as the procedures described in more detail here, in tests on over 200 different samples in both hemagglutination and hemagglutination–inhibition assays. This is the so-called "Microtiter System."*

When "blocking" antibodies are studied, the test is carried out in the same way except that a standard antiglobulin test (Section 16.B.5) is performed on the red cells after an ordinary incubation period after determination of titer of "saline" agglutinins.

The hemagglutination–inhibition test may also be modified by varying single steps of it. Thus the procedure may be "reversed" in that the "antireagent" is titrated and a constant amount of inhibitor is added to it. So-called "block" tests (Fig. 1) save time and decrease inaccuracy if dilutions of a given inhibitor are tested with a number of different sera and/or red cells or, alternatively, progressive dilutions of "antireagent" with a number of inhibitors. An amount of the reagent to be diluted, sufficient for all tests, is then titrated in larger tubes, and from each dilution a transfer is made to the corresponding tube of the test proper (Fig. 1). The other reagents are added as described.

[17] G. Takatsy, *Acta Microbiol. Acad. Sci. Hung.* **3**, 191 (1955).
[18] J. L. Sever, *J. Immunol.* **88**, 320 (1962).
* Available from Cooke Engineering Co., 735 N. St. Asaph St., Alexandria, Virginia.

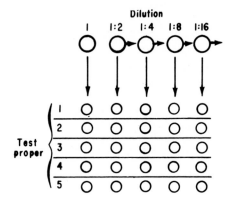

Fig. 1. Block titration. 1–5 are sample numbers.

h. Precautions in Interpretation of Results Obtained with the Hemagglutination–Inhibition Procedure

General precautions to be taken in all serological experiments have been adequately described elsewhere.[14] The limitations of the hemagglutination–inhibition procedure have been mentioned in the introduction of this section. In addition, it is necessary to pay particular attention in all hemagglutination–inhibition assays to false-positive and occasional false-negative reactions. Inclusion of appropriate controls and a standard in each test will guard against this being caused by faulty reagents. Some putative inhibitors, however, do not act by entering into a complementary reaction with the antibody combining site, but rather render the erythrocytes inagglutinable by changing their surface properties. Frequently, specificity or lack of it can be ascertained by sufficient dilution of the substance tested. However, some acidic polymers, lipids, or aldehydes will unspecifically prevent agglutination even at high dilutions.[19] Such an effect given by substances as different as the Vi antigen of gram-negative bacteria, formaldehyde, and some phospholipids can usually be recognized by the similar activity of these substances in a large number of different hemagglutination–inhibition systems. Other substances may unspecifically combine with certain classes of antibodies and thus prevent their attachment to specific structures on the erythrocyte surface.[20] False-negative reactions occur less frequently but may be caused by heavy metals and other cations if they are bi- or multivalent.[19] These false-negative reactions may be detected by incubation of red cells with the putative inhibitor; agglutination will then occur already in the absence of agglutinins.

[19] G. F. Springer, *Bacteriol. Rev.* **27,** 191 (1963).
[20] B. Pirofsky, M. S. Cordoba, and D. Rigas, *Vox Sang.* **9,** 653 (1964).

2. QUANTITATIVE INHIBITION OF HEMAGGLUTINATION (CELL-COUNTING METHOD)*

a. THEORETICAL CONSIDERATIONS

Rather simple methods can be used readily to screen compounds for inhibitory capability (Vol. I, Chap. 1.C.1.i). For precise quantitation, the HID_{50} value can be ascertained by the method given below. This value is defined as the amount of inhibitory substance required to lower the agglutinin activity until only 50% of the erythrocytes are agglutinated in the presence of 6 HD_{50} units of antibody (Section 16.A.3), a concentration that otherwise agglutinates 95 to 97% of the standard cell suspension.

Principle

The quantitative cell-counting hemagglutination technique of Wilkie and Becker[1] (Section 16.A.3) has been modified by Gibbs et al.[2] to provide a precise estimate of the inhibitory activity per unit weight of blood group substance.

When a standard dose of agglutinating antibody and a constant volume of test cells are allowed to react to equilibrium in the presence of various amounts of blood group substance as inhibitor, the relation between the proportion of cells agglutinated and the logarithm of the amount of substance used is sigmoidal in the region of partial inhibition (Fig. 2). The sigmoid curve is transformed into a linear curve by converting the proportions of cells agglutinated to probability units or probits. The 50% unit of inhibitory activity of the substance designated the HID_{50}, is obtained by interpolation on the log-probit assay curve or by computation from the linear equation (Section 16.A.3). The HID_{50} is defined as the amount of inhibitory substance required to inhibit a standard dose of agglutinin activity to 50% agglutination of the test cell suspension.

The method can be applied to any hemagglutination inhibition system in which the proportion of cells agglutinated is a sigmoid function of the concentration of inhibitory substance in the region of partial inhibition.

b. MATERIALS AND SPECIAL EQUIPMENT

Phosphate-buffered saline (pH 7.3), collection and treatment of sera, preparation of standardized concentrations of test cells, and special equipment are the same as given in Section 16.A.3.

---

* Section 16.C.2 was contributed by Mary B. Gibbs.

[1] M. H. Wilkie and E. L. Becker, J. Immunol. **74**, 192 (1955).
[2] M. B. Gibbs, W. S. Collins, and J. H. Ackroyd, J. Immunol. **87**, 396 (1961).

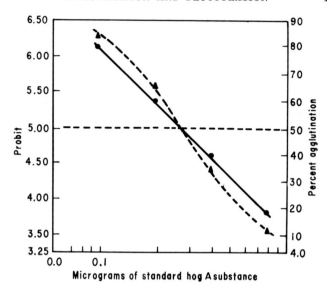

Fig. 2. The hemagglutination–inhibition assay curve and its transformation by probits.

Antisera from individuals immunized with blood group substances are recommended. These sera give inhibition assay curves with a steep slope; naturally occurring isoagglutinins give curves with low slopes.

Purified blood group substances are dried to a constant weight and made up in stock solutions (generally 10,000 μg per milliliter of buffered saline) and stored in small samples at $-20°$.

c. PRELIMINARY TESTS

Step 1. Prior to performance of the quantitative procedure, the HD_{50} unit of the antiserum is determined by the cell-counting method described in Section 16.A.3. Multiplication of the HD_{50} value by 24 gives the concentration of antiserum to be prepared for use in the assay procedure (24 HD_{50} units/ml or 6 HD_{50} units/0.25 ml serum dilution). This amount of agglutinin activity produces 95 to 97% agglutination of the standard cell concentration.

Step 2. The range of concentrations of inhibitor to be used in the assay procedure is determined from the results of a serial dilution titration performed with the standardized serum dilution (24 HD_{50} units/ml dilution) and the standard concentration of test cells. Twofold serial dilutions of the stock inhibitor solution are made in buffered saline. When the inhibitor is costly, 0.1-ml dilutions can be made directly in the tubes with 0.1-ml pipettes. To each tube is added 0.1 ml of these dilutions, 0.2 ml of cell suspension, and 0.1 ml of the antiserum dilution. The tubes are allowed to stand at room temperature for 2 hours, centrifuged at 600 g for 1 minute, and examined macroscopically for the end point of inhibition. The range of concentrations of inhibitor giving partial inhibition is located within a fourfold range above and below the substance concentration giving the end-point inhibition titer.

d. Procedure

Each hemagglutination–inhibition assay consists of four 2-fold concentrations of the blood group substance made by dilution of the stock substance solution in class A volumetric flasks. Duplicate 0.25-ml portions of each concentration of inhibitor are transferred to 12 × 40-mm test tubes, and 0.5 ml portions of the standard cell suspension are added to each tube. Each tube then receives 0.25 ml of the standardized serum dilution (a total of 6 HD_{50} agglutinin units). The tubes are stoppered and placed on a rotator for equilibration of test mixtures at room temperature. The procedure is the same as described in Section 16.A.3. A 5-hour period of rotation at 10 rpm assures equilibration of test mixtures with most antisera from immunized individuals. When shorter periods of rotation are desirable, the rate of the aggregation reaction must be determined for the antiserum. Saline control tubes containing 0.5 ml of saline and 0.5 ml of cell suspension are used to determine the total cell count. Additional antibody controls are set up consisting of 0.25 ml of the serum dilution 0.25 ml of buffered saline, and 0.5 ml of cell suspension. These positive controls should be agglutinated to the extent of 95 to 97%. The equilibrated test mixtures are then measured by enumerating free cells by one of the methods described in Section 16.A.3. The calculations of percentage of cells agglutinated and treatment of data are the same as given in Section 16.A.3, substituting concentrations of inhibitor for serum concentrations. Determination of the HID_{50} unit of inhibitory activity and the error of the estimate are the same as given for the HD_{50} unit of agglutinin activity. The same factors which influence the reproducibility of HD_{50}'s also influence the reproduction of HID_{50}'s.

e. Limitations

The only limitation with hemacytometry is the potency of the antiserum. When a given serum shows less than 24 HD_{50} units per milliliter, results are unsatisfactory. With electronic counting, the same limitations apply as with hemagglutination reactions (Section 16.A.3).

D. Bacterial Agglutination*

Antibodies to bacteria arise largely against surface antigens (cell walls, flagella, capsular material); under appropriate circumstances antibodies are formed to bacterial enzymes, antigenic metabolites, and exotoxins. Various methods have been applied to isolate and characterize antigenic structures of bacteria (Vol. I, Chap. 1.B).

For preparing agglutinating antisera, the "antigenic status" of the bacterial cells—culture phase, age, growth characteristics—must be taken into account, as well as any alterations incurred in preparing nonliving vaccines. The preparations of bacterial vaccines for immunization are summarized in Vol. I, Chap. 2.B.1 (Table II), and discussed in greater detail below. Immunization schedules are given in Vol. I, Chap. 2.B.1 (Table I, part 4).

Quantitative studies have been made of the interaction between certain bacterial species and agglutinating sera (pneumococci, hemolytic streptococci, staphylococci, *Haemophilus influenzae*, *Bordetella pertussis*, meningococci, gonococci, shigellae, and brucellae). In principle, for the purpose of quantitative determinations, carefully washed suspensions of bacteria of known content are added to a given volume of the antiserum or antibody solution. After appropriate incubation at 37° to assure optimal attachment of the antibodies to the surface of the bacterial cells, followed by holding at 4°, the bacteria are washed twice in the cold and analyzed for N. Agglutinin N is determined by subtracting bacterial N from total N of the sediment. Details are given by Kabat.[1]

Bacterial agglutination tests are employed both for identification of antibodies with known bacterial antigens and identification of bacterial antigens with known antisera. The bacterial suspension to be used must be "smooth" and not subject to autoagglutination; any antigens or other substances that would interfere with specific agglutination are to be eliminated if present; and "complete" rather than "incomplete" antibodies will be detected or employed unless the Coombs technique (Section 16.B.5) or similar procedures are utilized. Use of the term "bacterial antigen" (e.g., *Salmonella* O antigen), does not imply that the bacterial suspensions are free from additional antigenic determinants.

1. PREPARATION OF BACTERIAL ANTIGENS FOR AGGLUTINATION TESTS

Strains must be maintained in pure culture, and great care be taken to ascertain whether mutational changes affecting the antigenic structure

---

* Sections 16.D.1–3d and 4–6 were contributed by Erwin Neter.

[1] E. A. Kabat, *in* "Experimental Immunochemistry" (E. A. Kabat and M. M. Mayer, eds.), 2d ed., Chapter 3. Thomas, Springfield, Illinois, 1961.

have occurred in the course of artificial cultivation. The microorganisms may be grown on artificial or synthetic culture media, either fluid or solid; cultural conditions will vary depending upon the species of microorganisms used. Whole cultures, or bacteria centrifuged and resuspended in an appropriate diluent, may be used. Agar-grown microorganisms are suspended in a suitable diluent, preferably after being washed. It is important to take cognizance of the following points. (a) Certain media contain antigenic substances and conceivably may lead to erroneous interpretation of results when antibodies to such substances are present in the "antibacterial" serum. (b) Organisms grown on agar may adsorb material than can cross-react with blood group substances. (c) When bacteria are grown in a fluid medium and the whole culture is used in agglutination tests without washing, soluble antigenic excretion products may provide antigens in addition to those of the bacterial surface.

a. KILLING OF BACTERIA

Nonviable bacterial suspensions often are preferable to viable antigens. Killed suspensions avoid autolysis of bacterial cells, and the danger of infection of personnel with pathogens. Also, reduction of chance bacterial contaminants in the laboratory area is desirable. Depending upon the particular microorganisms and the particular antigens for study, killing may be effected by heat, one of several chemicals, or a combination of these procedures. Gram-negative enterobacteriaceae to be used for the study of heat-stable O antigens, for example, can be killed by heating in boiling water. Pneumococci and meningococci are killed by heating in a water bath at 60° for 45 minutes, the microorganisms preferably being suspended during heating in 0.5 or 1% formalin. Killing of these organisms can be effected also with use of 0.5% phenol in saline solution, but for many bacterial species this low concentration of phenol will require many days to kill.

b. PRESERVATION OF BACTERIAL SUSPENSIONS

Bacterial suspensions in 0.15 M (0.85%) saline can be preserved by adding some disinfectant, such as phenol, formalin, or Merthiolate. The choice depends upon the particular antigen; for example, phenol (0.5%) is recommended for *Brucella*, *Francisella* (*Pasteurella*) *tularensis*, and *Salmonella* O antigens, and formalin (0.6%) for *Salmonella* H and other enterobacterial H antigens.

c. DENSITY OF BACTERIAL SUSPENSIONS

Agglutination is commonly expressed in terms of "titer," the greatest dilution of a serum that gives a definitely positive, although feeble, agglutination of some bacterial or erythrocyte suspension. The reported end point depends upon the immunoglobulin concentration in relation to the available antigenic surface; the "titer" found with a given antiserum depends upon the density of test suspension, just as it does with antigen-coated erythrocytes employed for pattern agglutination (Section 16.B.2.b.i) or with formalinized red cells used in indirect hemagglutination (Section 16.B.3.c.ii). Similarly, the titer of sheep cell agglutinins in patients' serum that is accepted as being diagnostic for infectious mononucleosis varies markedly with the concentration of erythrocytes used in the test.

Standardization of bacterial suspensions varies widely in diagnostic laboratories, and "titers" will vary considerably within a laboratory, or among laboratories. Some workers use, as standard, the uncertain density of an "18-hour broth culture" or grade a suspension against the McFarland barium sulfate turbidity standards.*†

Several methods to grade turbidities more precisely have been devised by passing nearly monochromatic light through a suspended culture at either a 180-degree (turbidimetry) or 90-degree (nephelometry) angle to the recording instrument. (Such instruments are discussed in Vol. II, Chap. 10.B.) It will be noted that decrease in light passing through a suspension is not equivalent to *absorbancy* of monochromatic light and that differences in two suspensions are fundamentally not capable of mathematical treatment as are optical densities of some given solute. Over a *narrow* range of concentrations, however, "optical density" readings can be proportional to turbidity. Hence the method of choice in reading turbidities with a spectrophotometer is to compare dilutions of standard and unknown that are *closely approximate*. (For working beyond this range, it is possible to construct a standard curve, but it cannot be recommended for the present purpose.)

---

* McFarland barium sulfate standards consist of 10 suspensions made in chemically clean tubes and sealed by heat [J. McFarland, *J. Amer. Med. Ass.* **49**, 1176 (1907)]. The first tube receives 0.10 ml of 1% pure barium chloride in water, the next tube 0.20 ml, and so on. The "tube number" designates the number of these 0.10-ml units in the tube. The volume of each tube is brought to exactly 10 ml with 1% aqueous H_2SO_4. As a rough guide, tube 1 corresponds to a density of ca. 3×10^8 organisms per milliliter, tube 3 to ca. 1×10^9, and tube 5 to ca. 1.8×10^9. The McFarland standards 1, 2, and 3 represent the most used ranges in bacterial densities. Note that $BaCl_2$ is highly poisonous if ingested.

† In using "visual" opacity standards, the unknown suspension contained within a precisely similar tube is lined up between two of the standards. The three tubes are held close together. A straight edge, such as a 6-inch celluloid ruler pressed against the tubes, assists in estimating relative transparency, or newsprint may be read through the tubes.

The general formula, when closely matching suspensions are read, would be:

$$\text{Final volume of vaccine} = \text{present volume} \times \frac{OD_{sample} \times \text{dilution in which read}}{OD_{desired}}$$

The examination of living bacteria in their growth medium is made in a spectrophotometer at 530 nm for yellowish media or at 660 nm for brownish media. Examination of washed cultures (essentially colorless medium) is made more accurately at 420 nm, using the optical density scale and 15-mm round cuvettes, and diluting to give readings that fall between 0.150 and 0.400. If standard curves are constructed to avoid the nonlinearity outside of this range, curves must be drawn for each wavelength to be used.

The CDC Reference Opacity Preparation is intended to replace the McFarland standards with narrower range and much longer stability. It consists of a suspension of Pyrex glass particles (≤ 10 μm) in distilled water containing 1:10,000 Merthiolate and stored at 4°.[2] After being agitated by a magnetic stirrer and dispensed aseptically, it is diluted with water to a density of 10 IU, which is represented by the tabulated values when 15-mm Pyrex round cuvettes are used and the reference standard is resuspended *immediately* before reading.

Wavelength (nm)	Percent transmission	Optical density
420	47.5	0.324
530	54.0	0.268
650	60.0	0.222

In use, the 10 IU product can be diluted to a particular desired opacity and to 1 unit less and 1 unit greater. The three tubes are then used for direct visual tests like the McFarland opacity standards.

Conversion of McFarland barium sulfate standards to International Unit values is given for one preparation of McFarland Standards (the Coleman Junior spectrophotometer, Model 6A, was read at a wavelength of 530 nm).

International units	McFarland units
3.3	1
6.5	2
10.0	3
12.2	4
14.8	5

[2] U.S. National Communicable Disease Center, "Recommended Specifications for Microbiological Reagents," 3rd ed. U.S. Dept. of Health, Education, and Welfare, Atlanta, Georgia, 1968.

d. SPECIAL ANTIGENS

A variety of bacterial antigens used for identification and titration of the corresponding antibodies (as in the Widal and similar tests), e.g., *Salmonella typhi* O and H antigens, *Brucella* and *Proteus* antigens, are available from commercial sources, and recommended specifications for producing such reagents are made by the National Communicable Disease Center.[2]* Other antigens, and suspensions of strains for identification, are prepared as the occasion arises. There is no uniform procedure for preparing all bacterial antigens, since needed antigenic characteristics vary (Vol. I, Chap. 2.B.1, Table II). Recommendations are given for selected examples.

i. Flagellar H Antigens of Enterobacteriaceae[2-4]

Highly motile organisms are grown in infusion broth. For seeding the broth, it can be advantageous to select highly motile colonies by passages in semisolid agar (0.5%) media. An equal volume of 0.85% saline containing 0.6% formalin is added to the culture, and the suspension is then filtered through cotton or coarse filter paper, if this is necessary to remove larger particles. The suspension is kept at 22° for 24 hours. Alternatively, agar-grown cultures may be used, the growth being suspended in 0.5% formalin in phosphate-buffered saline. Sterility tests are made and the subcultures are examined for growth for several days. The density of the antigen depends upon its intended use (Section 16.D.1.c).

ii. Somatic O Antigens of Enterobacteriaceae[2-5]

A "smooth" strain—as opposed to one that is granular in growth (rough strain)—is grown on infusion agar for 18 to 24 hours at 37° and harvested in a small amount of physiological saline solution. It is preferable to wash the organisms once and to resuspend in saline. For stock antigens, add an equal volume of 95% ethyl alcohol gradually, with swirling; allow the well-mixed suspension to stand at 22° overnight; then add 1 volume of physiological saline solution for each 2 volumes of suspension, thus reducing the alcohol concentration to 33%. This concentrated antigen, to

---

* More recently, CDC was renamed the National Center for Disease Control.

[3] U.S. National Communicable Disease Center, Laboratory Branch, "Recommended Methods for Evaluation of Microbiological Reagents," 2nd ed. Public Health Service, D3-3. U.S. Dept. of Health, Education, and Welfare, Atlanta, Georgia, 1969.

[4] P. R. Edwards and W. H. Ewing, "Identification of Enterobacteriaceae," 3rd ed. Burgess, Minneapolis, Minnesota, 1972.

[5] A. C. Sonnenwirth and M. R. Castaneda, *in* "Gradwohl's Clinical Laboratory Methods and Diagnosis" (S. Frankel and S. Reitman, eds.), 7th ed., pp. 760–775. Mosby, St. Louis, Missouri, 1970.

which 0.5% phenol is added, may be kept for months. Prior to use it is diluted with saline solution to an alcohol concentration not greater than 12% and a turbidity corresponding to 10 IU (tube 3 of the McFarland nephelometer). Alternatively, cultures grown in broth may be used, for example, N-Z amine broth. The organisms are examined for purity and then killed by adding 0.5% phenol and holding for approximately 12 hours at 20°. When no viable bacteria remain (shown by culturing a reasonable sample of organism washed free of phenol), the organisms are harvested by centrifugation and treated with approximately 10 volumes of 95% ethyl alcohol. This suspension is allowed to stand overnight at 37°. The alcohol is removed and the cells are washed free of alcohol; the final concentrated suspension is made in diluent containing 20% glycerin and 12% sodium chloride, which is diluted further for use as slide test antigen. The density of the stock suspension is adjusted depending upon its use in slide or test tube tests (Section 16.D.1.c and Table I). Phenol and formalin should be avoided in the suspending medium.

For identification of unknown strains, growth from an agar slant can be used by suspending in 0.5 ml of physiological saline solution, heating in boiling water for 2 hours, and adjusting the density. Broth cultures can be used likewise after heating. In both cases, washing of the suspensions is recommended, with gentle resuspension, before conducting the agglutination test (Section 16.D.1).

iii. Pneumococcal Antigens[6]

A smooth strain is grown in infusion broth at pH 7.8. If volumes larger than the usual tube cultures are needed, 1-liter flasks containing 500 ml of infusion broth should be seeded with 5 ml each of an 18-hour-old culture and incubated at 37° for 8 to 18 hours. Check for contamination by Gram's stain. Add formalin (6 ml/500 ml of infusion broth) and hold the formalinized culture at room temperature for 24 hours. Centrifuge at 5° for 30 minutes at 1400 g. Resuspend the sediment in $M/20$ phosphate-buffered saline and add formalin to a final concentration of 0.1%.

iv. Staphylococcal Antigens[7]

An agar slant is seeded with a small portion of an 18-hour-old culture and incubated at 37°. Live bacteria from a 5-hour-old culture are used for slide agglutination tests. If the antigen is not satisfactory, a suspension from a 24-hour-old culture is used. Should autoagglutination be present, autoclaving at 120° for 2 hours may provide a satisfactory antigen.

[6] D. H. Campbell, J. S. Garvey, N. E. Cremer, and D. H. Sussdorf, "Methods in Immunology." Benjamin, New York, 1964.

[7] P. Oeding, *Acta Pathol. Microbiol. Scand.* **41**, 310 (1957).

v. Bacterial Spore Antigens[8]

Bacillus cereus is given as an example of an endospore antigen intended for preparation of antisera and for use in agglutination tests. Rigid precautions are needed to avoid contaminating the laboratory with spores.

Solid medium is used, prepared as follows: 1.75% agar, 0.5% peptone, 0.25% yeast extract, 0.125% dextrose, 0.01% K_2HPO_4, 0.0025% $CaCl_2$, 0.001% $MgSO_4 \cdot 7H_2O$, 0.001% $MnSO_4 \cdot H_2O$. Sporulated cultures are used for seeding. If the culture for seeding is not composed largely of spores, the suspension is subjected to "heat shock"—7 minutes at 56° or 5 minutes at 60°. The surface of agar in Blake bottles or *flat* whiskey or wine flasks is inoculated, and the cultures are grown for at least 2 weeks (incubate at 30°) to ensure a minimal residue of vegetative forms. Harvest the growth in sterile saline solution, sediment the spores by centrifugation, and wash 3 or more times with saline solution. Examine wet or stained specimens to determine the extent of contamination with vegetative forms. The density of the suspension is adjusted so that a 1:3 dilution will be equal to 10 IU of the density standard; i.e., undiluted suspension is comparable to density of tube No. 9 of the McFarland nephelometer.

vi. Mycobacterial Antigens[9]

Suspensions of certain atypical mycobacteria have been utilized in agglutination tests for serological analysis. The mycobacteria are grown in liquid Tween–albumin medium. [Special precautions against droplet (aerosol) dispersion are required in handling this medium.] The cultures are then plated in various dilutions onto oleic acid–albumin agar plates and incubated at 37° for 2 to 3 weeks. These atypical mycobacteria are collected by suspension in phosphate-buffered saline at pH 7.0 containing 0.5% phenol. The suspensions as used for agglutination tests and for immunization of rabbits are adjusted to an optical density of 0.3, measured in a Coleman Junior spectrophotometer at 525 nm (slightly more dense than 10 IU).

vii. Other Antigens

The reader is referred to special sources[2, 4, 10, 11] for the preparation of other bacterial antigens used in agglutination tests and for the production of antisera.

[8] C. Lamanna and D. Eisler, *J. Bacteriol.* **79**, 435 (1960).
[9] W. B. Schaefer, *Amer. Rev. Resp. Dis.* **92**, No. 6, Part II, 85 (1965).
[10] U.S. Dept. of the Army, "Laboratory Procedures in Clinical Serology," Technical Manual 8-227-1. Washington, D. C., 1960.
[11] Kwapinski, J. B., ed., "Methods of Serological Research." Wiley, New York, 1965.

2. BACTERIAL ANTISERA

Highly specific and potent antisera are needed for the serodiagnosis of unidentified bacterial strains. Immunizing antigens are selected with great care for antigenic characteristics, often reflected in part by morphology and uniformity of colonial growth (Vol. I, Chap. 2.B.1, Table II).

The desired antigenic characters (including selected phase-type antigens at times) should be maximal in relation to other antigens of the particular strains.[2,4] To keep the antibody response from becoming too broad, immunizing injections are commonly given only over a 3 to 4 week period,* and absorption of the antiserum is usually necessary in order to obtain a monospecific reagent. Recommended specifications have been compiled by the National Center for Disease Control[2]; a large number of diagnostic antisera are available from commercial sources. A few principles are indicated below.

Salmonella and *Escherichia coli* suspensions intended for immunizing rabbits to induce antibody response to heat-stable somatic O antigens are treated to inactivate the flagellar H antigen (6- to 8-hour broth cultures heated at 100° for 2.5 hours† before adding formalin to 0.3% or exposing to 95% alcohol for 4 hours). *Salmonella* and *E. coli* suspensions intended to develop antibody to the labile flagellar H antigen come from cultures highly selected for motility by migration through semisolid agar in a U-tube.‡ Cultures incubated 15 to 18 hours are killed and preserved with 0.3% formalin. (Note that flagellar antibodies are of high titer and are used at a dilution that does not give O-type agglutination.)

Staphylococcal antigen for immunization (5×10^9 bacteria per milliliter) consists of formalin-killed vaccine prepared from agar slant cultures that have been incubated at 37° for 18 hours.[7]

Spore antigen for immunization is the suspension with density of 30 IU described in Section 16.D.1.c. Note that the antigen can be viable.

---

* Immunizing schedules are given in Vol. I, Chap. 2. B.1, Table I, part 4.
† More advantageously, the heated organisms are sedimented and suspended in 95% alcohol for 4 hours at 37° and then are made into a stable, dry acetone powder [R. Roschka, *Klin. Med. (Vienna)* **5**, 88 (1950)] by two washes with acetone in capped centrifuge tubes. After drying on a sterile glass petri dish in a warm dry atmosphere, the dried material is ground finely in a mortar, collected, and stored in a stoppered tube at room temperature. It is suspended in saline for injection (see Vol. I, Chap. 2). Note that drying should not be carried out in an incubator used for other cultures, and that stringent precautions should be employed to avoid inhaling bacterial powder.
‡ Alternatively, lengths of glass tubing are placed in culture tubes to protrude above the surface of semisolid agar. Inoculation is made into the central well and seed cultures are fished from the peripheral agar. The first two passages may be made through agar at 0.1 to 0.2%, increased to 0.3 to 0.4% for subsequent passages.

(Indeed, when *Bacillus anthracis* spore suspensions are injected, 150,000 units of penicillin G are given to each rabbit with each of the first 4 spore injections to prevent death from anthrax.)

Antigenic suspensions of *atypical mycobacteria* are described above in Section 16.D.1.d.vi.

3. BACTERIAL AGGLUTINATION TESTS

a. TUBE AGGLUTINATION TESTS[12]

Dilutions of the antiserum are made in a volume of 0.5 ml in clean test tubes (10 × 75 mm or 13 × 100 mm) in 2-fold serial dilutions as from 1:10 to 1:5120 for determining antibody concentration, or in selected steps, say of 3-fold dilutions, when culture identification is sought with a known serum. The tubes are held vertically in a well-fitting nonrusting rack. Physiological saline solution usually is used as diluent. The bacterial suspension is prepared at a density (Table I) twice as great as that wanted in the tests. The preparation is kept uniformly suspended while 0.5-ml amounts are added to all test tubes, including one or more tubes containing only the diluent (control for spontaneous clumping). The density of the bacterial suspension which gives reproducible and optimal results depends upon numerous factors, such as the particular antigen, incubation period, and incubation time. Recommended densities and diluents are given in Table I. Positive controls (known antigen or antiserum as appropriate) should be included in every test. After mixing, the tubes are incubated at a suitable temperature, depending upon the particular antigen–antibody system under investigation (see Table II). The resulting agglutination is read grossly. (The "titer" is the *total* dilution of antiserum in the final tube that shows agglutination.) Flagellar agglutination is characterized by being rapid, with clumps which are loose, cloudy gray, and easily dispersed. O agglutination occurs more slowly; the resulting clumps are not as rapidly dispersed. The degree of agglutination may be recorded as follows:

4+ = All the organisms appear clumped and the supernatant fluid is clear
3+ = Approximately 75% of the organisms have agglutinated and the supernatant fluid is slightly cloudy
2+ = 50% of the organisms agglutinated and the supernatant fluid is moderately cloudy
1+ = 25% agglutinated and the supernatant fluid is cloudy
0 = Absence of agglutination, characterized by an even suspension of antigen–serum mixture

[12] Lederle Laboratories, "Diagnostic Agents for Laboratory Use," rev. ed. Lederle Laboratories, Pearl River, New York, 1964.

TABLE I
DENSITY OF BACTERIAL SUSPENSIONS RECOMMENDED FOR
AGGLUTINATION TESTS

Bacterial suspension	Stock concentrate	Diluent	Recommended density (IU) Tube agglutination	Recommended density (IU) Slide agglutination[a]
Enterobacteriaceae				
Unknown *E. coli*	—	Saline	3.3	300
Flagellar H antigens	0.5% formalin in saline	0.6% formalin	3.3	300
Somatic O antigens				
(a) Stock	33% alcohol plus 0.5% phenol in saline	0.5% phenol in saline (dilute to <12% alcohol)	3.3	300
(b) Broth cultures treated with 86% alcohol	20% glycerin +12% NaCl	0.5% phenol in saline	3.3	300
(c) Broth cultures or suspended agar growth held at 100°C for 2 hours	(temporary use)	0.5% phenol in saline	3.3	300
Pneumococci	0.1% formalin in $M/20$ buffered saline	0.1% formalin	—	300
Staphylococci				
5-hour growth	Use living	Saline	—	300
Autoclaved 24-hour growth	—	Saline		300
Mycobacteria	0.5% phenol in saline	0.5% phenol in saline	11	300
Francisella tularensis	0.5% phenol in saline	0.5% phenol in saline	6.5	300
Bordetella pertussis	Saline		—	300
Brucella	0.5% phenol in saline		3.5	300

[a] Not to be regarded as reliable unless very appropriate controls are used.

Agglutination tests can be carried out also with bacterial endospore suspensions. In the procedure used by Lamanna and Eisler,[8] spore suspensions are made up to an optical density of 0.6 as measured in a Coleman Junior spectrophotometer at 640 nm. Twofold serial dilutions of the

TABLE II

RECOMMENDED CONDITIONS FOR TEST TUBE AGGLUTINATION[a]

Antigen	Method	Time	Primary incubation Temperature (°C)	Time	Secondary incubation Temperature (°C)
Bordetella pertussis and *B. parapertussis*	Mechanical shaker	3 minutes	Room temperature	1 hour	37, water bath
Brucella	Water bath	48 hours	37	ND[b]	ND
Escherichia coli O	Water bath	16 hours	48–50	ND	ND
Escherichia coli OB	Incubator	2 hours	37	18 hours	4
Francisella (*Pasteurella*) *tularensis*	Water bath	20 hours	37	ND	ND
Salmonella O	Water bath	18 hours	45–50	ND	ND
Salmonella H (also *Citrobacter* H)	Water bath	0.25, 0.5 and 1 hour	48–50 coli H 45–50 50–52 Sal H	ND	ND

[a] U.S. National Communicable Disease Center, Laboratory Branch, "Recommended Methods for Evaluation of Microbiological Reagents," 2nd ed., Public Health Service, D3-3. U.S. Dept. of Health, Education, and Welfare, Atlanta, Georgia, 1969.
[b] Not done.

antiserum are mixed with equal volumes (0.1 ml) of the spore suspension. The mixtures are shaken vigorously for 30 to 60 minutes at room temperature. To each tube 0.8 ml of saline solution is then added, the agglutination reaction being read immediately after shaking and again after overnight storage at 4°. Attention is called to the relatively frequent occurrence of a prozone, in which the higher concentrations of antiserum may fail to cause clumping of the organisms.

Agglutination tests with certain mycobacteria are carried out as follows. The antiserum, in 2-fold serial dilution (0.5 ml), is mixed with an equal volume of the bacterial suspension (Section 16.D.3.a) in 12 × 75 nm tubes. The mixtures are incubated at 37° and the agglutination is read 3 to 5 hours later and after holding at 4° again the following morning.[9]

b. COVER SLIP AGGLUTINATION REACTION

Rapid identification of an unknown organism in the gram-negative Enterobacteriaceae class, including salmonellas, can be performed by placing one volume (as, one bacteriological loop) or a suitable dilution of the unknown bacterial suspension on each of two cover slips, and adding an equal volume of a suitable dilution of a diagnostic antiserum to one of these cover slips and a like dilution of a normal serum to the other, with mixing but without spreading the fluids laterally. Conversely, antibodies can be sought in patients' serum which react with suspensions of known organisms, such as typhoid (the Widal test, also termed the Gruber-Widal test).

Two cover slips are inverted over two depressions in a "hanging drop" slide and sealed at the rim with petroleum jelly or with a loopful of water to avoid evaporation. The unknown and the negative control are examined under "high dry" power of a microscope, with illumination reduced and focusing made at the *edge* of the drops. (Hanging drops are usually not appropriate to the focal planes demanded by phase-contrast microscopy.) As agglutination occurs, incipient aggregation may been seen despite the Brownian motion; the clumps will settle within the hanging drop so that its entire depth should finally be viewed at a lower power selected to allow sufficient clearance between cover slip and the objective lens.

c. MACROSCOPIC SLIDE AGGLUTINATION TESTS

By using very dense bacterial suspensions (Table I), agglutination can be observed macroscopically on slides. Owing to the large amount of bacterial surface presented, the diagnostic serum must be employed in correspondingly high concentration (1:5 or 1:10 dilutions), where the specificity of the agglutination is most suspect. It is extremely important with this test to employ appropriate positive and negative controls, for identification rests wholly on the potency and specificity of the reagents. Some commercial reagents are dilute and afford scant latitude.

The tests are performed on large glass plates, microscope slides or within petri dishes. Slides marked with ceramic rings or squares are commercially available, the most useful being rings with internal diameters of 0.75 or 1 inch. Bacterial suspensions may be prepared by suspending generous portions of growth from the agar slant in a small volume (as, 0.5 ml) of saline. The density of the suspension, diluted 1:30 on a side portion, should correspond to 10 IU (McFarland No. 3). Depending upon the particular antigen to be identified, boiled or unheated suspensions are used (Table I).

Approximately 0.05-ml amounts of the antiserum in proper dilution(s) and of bacterial suspension are allowed to fall within a ring (note that 0.05 ml is delivered as a single drop from a Kahn serological pipette of 0.2-ml capacity when held in a vertical position). The reagents, antigen and antiserum, should be properly mixed either with a sterile loop or a suitable applicator, and the slide, plate, or dish should be rocked and tilted. Agglutination is observed grossly by inspection over a lightbox against a dark background.† Strong agglutination reactions usually occur rapidly, generally within a minute. The degree of agglutination can be recorded as described in Section 15.D.3.a.

d. OTHER PROCEDURES

Occasionally agglutination is conducted in glass capillary tubes. For special purposes antiserum is added aseptically to culture medium in serial dilutions ("growth agglutination test"[11]). The tubes are seeded with the test organism, and agglutinated growth is recorded after incubation for 18 to 24 hours at 37°.

e. ENUMERATION OF BACTERIAL COLONIES IN LIQUID MEDIA*

A special technique that allows enumeration of bacterial colonies in liquid medium, rather than by plating in agar, was devised for nonmotile, "rough" (nonencapsulated) pneumococci by adding specific antiserum to the medium in dilutions of 1×10^{-3} to 10^{-2}. The procedure is described here, since it may be applicable to other systems in which nonmotile bacteria possessing a nondiffusible surface antigen is present, in instances in which the antibody does not interfere with colonial growth.

Antiserum which agglutinated nonencapsulated pneumococci but did not prevent their growth was used by O. T. Avery and co-workers[13,14] to sequester these cells and separate them in cultures undergoing mutation or transformation of capsular antigens. Hotchkiss[15,16] has used this type of antiserum or purified globulin fractions thereof, in a series of investigations to produce and enumerate bacterial colonies in liquid growth media.

When small numbers of cells or viable units (less than 100 per milliliter) are present and the antiserum is diluted as stated, the bacteria become coated with immunoglobulin but agglutination does not occur. Instead, growing units produce clones in which daughter cells remain clumped and form discrete colonies which settle to the bottom of the culture tube

---

† Various devices for dark field observation are described in Volume IV, Chap. 14.E.2.b.

* Section 16.D.3.e was contributed by Rollin D. Hotchkiss.

[13] M. H. Dawson, *J. Exp. Med.* **51**, 123 (1930).
[14] O. T. Avery, C. M. MacLeod, and M. McCarty, *J. Exp. Med.* **79**, 137 (1944).
[15] R. D. Hotchkiss, *Proc. Nat. Acad. Sci.* U.S. **40**, 49 (1954).
[16] R. D. Hotchkiss, *in* "Methods of Enzymology" (S. P. Colowick and N. O. Kaplan, eds.), Vol. III, p. 708. Academic Press, New York, 1957.

where they may be counted when held over a transilluminated ground glass viewing box. The system is insensitive to vibration or simple manipulation during the first hour or two of preparation when the small microclones are suspended in the liquid layer, and again at the time of counting (24 hours) when the colonies can no longer grow. A dental mirror facilitates counting the colonies.

4. ANTIGENS INHIBITING AGGLUTINATION*

In addition to flagellar antigens, the bacterial surface may contain other antigens.† It is important to recognize that certain of these, such as the Vi antigen of *Salmonella typhi* and related microorganisms, as well as the K antigens of other gram-negative bacilli, may interfere with agglutination by the respective O antibodies. It has been shown that the inhibitory effect of Vi antigen is due to interference with the clumping reaction itself rather than with antigen–antibody interaction, for Vi antigen does not interfere with complement-dependent lysis.[17]

In practice, the interfering effect can be abolished by heating the bacterial suspensions. Depending upon the nature of such interfering antigens, heating in boiling water for 1 hour or in the autoclave at 121° for 15 minutes is carried out. Accordingly certain Enterobacteriaceae which contain both O and K antigens should be tested as both heated and nonheated suspensions for agglutination with appropriate O and OK antisera in order to detect the presence of the two antigens.

5. INTERPRETATION

Agglutination tests must be interpreted carefully. When unknown strains of bacteria are being tested, the titer of the known antiserum should be substantially the same with the strain under study as with the standard strain. Since antigens often are shared by other groups within the same bacterial species or even by other species, agglutination alone does not provide unequivocal evidence of identity of strains.

Whenever antibody is detected in sera of patients or animals by agglutination tests with known strains, the titers observed must be considered in comparison with those of "normal" antibodies occurring in the

---

* Sections 16.D.4-6 were contributed by Erwin Neter.

† In the Kauffmann-White schema of antigens in the gram-negative, nonsporing rod forms of bacteria, cell-wall antigens are referred to as O antigens, surface or capsular antigens as K antigens (including the Vi antigen), and flagellar antigens as H antigens. [G. S. Wilson and A. A. Miles, *in* "Principles of Bacteriology and Immunity" (D. D. Topley and G. S. Wilson, eds.), 6th ed., Vol. I, pp. 918–955. Williams & Wilkins, Baltimore, Maryland, 1975.]

[17] E. Neter, *Nature (London)* **194,** 1256 (1962).

respective species. If antibodies are present in titers far exceeding those present in "normal" sera, the examination of a single serum specimen from a patient may aid in diagnosis. Often, a significant rise in antibody titer in two consecutive serum specimens provides more convincing evidence of a specific antibody response of the patient.

In all serological tests, the "negative control" tubes of *bacteria suspended in diluent* and *bacteria suspended in normal serum* must yield negative results; also it may prove useful to put up a tube containing only diluent and serum to rule out sedimentation of serum components.

It should be emphasized again that agglutination may fail to occur even though the bacterial cells contain a given antigen and the antiserum contains the corresponding antibody. Such false-negative reactions may be due to substances on the surface of bacterial cells that interfere with agglutination, such as Vi and K antigens in tests using enterobacteriaceae and specific O antisera, mentioned before. An erroneous interpretation can result from making readings when serum is not diluted sufficiently (prozone effects simulating negative results).

6. APPLICATIONS

The practical use of agglutination includes specific serodiagnosis of infectious diseases such as the Widal test for typhoid fever, the Vi agglutination test as an aid in detecting typhoid carriers, the Weil-Felix test (which employs strains of *Proteus* such as OX-19) for diagnosis of certain rickettsial diseases, and tests for agglutinins in diagnosing whooping cough and brucellosis. Second, agglutination tests are widely employed with bacteria isolated from patients for identifying the following as pathogenic agents—*S. typhi* and other salmonellae; shigellae; enteropathogenic *Escherichia coli; Haemophilus influenzae; Bordetella pertussis;* and others as well. Third, agglutination tests offer considerable help in epidemiologic studies, for example in tracing the chain of events leading to an epidemic that is caused by a given serotype of an enteric pathogen. Fourth, these procedures have been of considerable value in microbiological research. Various bacterial antigens and corresponding serotypes have been discovered; e.g., a thousand serotypes of salmonellae have been identified. Also, the existence of antigenically similar constituents in various species of taxonomically unrelated microorganisms have come to light, such as in *Haemophilus influenzae* type b and pneumococcus type 6.[18] In addition agglutination and specific inhibition of agglutination by soluble derivatives have been applied with advantage in studies of the composition of bacterial cell-wall antigens.

[18] E. Neter, *J. Immunol.* **46**, 239 (1943).

E. Immobilization of Motile Bacteria by Anti-Flagellar Antibody*

Many immunological studies have employed the immobilization of motile bacteria as a test for the presence of anti-flagellar antibody.[1-3] The immobilization of bacteria and their adherence to cells have been used to·measure antibody production by single cells, to identify antibody producing cells in mass cell cultures, and to titer the antibody content of sera and other fluids (see Vol. V, Section 26.C.4.b–d). The techniques described below have been used to study the anti-flagellar antibody response against whole salmonellae in mice.[4]

1. TEST CULTURE PREPARATION

Successful antibody titrations depend on the availability of uniformly motile test cultures. Bacteria are maintained at maximal motility by daily passage through a semisolid nutrient medium (0.4% agar, 8% gelatin in Difco Antibiotic Medium 3) in a petri dish.[5] Alternative techniques of selection for maximal motility (Craigie tubes, U tubes, 0.2% agar) are described by Stuart et al.[6] and by Lennette et al.[7] Organisms from the leading edge of such a culture are taken up with a 4-mm loop and inoculated into 5 ml of fresh liquid medium. This culture is then rotated for 2 to 3 hours at 37°. Cultures grown in this way are easily countable at 400 to 600 magnification without preliminary dilution (1 to 15 bacteria per microscopic field) and are routinely 95 to 100% motile. If heavier growth is allowed, the percentage of motile bacteria decreases. Background immobilization will be too high also if organisms are taken up too far behind the leading edge of the semisolid culture. Overgrown liquid cultures cannot be diluted successfully and should not be used. At this low concentration of test bacteria, there is no problem with agglutination, even if the original immunogen is used as the test culture.

---

* Section 16.E was contributed by Richard C. Blinkoff.

[1] G. J. V. Nossal, *Brit. J. Exp. Pathol.* **39**, 544 (1958).

[2] O. Mäkelä and G. J. V. Nossal, *J. Immunol.* **87**, 447 (1961).

[3] G. J. V. Nossal, A. Szenberg, G. L. Ada, and C. M. Austin, *J. Exp. Med.* **119**, 485 (1964).

[4] R. C. Blinkoff, *J. Immunol.* **97**, 727 (1966).

[5] J. Lederberg, *Genetics* **41**, 845 (1956).

[6] C. A. Stuart, K. M. Wheeler, V. McGann, and I. Howard, *J. Bacteriol.* **52**, 519 (1946).

[7] E. H. Lennette, E. H. Spaulding, and J. P. Truant, "Manual of Clinical Microbiology," 2nd ed., p. 933. Amer. Soc. for Microbiology, Bethesda, Maryland, 1974.

2. DILUTION PROCEDURE

Serial dilutions of immune serum are prepared in disposable plastic dishes with physiological saline. An equal volume of a test culture, still growing after 2 to 3 hours of incubation, is mixed with each dilution. Incubation for 20 minutes at room temperature is sufficient for maximum immobilization. Not too many dilutions should be tested at a time lest the test bacteria multiply or lose their motility before the end of the counting period. The inoculation of test bacteria can be so timed that cultures are 2 to 3 hours old at regular intervals. A group of 6 to 8 dilutions can be assayed every 45 to 60 minutes in this way.

The dilutions are most easily handled with 1-inch micropipettes drawn from capillary tubing (0.7 to 1.0 mm). Place separate pipettes in each cup of the disposable tray and allow them to fill by capillary attraction. The pipettes are easily dispensed with the aid of a bulb assembly (Drummond Scientific Co., Broomall, Pennsylvania) attached to a piece of rubber tubing held in the operator's mouth. Spread a thin layer of mineral oil over the surface of a clean glass cover slip (22 × 50 mm). With the bulb assembly as many as 15 microdroplets can be evenly spaced under the layer of oil.

3. THE COUNTING CHAMBER

A simpler counting chamber than that used in previous studies[1, 8] can be constructed of wax instead of brass rods. On a 3- by 1-inch glass microscope slide, outline a rectangular area slightly smaller than the cover slip on three sides with molten wax (paraffin:petroleum jelly, 2:1). Invert the cover slip on this chamber after the wax has hardened and fill any empty space beneath it with additional mineral oil. This method gives chambers of varying depths depending on the thickness of the wax, but this does not affect the experimental results. The chamber has the advantage of being entirely disposable when the counting is finished. The resolution by phase contrast microscopy is better if the microdroplets are in contact with both the top and the bottom of the chamber. With practice, the height of the chamber and the volume of the droplets can be controlled so that the droplets spread slightly without coalescing when the cover slip is inverted.

4. END-POINT DETERMINATION

Observe the microdroplets with a 40× phase contrast objective. Since the immobilization is not an all-or-none phenomenon, at intermediate

[8] P. de Fonbrune, "Technique de Micromanipulation." Masson, Paris, 1949.

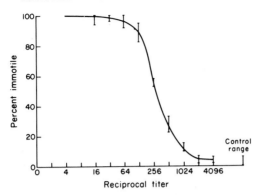

Fig. 1. The immobilization of motile test bacteria by a specific antiserum. See text for explanation.

dilutions some bacteria exhibit spinning and sporadic forward motion. As a general rule, it is best to classify bacteria showing any movement other than Brownian motion as motile. Count 50 to 100 bacteria in each droplet and calculate the percentage immobilized. Take care always to count throughout the depth of the droplet, as there may sometimes be more immotile bacteria toward the bottom.

A typical titration curve is shown in Fig. 1. There are four to five doubling dilutions between complete immobilization and complete motility. The spread of values at the same dilution is less than 15%. The immobilization of controls is always well within the range indicated. In studies by this author, the end point of a titration has been taken as the greatest dilution containing more than 25% nonmotile bacteria, or 1/256 in the illustration shown. On repeated titration of the same serum, the standard deviation of end points has always been less than one doubling dilution. The counting procedure was chosen instead of the estimation of a 90% immobilization end point used by other authors because it gave more reproducible results in duplicate tests employing both methods. In actual practice, counting takes only slightly more time than scanning, and only 3 to 4 dilutions of an unknown serum need be counted to determine the end point. The determination of end points by this method is free of subjectivity to a high degree, and results are easily duplicated by various persons in the laboratory. The immobilization of motile bacteria provides an easy, precise, and highly sensitive technique for antibody titration.

F. Agglutination of Spermatozoa*†

1. INTRODUCTION

Spermagglutination presents several kinds of problems that are not likely to be encountered in phenomena such as hemagglutination and bacterial agglutination. Two types of problem are generally explored by this method: (1) a search in human males and females for antibodies against human spermatozoa, with the purpose of explaining infertility; (2) studies with anti-sperm antibodies raised deliberately in other species (heteroagglutinins) or in the same species (autoagglutinins). The complexity of the spermatozoon is evident from Fig. 1; data at hand show that antibody-containing sera can cause head-to-head, tail-to-tail, or end piece-

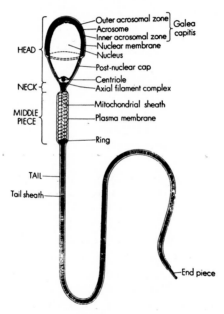

FIG. 1. Diagrammatic representation of a spermatozoon. From T. Mann, "Biochemistry of Semen and of the Male Reproductive Tract." Barnes & Noble, New York, 1964.

* Section 16.F was contributed by Sidney Shulman.

† This work was aided by a research grant from The John A. Hartford Foundation, Inc. and a Contract (NO1-HD-4-2824) from the National Institute of Child Health and Human Development, and a General Research Support Grant (RR-05398) from the General Research Support Branch, Division of Research Resources, National Institutes of Health.

to-end piece agglutination, among other possibilities. Indeed, by means of fluorescent antibody procedures, differential coating has been shown for the acrosome, postnuclear cap, equatorial segment, and tail sheath, at least.

Most studies of spermagglutination have shown that the cells must be quite actively motile to give high titers, hence seminal plasma cannot be removed, but only diluted. With heteroagglutinins or induced autoagglutinins, however, washed and immotile sperm can serve well (Section 16.F.5.c). The reactions of human antibodies with human sperm cells may well differ in some ways from the agglutination of such sperm by deliberately induced hetero- or autoantibodies. With further experience, development of additional methodology can be expected. Several varieties of spermatozoa can be studied, and these differ antigenically. Ejaculated sperm, for example, differ from epididymal sperm in that the former have acquired an outer layer of sperm-coating antigen during passage through the urethra. In addition, these forms differ considerably in the degree of difficulty in their study.

Certain human sera do indeed agglutinate human spermatozoa. Much indirect evidence has accumulated in recent years to show that infertility in either sex is sometimes related to the presence of sperm antibody. Many of these sera act by reason of one or more types of sperm antibody, yet some others cause clumping by non-antibody factors, and the distinction becomes important.

In general, the cells must be quite actively motile in almost every procedure of spermagglutination, to give a high titer for the antiserum. As a result, the cells cannot be washed before being used in a test, since this manipulation can readily lead to loss of motility. Whole semen is therefore generally used, with adjustments made in sperm concentration and the possibility of adding certain ingredients. The vagaries of the composition of seminal plasma must be accepted; hence, known positive and negative control sera must always be included in every test series. An additional problem is that nonspecific agglutinating factors may be present. These are sometimes called "natural antibodies," sometimes "non-antibodies" or a similar term, sometimes merely "factors."

More extensive reviews on the general subject of sperm antigens and antibodies, including several kinds of autoimmunity, have appeared elsewhere.[1-6]

[1] S. Shulman, *Deut. Aerztebl.* **67**, 3342 (1970).
[2] S. Shulman, *Clin. Exp. Immunol.* **9**, 267 (1971).
[3] S. Shulman, *Contraception* **4**, 135 (1971).
[4] S. Shulman, *CRC Crit. Rev. Clin. Lab. Sci.* **2**, 393 (1971).
[5] M. W. Chase, *Biol. Reprod.,* **6**, 335 (1972).
[6] S. Shulman, *Obstet. Gynecol. Survey,* **27**, 553 (1972).

2. NATURAL ANTIBODIES AND NONSPECIFIC FACTORS

There is a long history of reports on nonspecific agglutination of spermatozoa, studied most frequently in cattle, i.e., agglutination evidently not related to sperm-specific immunoglobulins. One theory held that two factors were involved, an agglutinating factor and a stabilizing "antagglutin" or "sperm antagglutin," both factors being present in seminal plasma. Details of the original observations are given elsewhere.[4, 6] Yet "natural" sperm agglutinins may well exist, analogous to the "natural" agglutinins for gram-negative bacteria found in serum of so many species.[7, 8] Johnson[9] showed, rather convincingly, that normal guinea pig serum contained a specific complement-fixing, γ-globulin antibody, directed against the acrosome of the spermatozoon. In other studies, a potent agglutinating substance was isolated from the semen of one particular rabbit; it caused massive head-to-head agglutination of its own ejaculated spermatozoa and also of spermatozoa from other rabbits.[10] This activity, apparently not complement-dependent, was seemingly due to a special substance, rather than to the absence of "antagglutins." It had already been accepted that there is a tendency for washed spermatozoa to agglutinate in the head-to-head fashion. This nonspecific clumping is even more likely to happen if the spermatozoa are suspended in normal serum of the same or another species.[11] On the other hand, it had been the impression for some time that tail-to-tail agglutination occurs only when there is antibody present. However, nonspecific tail-to-tail agglutination of rabbit spermatozoa can occur, but only under certain circumstances—for example, when the spermatozoa are placed in isotonic sucrose, glucose, or fructose, with little or no electrolyte. In general, there are striking differences among the species concerning these non-antibody agglutinations, guinea pig sperm being rather readily agglutinated, and human sperm (at the other extreme) being rarely agglutinated.[4, 6]

Nonspecific clumping is thus most apt to occur with cell suspensions in saline media containing serum, or in low-electrolyte isotonic sugar solutions; also by di- and trivalent salts. (Di- and trivalent ions also cause bacterial agglutination.) Agglutination is caused by *Pseudomo-*

[7] R. G. Edwards, *J. Reprod. Fert.* **1**, 268 (1960).
[8] R. G. Edwards, *in* "Immunology of Spermatozoa and Fertilization" (Proc. Int. Symp., Varna, Bulgaria, 1967) (K. Bratanov, ed.), p. 27. Bulgarian Acad. Sci. Press, Sofia, 1969.
[9] M. H. Johnson, *J. Reprod. Fert.* **16**, 503 (1968).
[10] J. M. Bedford, *J. Reprod. Fert.* **22**, 193 (1970).
[11] J. M. Bedford, *Exp. Cell Res.* **38**, 654 (1965).

nas,[12] mycoplasma,[13] and certain viruses.[14] Viral agglutination is of special interest because comparison can be made with the hemagglutination produced by the same agents. As examples, bovine and rooster spermatozoa are agglutinated by the viruses of influenza, Newcastle disease, and mumps. For viral agglutination, sperm must be motile,[14] but for the effects of mycoplasma, they can be immotile.[13]

3. VARIETIES OF SPERM ANTIGENS

Sperm antigens fall into several categories. Distinct antigens have been demonstrated in a number of different regions of the cell, as already mentioned. Besides questions of species specificity and the sperm-specific antigens, one must deal with spermatozoa-coating antigens from the seminal plasma, and the presence of blood group antigens and transplantation antigens. A schematic representation of a sperm cell is shown in Fig. 1, illustrating many of the detailed morphological structures. Many details on the anatomy and function of the primary and accessory glands of the male reproductive system have been presented elsewhere,[15] along with the chemical structures and interactions that are involved in the semen and its production.

a. SPERMATOZOA-COATING ANTIGENS

In 1960, Weil and his colleagues revealed the occurrence on spermatozoa of an antigen of seminal plasma, termed the spermatozoa-coating antigen (SCA). They demonstrated this activity in both the rabbit[16] and man.[17] Antisera prepared in a foreign species against ejaculated spermatozoa will show strong positive reactions with ejaculated spermatozoa—generally by means of complement fixation tests—but they will be completely negative when tested with epididymal spermatozoa. Second, antisera can be prepared against the seminal plasma, and these antisera also give strong positive reactions with ejaculated spermatozoa and are totally negative with epididymal spermatozoa. This kind of study shows that the antigenic composition of epididymal spermatozoa and ejaculated spermatozoa are significantly different, the epididymal spermatozoa acquiring an additional antigenic property while traveling through the urethra.

---

[12] E. B. Bell, *J. Reprod. Fert.* **17**, 275 (1968).
[13] D. Taylor-Robinson and R. J. Manchee, *Nature (London)* **215**, 484 (1967).
[14] B. A. Peleg and M. Ianconescu, *Nature (London)* **211**, 1211 (1966).
[15] T. Mann, "Biochemistry of Semen and of the Male Reproductive Tract." Barnes & Noble, New York, 1964.
[16] A. J. Weil, *Science* **131**, 1040 (1969).
[17] A. J. Weil and J. M. Rodenburg, *Proc. Soc. Exp. Biol. Med.* **105**, 43 (1960).

Antigenic analysis of seminal plasma by immunoelectrophoresis revealed nine components, of which the SCA was shown to be one of the faster migrating components, but not the major component.[18-20] The SCA was in fact shown to be lactoferrin, a major component of milk.[19] Additional studies on human seminal plasma have been presented elsewhere.[21, 22] It has been argued that actually two or three antigens in man show SCA activity, and even a larger number in the rabbit. If several SCA antigens exist, these antigens may well function in some of the spermagglutination phenomena.

b. BLOOD-GROUP ANTIGENS

Sperm cells have been examined for the presence of antigens of the ABO blood group system. Landsteiner and Levine in 1926 showed that A and B antigens were present on human spermatozoa obtained from semen,[23] a fact confirmed in 1961.[24] The studies of certain workers, as reviewed elsewhere,[4, 6] have led them to conclude that the A and B factors are inherent components of the sperm cells. However, other investigators have indicated rather convincingly that the A and B substances are actually secreted into the seminal plasma, from which they adhere to the sperm cells. The methods used for the detection of the antibody seem to explain the continuing dispute. A decision might be reached by determining whether the blood group substance exists on sperm in the form of glycolipid (the erythrocyte type) or glycoprotein (the water-soluble, secretory form), as described in Volume I, Chap. 1.C.

c. TRANSPLANTATION ANTIGENS

Spermatozoa do carry histocompatibility antigens. In 1969, Vojtíšková,[25] using antisera prepared by immunizing strains of mice with the sperm cells from other strains, showed that the H-2^d antigens occur on mouse spermatozoa. By means of hemagglutination inhibition the spermatozoa were found to absorb the hemagglutinating antibody from the

[18] A. Hekman and P. Rümke, in "Immunology of Spermatozoa and Fertilization" (Proc. Int. Symp., Varna, Bulgaria, 1967) (K. Bratanov, ed.), p. 107. Bulgarian Acad. Sci. Press, Sofia, 1969.

[19] A. Hekman and P. Rümke, Fert. Steril. 20, 312 (1969).

[20] S. Shulman and P. Bronson, J. Reprod. Fert. 18, 481 (1969).

[21] S. Shulman, in "Immunology and Reproduction" (R. G. Edwards, ed.), p. 111. Int. Planned Parenthood Fed., London, 1969.

[22] S. Shulman, "Tissue Specificity and Autoimmunity," p. 71. Springer-Verlag, Berlin and New York, 1974.

[23] K. Landsteiner and P. Levine, J. Immunol. 12, 415 (1926).

[24] P. Levine and M. J. Celano, Vox Sang. 6, 720 (1961).

[25] M. Vojtíšková, Nature (London) 222, 1293 (1969).

indicated antisera. Later studies[26] showed that several antigens were expressed, corresponding to a number of the histocompatibility alleles. H-2 antigens have been demonstrated on mouse spermatozoa also by a special cytotoxicity method.[27] Histocompatibility antigens have been demonstrated also on the spermatozoa of man.[28] Fellous and Dausset concluded that these antigens are segregated to represent the haploid genome, that is, that they express postreductional gene action. This interesting claim awaits further confirmation.

4. PREPARATION OF HETERO- AND AUTOSPERMAGGLUTININS

For preparing an antiserum containing heteroantibodies against human sperm cells, one procedure that has been found satisfactory is as follows: New Zealand White rabbits are injected with a well-washed sperm suspension emulsified with an equal volume of Complete Freund's Adjuvant (CFA). The antigen dose should be approximately 10 million cells per milliliter of final emulsion. This is injected in a number of intradermal sites. Similar injections are repeated at intervals of 2 weeks for a total of 4 or 5 injections, often with reduction or elimination of the mycobacterial dose. Trial bleedings are taken at intervals for the evaluation of the antibody response.

Spermatozoa are antigenic for the individual animal of origin when given parenterally; most notably, guinea pig spermatozoa, included in CFA, will give rise to induced autoantibodies.[4, 6]

5. PROCEDURES AND PROBLEMS IN THE SPERMAGGLUTINATION METHODS

Agglutination methods were rarely used during the early years of study of sperm antibodies. The technique of spermagglutination does not easily give unambiguous results. A suspension of spermatozoa may exhibit clumping and settling by itself, particularly in the presence of normal serum. Special precautions must be taken to avoid confusing such clumping with antibody effects. To have a sensitive degree of agglutination when antibody is present, yet to avoid nonspecific agglutination when antibody is absent, requires careful adjustment of the test conditions.

Methods for observing agglutination finally were developed in two major forms—viewing the reaction under the microscope, and direct macroscopic observation.

The first successful effort to avoid the difficulty of spontaneous aggluti-

[26] M. Vojtíšková, M. Poláčková, and Z. Pokorná, *Folia Biol. (Prague)* **15**, 322 (1969).
[27] E. Goldberg, T. Aoki, E. Boyse, and D. Bennett, *Nature (London)* **228**, 570 (1970).
[28] M. Fellous and J. Dausset, *Nature (London)* **225**, 191 (1970).

nation in saline or in serum, as seen in macroscopic procedures, was made by Mudd.[29] Mudd suggested centrifuging the tubes after incubation and then resuspending the sediments by shaking until an even suspension was obtained in the control tubes. Specific agglutination could be discerned by differences in the ease of breaking up the clumps. Yet sometimes, loose clumps of spermatozoa were easily broken up by the agitation. Kibrick, Belding, and Merrill[30, 31] developed several successive modifications in the procedure. First, narrow-bore tubes (5 × 65 mm) were used to permit resuspension by inverting the tubes three times gently instead of by shaking. The more loosely bound of the specific clumps would not break up. They also emphasized the importance of an appreciable dilution of the semen, by selecting donor semen samples having a high initial sperm count—at least 80 or 100 million cells per milliliter.* Adjustment to the initial test level of 40 million cells per milliliter then reduces the seminal plasma. Also, the sperm cells must be motile†; otherwise, much lower titers will be found. Finally, incubation was to be done at 37° for 2 hours; a shorter time should be used if the controls began to show granular sedimentation.[30]

Yet the test was not sufficiently sensitive, and a gelatin agglutination test[31] was introduced, which is now often designated the Kibrick method; we may also term it the K-B-M method. By suspending the sperm cells

---

[29] S. Mudd, *J. Immunol.* **13**, 113 (1927).

[30] S. Kibrick, D. L. Belding, and B. Merrill, *Fert. Steril.* **3**, 419 (1952).

[31] S. Kibrick, D. L. Belding, and B. Merrill, *Fert. Steril.* **3**, 430 (1952).

* The original recommendation called for 100×10^6 cells per milliliter, or at the very least, 80×10^6 cells per milliliter. Even with the situation of selecting donor (human) samples, one may need to be fortunate to find many with such high counts. If the situation is one of searching for antibodies against the sperm cells of a given male patient (or a female patient's husband), a lower figure may have to be accepted, with the risk of lower titers or a false-negative result.

† Motility is an important but elusive variable. In the original proposals, the requirement was stated only in qualitative terms, such as that they be "actively motile" [S. Kibrick, D. S. Belding, and B. Merrill, *Fert. Steril.* **3**, 419 and 430 (1952)]. Some later investigators have stipulated that a motility of 90% should be considered as a useful minimum. Again, it is difficult to find such samples; even a 70% minimum would require much screening of semen donors. In the actual situation with human patients, a compromise will frequently be required and samples of only 50% motility may be risked, with the understanding that poor agglutination may be the result. Yet in the original study, immotile (or sluggish) spermatozoa were not found to give no agglutination at all, but merely to yield lower titers; the difference from high-motility samples was given as a 4-fold factor in the titer (Kibrick *et al.*, 1952, p. 419). The motility requirement has been repeatedly emphasized in agglutination methods of all sorts. Such a requirement limits stockpiling of antigenic material to be used for test purposes. The requirement for motility has been debated, but it remains unexplained.

in a gelatin solution, the problem of disruption of weak unions was further minimized. No inversion of the tubes was necessary. The distinction between positive and negative agglutination could readily be seen in the small test tubes. The gelatin modification gave titers that were in general 32-fold higher than those obtained by their first modification, and about 100-fold higher than in other agglutination methods.

a. EXAMINATION OF THE SEMEN

While detailed and complete evaluation of a semen sample requires some considerable training and experience in this special technique, the few parameters that need be checked to judge and prepare the sample for agglutination studies can be readily learned for this purpose.

The sample should be examined while quite fresh, preferably within 2 hours of ejaculation; however, one should not attempt to study it before 30 minutes has elapsed, since the initial gel formation requires approximately this time for redissolving. The semen sample should be maintained at room temperature and should not be cooled or kept refrigerated, since sperm can undergo damage at reduced temperature.

Preparations of epididymal sperm can be examined by the methods described below, but without any concern for gelation and redissolving, and with less concern for cellular contamination, although there may be some admixed cell types.

i. Determination of Sperm Motility

A drop of the semen is placed on a slide and surmounted with a cover glass. It is then examined under high power, such as a $\times 430$ magnification. An estimate is made to the nearest 10% of the percentage of actively motile cells, after several fields have been explored. This is a rather subjective measurement, but it should become reasonably reliable after some experience.

At the same time, notice should be taken of the additional cells and the cellular debris that may be seen; unusually large amounts of such contaminants should be noted in the semen description. Any sign of sperm autoagglutination should be carefully checked, but the clumping that may be seen as a result of sticking to the debris must be distinguished from the clumping of sperm cells with each other.

ii. Determination of Sperm Count

Mix the semen sample thoroughly. If the semen seemed quite dense (in the motility examination), it will be well to dilute it 1:10 with saline or buffer. Fill a white cell pipette to the 0.5 line with the sperm suspension and to the 11 line with the diluting-counting fluid (4.0 gm of $NaHCO_3$ + 1.0 gm of phenol in 100 ml of water).

Shake the pipette for 1 minute. Place a cover glass on the hemacytometer (or counting chamber). The improved Neubauer grating is useful.

After discarding the first few drops from the pipette, fill the counting chamber by letting a drop be drawn under the cover glass on each slide. The moats of the hemacytometer must remain dry. If the fluid is drawn into the moats, clean the hemacytometer and refill counting chamber. Allow the cells to settle for about 2 minutes.

In the hemacytometer, count sperm cells in two diagonally opposite large squares (consisting each of 16 subdivisions). Sum the number of sperm cells counted in each square, and take the total. Multiply the number of sperm cells counted by 10^5 (and by any preliminary dilution factor) to obtain the concentration, provided that the proposed grating was used; an alternative computation may be readily derived. The concentration is then expressed as the number of sperm cells per milliliter.

b. Macroscale: The Kibrick Method

i. Performance of the Kibrick (K-B-M) Method*

For human sperm cells, a fresh ejaculate should be used in order to have maximum motility. It is preferable that the sperm count in the original semen be at least as high as 80×10^6 cells per milliliter, with motility of at least 50%; however, compromise in these requirements must at times be risked with samples that need to be examined regardless of their marginal quality.

The reagents needed are Baker's buffer,[32] saline, and gelatin. Baker's buffer has the following composition: glucose, 30.0 gm; $Na_2HPO_4 \cdot 7H_2O$, 4.6 gm; NaCl, 2.0 gm; KH_2PO_4, 0.1 gm; with water to 1000 ml. The gelatin (Difco) is a 10% solution in Baker's buffer, conveniently made up in 250-ml quantities, with storage in 5-ml portions; each portion will generally be suitable for 1 day's work. The gelatin and the buffer are to be kept in the refrigerator until needed. Neither reagent should become more than 2 months old.

The serum (or antiserum) under investigation is inactivated prior to use by heating at 56° for 30 minutes, to destroy complement activity that may otherwise cause (with the antibody) sperm immobilization or

---

* This detailed description is intended primarily for the study of human sperm cells. For other species, some of the parameters may be different as described in the text.

[32] J. R. Baker, *J. Hyg.* **32**, 171 (1932).

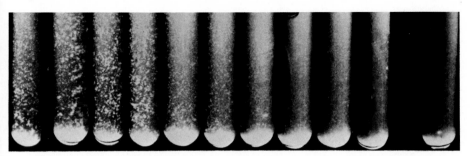

FIG. 2. Test-tube spermagglutination, as done in the Kibrick method. Twofold serial dilutions of a positive serum, incubated with semen–gelatin mixtures. First tube: 1:2 dilution. Last tube: saline control. From P. Rümke, *Immunopathol., Int. Symp. 1st, 1958*, p. 145 (1959).

because there might be nonspecific agglutination due to normal fresh serum.

The fresh semen (or, if such is studied, the epididymal suspension) is diluted with Baker's buffer to a concentration of 40 million cells per milliliter. This diluted sperm suspension is warmed to 37° and mixed with an equal volume of fluid 10% gelatin in Baker's buffer (also at 37°), and allowed to cool. This provides the test antigen. The antigen is then mixed with an equal volume of an appropriate dilution of the serum or antiserum in Baker's buffer, starting with 1:4. The final concentrations are 2.5% gelatin and 10×10^6 sperm cells per milliliter.

The mixtures are agitated gently and transferred to small tubes of 3 mm (inner) diameter and about 3 cm in length.* These tubes are incubated at 37° and examined after 1 hour and after 2 hours, against a dark background and in front of a strong light. Positive results are judged by observing the presence of clumps and intervening clear fluid. The actual appearance of a row of such tubes is illustrated in Fig. 2.

Sera which show a positive result at such a dilution of 1:4 are studied again, in dilution series. The highest dilution that shows a positive result, expressed as the reciprocal of this dilution, is taken as the titer.

Control sera, both positive and negative, are always tested in parallel, not only for the usual technical reasons, but especially to evaluate the

---

* These tubes are most readily prepared from glass tubing, which is cut into 3-cm lengths. One end is sealed in a flame. To provide a test tube rack, it is convenient to obtain a block of styrofoam or similar plastic of comfortable dimensions for holding in the hand, such as 9 cm × 9 cm × 5 cm in height. In the top surface of such a block, a pattern of short holes can be drilled to accommodate these tubes.

particular semen samples used in the test. Thus, if several semen samples are being employed on a particular day, each of these is to be tested with the control sera, in addition to whatever test sera are involved. If either type of control serum gives an unexpected reactivity, all the tests with that semen sample must be disregarded.

ii. Application to Human Spermatozoa

This gelatin method has been used extensively by Rümke et al. for human clinical studies.[33-35] All the early work was done with human antigen, which means that only ejaculated spermatozoa were used. These studies were the first application of this method to the human clinical situation of unexplained infertility. A very conservative judgment was made as to whether a serum sample was positive or not: A titer of 1:32 or higher was required in order to have a positive result, since serum of normal individuals sometimes gave weak agglutination with titers between 1:4 and 1:16. A 1:4 dilution was the most concentrated serum that was routinely studied. It has been emphasized that one should be careful to use fresh gelatin solutions.[35, 36] The gelatin becomes less viscous after it is kept too long at room temperature, and the pH also decreases. In a system with a pH lower than 7, spermatozoa suffer a loss of motility.

The Kibrick method has been applied to human spermatozoa and human antibodies by many other workers, as reviewed elsewhere.[4, 6] Flocks et al.[37] used 10% agar in place of the 10% gelatin. The possibility that the ABO blood groups, if present as antigenic components on the sperm cells, might be reactive in Kibrick testing was ruled out by Fjällbrant,[38, 39] who showed that the ABO blood groups had no bearing on the agglutination results. Furthermore, absorption of the sera with blood group substances did not decrease the sperm antibody activity of the sera.

In Kibrick testing, the agglutinins seem to be specific for spermatozoa, since erythrocytes, leukocytes, and platelets did not react with the positive sera. To prove that the agglutination was indeed caused by an antibody, Rümke[33] tested eluates after paper electrophoresis of positive serum, and indeed only the γ-globulin fraction gave any appreciable agglutination with a semen sample.

[33] P. Rümke, Vox Sang. 4, 135 (1954).
[34] P. Rümke, Ann. N. Y. Acad. Sci. 124, 696 (1965).
[35] P. Rümke and G. Hellinga, Amer. J. Clin. Pathol. 32, 357 (1959).
[36] P. Rümke, Immunopathol., Int. Symp. 1st 1958, p. 145 (1959).
[37] R. H. Flocks, K. Bandhaur, C. Patel, and B. J. Begley, J. Urol. 87, 475 (1962).
[38] B. Fjällbrant, Acta Obstet. Gynecol. Scand. 47, 89 (1968).
[39] B. Fjällbrant, Acta Obstet. Gynecol. Scand. 48, 131 (1969).

iii. Application to Nonhuman Spermatozoa

The gelatin agglutination method has also been used in studies of non-human spermatozoa. In such work epididymal spermatozoa are often used, although not invariably. Otani and Behrman studied guinea pig epididymal spermatozoa vs guinea pig antibodies.[40] Readings had to be made rather early, since agglutination occurred in 10 to 20 minutes in normal guinea pig serum. Collecting the sperm suspension by flushing the epididymis requires more time and could tend toward spontaneous agglutination. A procedure of mincing the tissue and thus obtaining cells quickly might be preferable, as suggested in other studies with this same system where the mixture with normal serum always remained negative for at least 2 hours.[41] Guinea pig ejaculated spermatozoa gave results closely similar to those for the epididymal variety.

The Kibrick procedure has been applied to rat spermatozoa, using rat antibodies obtained as a consequence of vasectomy or vasoligation done in these animals.[42] Major changes in technique were found to be required, namely, omission of gelatin from the test mixture and incubation of the mixtures at 30° instead of the customary 37°. In this species, gelatin caused a loss of motility. With these alterations, the test worked well. Readings were taken after 1 and 2 hours and, in the case of the weaker antisera, also at 3 hours.

The Kibrick method has been applied to rabbits and to cattle; sperm antibodies could be detected conveniently.[43-45]

iv. Comments

Although the Kibrick procedure applies to human spermatozoa and particularly with human anti-sperm antibodies, the requirements for study of human sperm with heteroantibodies and for study of sperm cells of other species with heteroantibodies or induced autoantibodies might very well differ in certain aspects. A number of factors, particularly sperm count, motility, and the opportunity of separating the cells from the seminal plasma are of prime importance and must vary with the particular test pair.

The sperm count should be high if a semen sample (rather than epididymal sperm) is studied, permitting dilution of the seminal plasma and of whatever cellular debris may be present.

[40] Y. Otani and S. J. Behrman, *Fert. Steril.* **14**, 456 (1963).
[41] S. Shulman, A. Hekman, and C. Pann, *J. Reprod. Fert.* **27**, 31 (1971).
[42] P. Rümke and M. Titus, *J. Reprod. Fert.* **21**, 69 (1970).
[43] A. C. Menge, W. H. Stone, W. J. Tyler, and L. E. Casida, *J. Reprod. Fert.* **3**, 331 (1962).
[44] A. C. Menge, *Proc. Soc. Exp. Biol. Med.* **127**, 1271 (1968).
[45] A. C. Menge, *J. Reprod. Fert.*, Suppl. 10, 171 (1970).

Readings should be taken at 1 and 2 hours (for some others, such as rat sperm studies, 3 hours) after starting the incubation. However, if the negative control serum had indicated a positive result by the second hour, then the first-hour readings should be accepted. Furthermore, the early observations may be needed even if the 2-hour readings can be used, since strongly reactive mixtures may by then have all the clumped material on the bottom of the tubes and be more difficult to judge, although the clearer condition of the fluid should indicate the positive reaction.

c. SEMI-MICROSCALE: THE CAPILLARY METHOD

i. General Considerations

A procedure has been developed recently that is simpler than the Kibrick procedure and does succeed in making possible the use of immotile human sperm so long as heteroantibodies are used.[41, 46] Thus, it increases greatly the usability of accumulated semen donations, which is always a problem, especially with human sources. It involves the formation of visible agglutinates inside capillary tubing. The method has been found to work well with guinea pig spermatozoa also, with either rabbit heteroantibodies or guinea pig autoantibodies, although somewhat different conditions are needed for spermatozoa of this species.

Two major conditions seem to be effective in preventing nonspecific agglutination from occurring as fast as the specific reaction. One factor is the very narrow bore of the relatively tall capillary tube; this geometric factor may also make the specific reaction more sensitive by increasing the number of contacts and collisions during the longer falling time within such tubes, as compared to events in shorter and wider tubes. The second factor is the temperature of incubation, which is lower than in other agglutination procedures.

ii. Performance of the Capillary Method

For guinea pig sperm cells, the initial sperm cell concentration should be 10×10^6 cells per milliliter (final concentration, 5×10^6 cells per milliliter). For human spermatozoa, 40×10^6 cells per milliliter should be used (final concentration, 20×10^6 cells per milliliter). Motility and washing of the sperm are discussed below.

Two drops each (Pasteur pipette) of sperm suspension in Baker's buffer—no gelatin is needed—and inactivated antiserum are mixed in a small test tube, and this is taken up in a capillary tube of about 1 mm inner diameter. This is easily done by inserting the capillary tube and

[46] S. Shulman and A. Hekman, *Clin. Exp. Immunol.* **9,** 137 (1971).

tilting it and the container. Various dilutions of antiserum can be used, as well as normal serum for negative control mixtures.

Two kinds of capillary tubing have been used satisfactorily: (1) Kimax capillary melting point tubes (Kimble Products, Owens-Illinois, Toledo, Ohio), with a diameter of 1.6 to 1.8 mm (o.d.) and length of 100 mm; (2) Blu-tip capillary tubes (Sherwood Medical Industries, Inc., St. Louis, Missouri), with a diameter of 1.1 to 1.2 mm and length of 75 mm. The Blu-tip tubes are somewhat to be preferred, especially since they are shorter and thus easier to fill completely, eliminating any problem of trapping air bubbles.

The various capillaries are positioned on a putty plate, either after sealing each bottom end with a small bit of soft putty, or by placing the end carefully into the putty of the plate, taking pains to avoid any leakage. One can easily line up 9 or 10 tubes in each of two rows per plate. An experimental arrangement is illustrated in Fig. 3.

The plates are then incubated at an appropriate temperature and observed after 1 and 2 hours. For guinea pig spermatozoa, this temperature is 4°; for human spermatozoa, it is 23° to 25°.

Positive results are readily seen as a formation of clumps and intervening clear fluid inside these capillaries, whereas the negative systems retain a uniform turbid appearance. Nonspecific agglutination is considerably

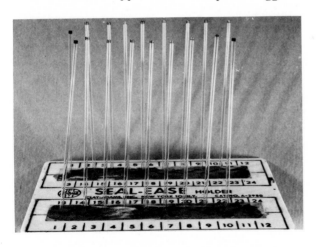
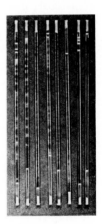

Fig. 3. Arrangement and results in the capillary test for spermagglutination. Left: Setup of the tubes containing antiserum–spermatozoa mixtures, as arranged on the putty plate (Seal-Ease Holder, Clay-Adams, New York, N.Y.). Right: Selected capillary tubes, after incubation. The two tubes on right contain normal serum. The other six tubes show a dilution series, from left to right, starting with a 1:4 dilution of the antiserum. From S. Shulman, A. Hekman, and C. Pann, *J. Reprod. Fert.* **27**, 31 (1971).

inhibited, whereas the anticipated agglutination by antiserum proceeds well.

iii. Comments

With this capillary method, immotile spermatozoa may give a better titer with heteroagglutinating (rabbit) or even autoagglutinating (guinea pig) antiserum than do motile spermatozoa. This fact removes many problems, since spermatozoa that are freshly available can be readily immobilized. It has been found, for example, that the addition to guinea pig spermatozoa of an equal volume of a solution of 1% sodium bicarbonate is effective. As another alternative, the sample may be refrigerated overnight, this procedure also yielding immotile spermatozoa. For human spermatozoa, centrifuging causes a decrease in motility, and upon washing, they generally become immotile. The capillary procedure can then be used with satisfactory results. The capillary method would therefore seem to have a greater potential versatility than do the other agglutination procedures.

Further studies with this method made with human spermatozoa[47] have shown much better activity with the use of well-washed spermatozoa, owing apparently to the removal of the large amounts of seminal plasma antigens, some of which may inhibit the reaction with spermatozoa. Such a consideration would not apply to the guinea pig epididymal sperm suspensions but would apply to ejaculates, since they include secretions from the accessory glands. Use of room temperature for incubation of human sperm and of 4° for guinea pig spermatozoa gave titration results with the capillary method which were quite comparable to Kibrick tests, although the capillary method employed heteroantibodies to human sperm. Efforts to use human antibodies to human spermatozoa in this method have so far been disappointing, but such procedures may still be developed for testing by the capillary method, thus allowing utilization of immotile sperm as a standard reagent.

d. MICROSCALE: MICROSCOPE OBSERVATION METHODS

i. General Considerations

In 1938, Henle et al.[48] used a "slide agglutination reaction." Mixtures were prepared from one drop each of sperm suspension and antiserum dilution placed on a slide, covered, and examined immediately under the microscope. Essentially similar procedures, described elsewhere,[4, 6] have

---

[47] S. Shulman and J. F. Shulman, *Fert. Steril.* **22**, 633 (1971).
[48] W. Henle, G. Henle, and L. A. Chambers, *J. Exp. Med.* **68**, 335 (1938).

been used for several sperm species. In some procedures, the mixtures were examined under the microscope after 15 or 30 minutes. Agglutination was predominantly by the tail or the middle piece. With a procedure using human spermatozoa, a semen count of 60×10^6 cells per milliliter[37] or 40×10^6 cell per milliliter[49] was the initial level, being mixed with equal volumes of antiserum dilutions. The mixtures were examined on slides upon incubation at room temperature after 5, 10, and 15 minutes. Agglutination was predominantly by the tail, although mixed agglutination was said to occur also. In a rather similar way, microscopic observation of human sera and spermatozoa had been utilized by several workers.[50, 51]

These studies opened the concept of human autoantibody in relationship to infertility. For example, three patients showed spontaneous sperm agglutination in their semen ejaculates, as seen under the microscope in wet films,[50, 51] including head-head, tail-tail, or mixed forms in early stages of the reaction, although tail agglutination predominated in the larger and later clumps. Agglutinating activity was found also in the serum and the seminal plasma of these men when these fluids were mixed with fresh normal donor semen. The agglutination was seen only in the presence of motile spermatozoa. These clumps could be completely dispersed by mechanical agitation, but the spermatozoa would subsequently reagglutinate, even though not quite to the original extent. This rather easy breakup is a recurring theme in a good deal of the literature on the agglutination of spermatozoa.* The speed of agglutination varied between 1 minute and 1 hour, depending upon titer, temperature, and quality of the sperm motility; yet clumps continued to grow so long as sperm motility was preserved. However, even after 24 hours, with use of a petroleum jelly-sealed cover glass, a few motile spermatozoa remained unclumped. The agglutinating activity withstood the inactivation of complement. The antibody could be removed by absorption, a procedure that unfortunately was not described. With sera that had been found positive with the test tube (Kibrick) method in other studies,[35, 36] wet films made with equal portions of inactivated serum and a sperm suspension showed agglutination in several forms: (1) head-to-head, (2) tail-to-tail, at the tip *or* end piece, (3) tail-to-tail, in the main part, (4) mixed, in which both head and tail types were seen. The tail type, especially with the

---

[49] K. Bandhauer, *Klin. Med.* (*Vienna*) **18**, 204 (1963).
[50] L. Wilson, *Proc. Soc. Exp. Biol. Med.* **85**, 652 (1954).
[51] L. Wilson, *Fert. Steril.* **7**, 262 (1956).
* The situation recalls the necessity of reading "pattern" agglutination, without disturbing agglutinated sediments, in testing for Rh-positive cells and for passive (indirect) hemagglutination with various antisera (Section 16.B.2.c).—Eds.

main part of the tail involved, was the one most frequently seen, a fact that is important for comparison with all later observations of the type of microscopic clumping seen in infertility studies. Figure 4 shows these aspects of cellular attachment, as they were first shown in those studies.

Figure 5 shows other examples of agglutination, as seen by phase contrast microscopy, under conditions similar to those of a Kibrick test, but without use of gelatin. These two forms, head-to-head and end piece-to-end piece, are thought to be not the most common types in the reactions of infertility sera.[52] Nonetheless, such agglutination patterns are illustrative and may bear especially on possible observations in other species.

A variant of the microscope procedure, utilizing a hanging-drop technique, has been used.[53] Semen was adjusted to a concentration of about 20×10^6 per milliliter, and one drop of this was mixed with one drop of serum in various dilutions. Hanging-drop preparations were sealed and incubated at 37° for 0.5 hour. (The use of a hanging drop, rather than a cover-slip wet film, is rather unusual among the various microscope procedures that have been proposed.) A serum sample was considered to be positive only if the titer was 1:80 or more. This seems to be a very severe criterion. The behavior of normal serum samples, however, was not discussed adequately.

A totally different approach was introduced by Franklin and Dukes,[54, 55] then adopted by Schwimmer et al.,[56] for study of antibodies in women's serum. In this test, which we now term the F-D method, suspension mixtures in tubes are examined periodically by making slide preparations at various times between 0.5 and 4 hours.

Very recently, another microscopic method has been developed by Friberg.[57] This procedure will not be described here in detail, since it has not been compared with the customary procedures, but it will deserve much interest in the future. This method is done in disposable microchambers of the sort that are used in tissue typing studies. The samples of semen and serum are mixed in microliter quantities, in circled areas on the plate. In this technique, as many as 200 to 300 sera may be tested simultaneously, using a single semen sample. A positive result is judged by a single examination under an inverted microscope. The type of agglutination can also be observed, and two main types were noted, namely, head-to-tail (H-T) and head-to-head (H-H).

[52] P. Rümke, personal communication, 1972.
[53] A. M. Phadke and K. Padukone, *J. Reprod. Fert.* **7**, 163 (1964).
[54] R. R. Franklin and C. D. Dukes, *Amer. J. Obstet. Gynecol.* **89**, 6 (1964).
[55] R. R. Franklin and C. D. Dukes, *J. Amer. Med. Ass.* **190**, 682 (1964).
[56] W. B. Schwimmer, K. A. Ustay, and S. J. Behrman, *Fert. Steril.* **18**, 167 (1967).
[57] J. Friberg, *Acta Obstet. Gynecol. Scand.*, Suppl. 36, 21 (1974).

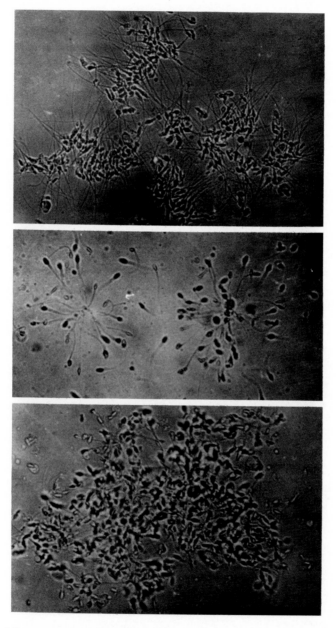

Fig. 4. Microscope view of agglutination of human spermatozoa, after mixing with sera from different men. *Top:* Head-to-head agglutination. *Middle:* Tail-to-tail agglutination by tip of the tail. *Bottom:* Tail-to-tail agglutination through the main part of the tail. From P. Rümke, *Immunopathol., Int. Symp. 1st, 1958,* p. 145 (1959).

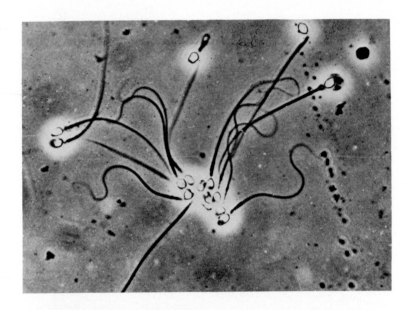

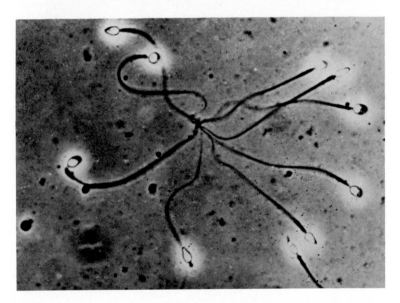

FIG. 5. Phase contrast view of agglutination of human spermatozoa, after mixing with sera from different men. *Top:* Head-to-head agglutination. *Bottom:* Tail tip-to-tail tip agglutination. From P. Rümke, personal communication (1972).

ii. Performance of the F-D (Franklin–Dukes) Method*

The fresh human ejaculate is adjusted to 50×10^6 cells per milliliter, and 0.05 ml of semen is then mixed with 0.5 ml of the serum sample, thus giving a rather high (1:11) dilution of the sperm cell suspension, or only 4.5×10^5 cells per milliliter. Mixtures are incubated at 37° for 4 hours, by the original description. At the end of 0.5, 1, 2, and 4 hours of incubation, a drop is taken from each tube and placed on a microscope slide for observation.† Figure 6 shows a typical picture.

iii. Comments

Franklin and Dukes in 1964 reported a remarkably high incidence of spermagglutinating activity in females with unexplained sterility.[54, 55] They reported at first an incidence of positive results in about 80% of such women,[54] yet this remarkably high figure has not been confirmed. Schwimmer et al., using the same technique, reported an incidence of approximately 40% positive in their group of women.[56] This is still a high number, especially so since 20% of women in their control groups were found to be positive. More recent reports suggest an incidence on the order of 10 to 30%. In all these reports, the original Franklin–Dukes method was used routinely. There is reasonable doubt concerning the degree of specificity of agglutination in this method.

In view of the lack of study given to development of the technique and to proper dilutions of serum, this method is not presently recommended for research purposes. The method is in widespread vogue for clinical application, but even here a carefully modified procedure (such as that described above) should be followed.

6. COMPARISONS OF THE RESULTS FROM THE VARIOUS AGGLUTINATION METHODS

It has been stated that the Kibrick test is based on the activity of immunoglobulins IgG or IgM, whereas in serum samples from several

---

* This procedure has been applied exclusively to the study of human sperm cells and human antibody.

† In our own modification of this F-D method, we routinely use a 1:4 dilution of the serum, rather than the undiluted serum, and generally read at only two times intervals, usually at about 1 and 2, or 2 and 3, hours. The sperm cells are counted in each of 12 high-power fields, counting only the motile cells, and noting, for each field, the number of free cells, the number of cells in clumps, the number of clumps, and the manner of clumping—whether head-to-head, tail-to-tail, or in some other fashion. The total number of clumped cells, divided by the total number of all motile cells, gives a percentage figure, which serves as an index of the degree of reaction. A minimum agglutination of 10% is required for a positive result.

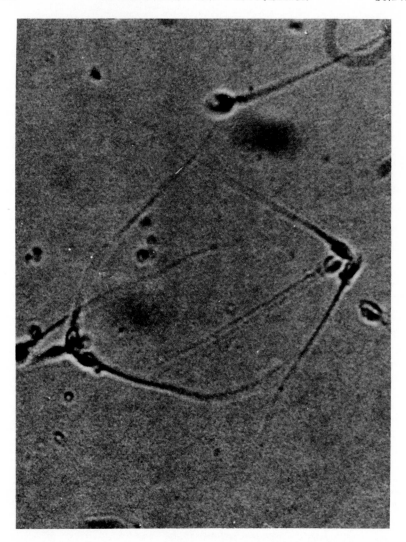

Fig. 6. Microscope view of human sperm cells showing agglutination (head-to-head) in consequence of action of human (male) serum containing spermagglutinating autoantibody. ×800, approx. From S. Shulman, *Clin. Exp. Immunol.* **9,** 267 (1971).

women, positive only in F-D, activity was claimed to be based on nonimmunoglobulin.[58] In comparing the results from these two methods, we note that the F-D method was at first applied only to human females

---

[58] B. Boettcher, D. J. Kay, P. Rümke, and L. E. Wright, *Biol. Reprod.* **5,** 236 (1971).

and the K-B-M method only to human males—and to various experimental animals. In addition, different laboratories have seemed to choose only one method or the other. The two methods were recently compared directly, in an investigation of human infertility, making parallel studies on a number of human sera.[47] Of 24 pairs of husband–wife serum specimens, there was agreement in 12 between the 2 methods, although in one case the determination is by titer, and in the other the decision is by a percentage (*or* index) of motile sperm agglutinated. In 4 cases of disagreement, the Kibrick test was negative, while the F-D test was positive. Evidently, values must be selected for the minimum level of activity which is to be considered positive in each test.[57] It was proposed that a minimal dilution of 1:4 be used in the K-B-M method[47] and minimal agglutination of 10% in the F-D method.[59-61] It is quite important to note that, in general, both of these test methods can be performed with the use of either a husband-semen or a donor-semen, and the same result will be observed.[60] Recent compilations of the incidence of positive findings with these two methods, as applied to a large group (about 150) of infertile couples, indicated an incidence of 23% for women and 10% for men, by the Kibrick method, and 16% for women and 5% for men, by the F-D method.[61, 62] While these values will probably be revised somewhat when larger populations have been studied, the present figures may be valid indications of the actual distributions, and they also emphasize that these two methods do measure different sorts of sperm-agglutinating activity. Many additional details of these methods, as well as related methods and concepts, have been published elsewhere.[63]

[59] S. Shulman, J. F. Shulman, and E. Lewin, *in* "Second International Symposium on Immunology of Reproduction, Varna, Bulgaria, 1971" (K. Bratanov, ed.), p. 325. Bulgarian Acad. Sci. Press, Sofia, 1973.

[60] S. Shulman, *Amer. J. Obstet. Gynecol.* 117, 233 (1973).

[61] S. Shulman, *in* "1st International Congress on Immunology in Obstetrics and Gynaecology" (A. Centaro, N. Carretti, and G. M. Addison, eds.). p. 41. Excerpta Med. Found., Amsterdam, 1974.

[62] S. Shulman, H. Jackson, and M. L. Stone, *Amer. J. Obstet. Gynecol.* 123, 139 (1975).

[63] S. Shulman, "Reproduction and Antibody Responses." Chem. Rubber Co. Press, Cleveland, Ohio 1975.

G. Agglutination with Antigen on Inert Particles

1. LATEX FIXATION TECHNIQUES*

The latex carrier, by adsorbing the antigen, presents it as a particulate agglutinogen and serves to indicate interaction between antigen and dilute

* Section 16.G.1 was contributed by Stephen D. Litwin.

antibody. The method has proved particularly useful in a variety of anti-gen–antibody systems.

In 1956 Singer and Plotz[1] demonstrated that human γ-globulin coated on polystyrene latex particles provided a sensitive method for the detection of rheumatoid factors (RF) in human serum. The latex fixation technique has since become increasingly popular as a serological method.

In general, it may be stated that if the same method is used on each performance of the test, latex fixation techniques have proved to be reproducible and the results reasonably comparable from one test to another. When the basic mechanics of agglutination are considered and the limitations of the system understood, latex fixation offers a flexible and sensitive tool for both experimental and routine studies.

a. PROPERTIES OF POLYSTYRENE LATEX PARTICLES

The spherical latex particle is a polymer of styrene. The latex particle in aqueous solution behaves like a lyophobic colloid with a negative surface charge, forming a suspension which is colloidal, relatively stable, chemically inert, and easily stored. These particles are closely uniform in size and have served in the past as standards of size in electron microscopy. The serological usefulness of this particle is directly due to the ease with which many proteins and other materials may be adsorbed to its surface. Although particles 0.1 to 1.2 μm in diameter have been shown to be effective particulate carriers,[1-3] the routine latex fixation test employs latex particles of 0.81 μm diameter.*

b. STANDARDIZATION OF LATEX PARTICLES

The concentrated latex suspension, approximately 27% by weight, must be diluted and standardized to serve as a *stock suspension*. As described originally, the semisolid latex is diluted in distilled water to the point where 0.1 ml mixed with 9.9 ml of water will match the light transmission of a standard barium sulfate solution when examined in a spectrophotometer at 650 nm. (The suspension then contains ca. 4.5×10^8 latex particles per milliliter.[3]) The standard barium sulfate solution is made by adding 3 ml of 0.1 N barium chloride to 3 ml of a $\frac{2}{3}$ N sulfuric

---

[1] J. M. Singer and C. M. Plotz, *Amer. J. Med.* **21,** 888 (1956).

[2] J. M. Singer and C. M. Plotz, *Arthritis Rheum.* **1,** 142 (1958).

[3] J. M. Singer, G. Altmann, A. Goldenberg, and C. M. Plotz, *Arthritis Rheum.* **3,** 515 (1960).

* Latex particles are available commercially from the Dow Chemical Co. or Monsanto Chemical Company (Lytron). A diluted, standardized suspension termed Bacto-latex is available from Difco Laboratories, Detroit, Michigan.

acid solution and heating at 56° for 1 minute.* Alternatively, commercially prepared standard latex suspension can simply be diluted according to the manufacturer's instructions. The standardized latex stock suspension can be stored for several months at 4° until used.

c. COATING OF THE LATEX PARTICLES

The following principles are applicable: polystyrene latex particles are unstable from pH 5 to pH 8. Glycine buffer pH 8.2 is quite suitable.† Borate buffer at pH 8.2 has been used effectively also.[1] The colloidal suspension is stabilized further by serum proteins of the test sera.[4] At high dilutions of serum, for example, the test may appear to be weakly positive; this nonspecific effect can be distinguished as such in two ways: (a) The higher concentrations of the test sera give no agglutination, but mildly positive reactions are found with the most diluted samples; (b) the extent of flocculation is less than a true one-plus reaction. When materials other than serum are being tested, these characteristics of the latex suspension must be kept in mind. Suitable controls are always necessary.

Different substances adsorb to latex particles in quite different degrees. The optimal quantity of reactant which gives the highest end-point titer yet does not lead to nonspecific reactivity must be determined experimentally for each system. Studies with radioactive tracers indicate that human serum albumin, for example, is adsorbed approximately half as well by weight as γ-globulin.[5] The amount of adsorbed material influences the stability of the system as mentioned.

d. LATEX FIXATION TEST FOR ANTI-γ-GLOBULINS

i. Sensitization of the Latex Particles with γ-Globulin

The use of latex for detecting rheumatoid factors (RF) in human serum was first demonstrated in 1956.[1] The latex is prepared as *working latex*

---

* The standard for determining opacity is akin to the McFarland barium sulfate standards (Section 16.D.1.c), for determining bacterial density.

† Glycine buffer, pH 8.2 with 0.15 M NaCl is prepared by diluting 97.5 ml of 1.0 M glycine (75.07 gm/liter) and 2.5 ml of 1 N NaOH to a liter with distilled water and adjusting the pH to 8.2. Ten grams of sodium chloride is added to each liter of buffer. At this pH, glycine has only meager capacity to resist acid shift (Vol. II, Appendix II, buffer 26).

[4] J. M. Singer, G. Altmann, I. Oreskes, and C. M. Plotz, *Amer. J. Med.* **30**, 772 (1961).

[5] C. J. van Oss and J. M. Singer, *J. Reticuloendothel. Soc.* **3**, 29 (1966).

suspension by mixing in the proportions 0.5 ml of 1% solution of human γ-globulin (Cohn's fraction II) in glycine buffer of pH 8.2 (described in footnote to subsection c above), 0.1 ml of the stock latex suspension, and 9.4 ml of glycine buffer. The mixture is swirled vigorously for several minutes at room temperature.[3] The protein concentration in the standard test is about 80 μg of protein N per milliliter. When the concentration of γ-globulin used to sensitize the latex is less than 1 μg of protein N per milliliter, the particles are unstable. Again, when the concentration is much greater than 100 μg of protein N per milliliter,[3] agglutination titers are decreased.

Evidence indicates that the proteins undergo alterations in adsorbing to the surface of the latex particles. Such changes induced in the reactant γ-globulin are believed to be responsible for the fact that excess free γ-globulin in solution cannot block the agglutination of sensitized latex particles by rheumatoid factors. Studies on the dynamics of the adsorption of γ-globulin to latex particles has helped to clarify several aspects of latex γ-globulin interaction.[6]

Although commercial preparations of human FII γ-globulin vary in the amount of aggregated material present, any reliable source of human FII is probably suitable. Under the conditions of this test, the end-point titers of sixteen commercial preparations were the same with a panel of high-titer rheumatoid sera.[3]

A suspension of sensitized latex particles will be stable for several hours after its preparation. A moderate degree of "settling" of the suspension can be easily reversed by simple swirling. A modified serological procedure has been reported in which the particles are washed free of excess protein after sensitization. Such modified particles may be stable up to one year.[7] (Washing, however, is said to render thyroglobulin–latex complexes ineffectual for agglutination.[*])

ii. Agglutination of γ-Globulin-Coated Latex Particles

Sera to be tested are diluted appropriately, and 0.5-ml volumes are placed in clear, round-bottom test tubes, e.g., 12 × 75 mm. It is not usually regarded as necessary to decomplement the sera prior to testing, yet

[6] S. Kochwa, M. Brownell, R. E. Rosenfield, and L. R. Wasserman, *J. Immunol.* **99,** 981 (1967).

[7] J. M. Singer, C. M. Plotz, and R. Goldberg, *Arthritis Rheum.* **8,** 194 (1965).

[*] See H. C. Goodman and J. Bozicevich *in* "Immunological Methods" (J. F. Ackroyd ed.), p. 107. Blackwell, Oxford, 1964.

heating can be advantageous in destroying factors of complement which can play an inhibitory role.[8] To these tubes are added 0.5-ml portions of the *working latex suspension* coated with γ-globulin. As controls, a similar set of serum dilutions receives 0.5-ml portions of a suspension of nonsensitized latex particles, and one tube is made with latex particles in buffer. The tubes are shaken and incubated at 56° for 90 minutes and at 4° overnight. The next day the tubes are centrifuged at 2300 rpm for 3 minutes and read with the naked eye. A bright artificial light source placed to one side of the observer provides excellent illumination. Each tube is read individually, by slowly tapping it until the button of packed latex particles is dislodged. A negative reaction is recognized by a smoothly rising, curling swirl of fine particles resembling smoke, and solitary agglutinates are absent. A positive reaction is marked by visible agglutinates observed upon tapping, in the absence of the "smoke puff." Agglutination is graded from one-plus to four-plus depending on the size and number of agglutinates present. Care must be exercised, for overly vigorous shaking can disperse even large agglutinates of latex particles.

In the performance of the FII latex particle test, some sera have exhibited prozones when relatively concentrated. If the first serum dilution is 1:20, prozones will generally not be encountered.

The rapidity with which serum proteins fix to latex particles leads to adsorption of proteins from the test sera during the course of the reaction, by partially coated or even maximally coated latex particles. Some workers believe that this property is responsible for the high incidence of positive reactions observed when sera are tested with uncoated latex particles. It is hypothesized that the patient's own serum γ-globulin adsorbs on the uncoated particle and serves as the "antigen" with respect to his own rheumatoid factors.[9] Serum complement is also involved in giving prozone effects.[8] Singer has demonstrated that a patient's γ-globulin may serve as a sensitizing agent for latex particles.[10] Accordingly, it is important to include uncoated latex particles as a control in any test system in which latex particles are in contact with proteins other than known reactants and wherever there is some uncertainty as to what the specific reactant is.

Radioactive labeling has permitted partial quantitation of the reaction between adsorbed γ-globulin and rheumatoid factors. It is estimated that sensitized latex particles carry adsorbed to their surfaces several thousand protein molecules, constituting complexes which may be completely ag-

[8] K. L. Brine, R. J. Wedgwood, and W. S. Clark, *Arthritis Rheum.* **1**, 230 (1958).
[9] G. M. Edelman, H. G. Kunkel, and E. C. Franklin, *J. Exp. Med.* **108**, 105 (1959).
[10] J. M. Singer, *Amer. J. Med.* **31**, 766 (1961).

glutinated by as few as 7 to 8 molecules of rheumatoid factor fixed per particle.

e. Latex Fixation of Antigens Other Than γ-Globulin

Further applications of direct latex agglutination include tests for histoplasmosis,[11] trichinosis,[12] hydatid disease,[13] C-reactive protein,[14] antinuclear factors (particularly in disseminated lupus erythematosus[15–17]), thyroglobulin antibody,[18] autoantibody to human kidney,[19] and human growth hormone.[20] The test for serum antibody to thyroglobulin was converted into a capillary tube test in which the volume of agglutinated latex was measured.[18]

The techniques discussed above are *passive* agglutination reactions in which antigen-coated latex particles are used to test for antibody activity. Other adaptations of the methodology have been described.

Inhibition testing for excess soluble antigen can be performed with antigen-coated latex–antibody systems (Sections 16.B.2.c.ii and 16.B.5.c.) It is possible to test for pregnancy by detecting human chorionic gonadotropin (HCG) in urine. This test, available commercially,* employs prestandardized latex particles coated with HCG and specific anti-HCG antisera. Sufficiently high concentrations of HCG in urine will inhibit the antigen-antibody system: for testing, undiluted urine, cooled and filtered cold, is used. The HCG inhibition test can also be done with HCG-coated formalized tanned cells (Section 16.B.2.c.ii).

[11] H. N. Carlisle and S. Laslow, *J. Lab. Clin. Med.* **51,** 793 (1958).
[12] F. Innella and W. J. Redner, *J. Amer. Med. Ass.* **171,** 885 (1959).
[13] A. Fischman, *J. Clin. Pathol.* **13,** 72 (1960).
[14] J. M. Singer, C. M. Plotz, E. Pader, and S. K. Elster, *Amer. J. Clin. Pathol.* **28,** 611 (1957).
[15] C. L. Christian, R. M. Mendez-Bryan, and D. L. Larson, *Proc. Soc. Exptl. Biol. Med.* **98,** 820 (1958).
[16] P. Miescher and R. Strassle, *Immunopathol., Int. Symp., 1st, 1958,* p. 454 (1959).
[17] W. J. Fessel, *Ann. Rheum. Dis.* **18,** 255 (1959).
[18] J. R. Philp, D. M. Weir, A. E. Stuart, and W. J. Irvine, *J. Clin. Pathol.* **15,** 148 (1962).
[19] N. C. Kramer, M. F. Watt, J. H. Howe, and A. E. Parrish, *Amer. J. Med.* **30,** 39 (1961).
[20] D. K. Keele and J. Webster, *Proc. Soc. Exp. Biol. Med.* **106,** 168 (1961).
* Such a product is Ortho Research Foundation's "Gravindex," used chiefly as a slide inhibition test.

2. THE BENTONITE FLOCCULATION TEST*

Bentonite belongs to the group of argils (potters' clay) and kaolins. It is a distinctive type of aluminum silicate clay found near Fort Benton, Wyoming.

* Section 16.G.2 was contributed by J. Bozicevich.

Sodium bentonite (Wyoming or Western bentonite) is a clay from which uniform particles measuring 0.3 to 0.5 μm can be separated by differential centrifugation. When the bentonite sheets are placed in water, they separate and expand to 15 times in volume, and the sodium ion is the predominant exchangeable ion. It has been calculated that 1 gm of sodium bentonite has a specific surface area of 250 to 500 square meters. (The calcium type, "Southern bentonite," does not expand in water to the extent of the sodium type.) The net balance electrical charge is negative, and the particles of sodium bentonite, when placed in water, are repelled from one another, and so remain in suspension. Bentonite provides an ideal inert substance on which to adsorb antigens[1-4] or antibodies[5] for serological and immunological methods. It has also been used for adsorbing proteins[6] and for immunization as a protein-carrier complex (Vol. I, Chap. 2.A.2.e). The bentonite flocculation test has been used successfully with *Trichina spiralis* antigens,[1] with *Echinococcus* cyst fluid antigens,[1] with DNA to study antibodies in lupus erythematosus,[7] and with thyroglobulin,[8, 9] also, the test using bentonite coated with human globulins (Cohn fraction II), has served to detect rheumatoid factor.[2,10]

a. PREPARATION OF STOCK BENTONITE SUSPENSION

In glassware washed free of detergents by three final rinses with distilled water, suspend 0.5 gm of Wyoming bentonite* in 100 ml of distilled water, and let run in a Waring Blendor for 1 minute; repeat for 1 minute after waiting for 5 minutes. Transfer to a glass-stoppered 500-ml cylinder

[1] J. Bozicevich, J. E. Tobie, E. H. Thomas, H. M. Hoyem, and S. B. Ward, *Pub. Health Rep.* **66**, 806 (1951).
[2] J. Bozicevich, J. Bunim, J. Freund, and S. B. Ward, *Proc. Soc. Exptl. Biol. Med.* **97**, 180 (1958).
[3] J. Bozicevich, J. P. Nasou, and D. C. Kayhoe, *Proc. Soc. Exp. Biol. Med.* **103**, 636 (1960).
[4] S. M. Wolff, S. B. Ward, and M. Landy, *Proc. Soc. Exp. Biol. Med.* **114**, 530 (1963).
[5] J. Bozicevich, H. A. Scott, and M. M. Vincent, *Proc. Soc. Exp. Biol. Med.* **114**, 794 (1963).
[6] N. Oker-Blom and E. Nikkilö, *Ann. Med. Exp. Biol. Fenn.* **33**, 190 (1955).
[7] I. G. Kagan, L. Norman, D. S. Allain, and C. G. Goodchild, *J. Immunol.* **84**, 635 (1960).
[8] J. A. M. Ager, M. S. R. Hutt, and G. Smith, *Nature (London)* **184**, 478 (1959).
[9] P. R. B. McMaster, E. M. Lerner, and E. D. Exum, *J. Exp. Med.* **113**, 611 (1961).
[10] K. J. Bloch and J. J. Bunim, *J. Amer. Med. Ass.* **169**, 307 (1959).
* American Colloid Company, 5100 Suffield Court, Skokie, Illinois. Purchase one-half pound amounts of BC micron or No. 200 standard Volclay. Note that Difco Laboratories, Detroit, Michigan, offers Bacto-Bentonite graded as described to reconstitute to 10 ml of suspension (item 3109-59) or units of 6 vials (item 3109-60).

and bring to 500 ml with distilled water. Shake thoroughly and let settle for 1 hour. Decant the *supernatant* into six 100-ml Pyrex centrifuge tubes (heavy duty), and centrifuge for 15 minutes at 500 g.* (Discard the 500 g sediment.) From the supernatant, recover the particle size that sediments on further centrifugation for 15 minutes at 750 g. Discard the supernatant. Suspend entire sediments in 100 ml of distilled water, and let run in the Waring Blendor for 1 minute. This stock bentonite suspension, if preserved with 1% by volume of 5% thymol in ethyl or isopropyl alcohols and held at 5°, will remain stable for at least 6 months without losing its absorptive properties.

b. Preparation of Substances for Adsorption

i. Buffers for Adsorption

Most proteins (either antigen or antibody) are adsorbed optimally between pH 7.2 and 7.5. Our usual buffered saline (PBS) is 0.025 M phosphate, pH 7.5, containing per liter 8 gm of NaCl, 0.5 gm of NaH_2PO_4 (anhydrous), and 3 gm of Na_2HPO_4 (exsiccated). Some proteins require a more alkaline pH in order to keep the adsorption complex from flocculating spontaneously. Fraction II (γ-globulin), for example, is adsorbed usefully at pH 8.6 for this reason.†

ii. Protein Concentration for Adsorption

The amount of protein material that is adsorbed completely by one unit of bentonite described below (particles from 5 ml of stock suspension concentrated to 1 ml) varies from 0.5 to 1 mg per milliliter in an appropriate buffer. Only 15 μg of highly polymerized deoxyribonucleic acid (DNA) will be adsorbed, and other substances, also, fall in this range.‡

c. Preparation of Antigen-Sensitized Bentonite Particles

Step 1. Shake the stock bentonite suspension thoroughly to distribute the bentonite particles evenly. Transfer 10 ml of the uniformly dispersed suspension to a 15 × 200 mm test tube. Centrifuge at 750 g for 5 minutes and decant the supernatant.

---

* H. N. Claman, using the No. 240 head International centrifuge, size 2, uses 1300 rpm for the first centrifugation in which heavy particles are discarded and 1600 rpm for the final centrifugation in which the desired particle size is sedimented (Vol. I, Chap. 2.A.2.e.i). Claman keeps the stock solution in 0.15 M NaCl at an optical density of 0.7 at 655 nm (Coleman colorimeter with 8-215 filter).

† Use 0.06 M ($\Gamma/2 = 0.054$) barbital buffer, pH 8.6, consisting of 1.84 gm of barbital and 10.3 gm of barbital sodium per liter.

‡ The adsorption of protein to bentonite is discussed also in Vol. I, Chap. 2.A.2.e.ii.

Step 2. Resuspend the bentonite particles in 1 ml of distilled water by agitating the tube.

Step 3. Add 1 ml of the desired antigen or antibody to be absorbed onto the bentonite and mix gently by inverting the tube several times. Allow the suspension to stand 1 hour at room temperature to permit adsorption. (Some materials require longer adsorption periods, even overnight.) Add 15 ml of buffer and mix gently again.

Step 4. Add to this suspension 1 ml of 0.1% aqueous methylene blue dye, shake. (While methylene blue has been used extensively, other dyes may be employed—such as 0.25 ml of 0.1% thionin—if one has color preference or the blue color interferes in reading the test.) After dye has been taken up, dilute with 10 ml of water and proceed.

Step 5. Centrifuge for 5 minutes at 750 *g*. Decant the supernatant. Resuspend the sediment first with 5 ml of buffer, shaking thoroughly, then add another 10 ml of buffer and shake.

Step 6. Repeat step 5. Decant the final supernatant.

Step 7. Resuspend the sediment in 10 ml of buffer, and centrifuge as in step 5. Decant the supernatant.

Step 8. Add 5 ml of buffer to the sediment, than add 0.1 ml of a 1% solution of a surface active agent. One of the following may be employed, the choice depending to some extent on the substance which was used to sensitize the bentonite particles. (a) Tween 80 (polyoxyethylene sorbitan monooleate*; (b) crystalline bovine albumin†; (c) polyvinylpyrrolidone (PVP) Grade K-30.‡

Step 9. To assure optimal stability of the sensitized particles, add one of the following preservatives for each 5 ml of completed bentonite suspension, either 0.1 ml of a 3% solution of Merthiolate or 0.1 ml of a 5% solution of thymol in either isopropyl alcohol or ethyl alcohol.

d. PERFORMANCE OF THE TEST FOR DETECTION OF ANTIBODIES

Serum to be tested should be heat-inactivated for 30 minutes at 56°. Microscope slides (3 × 2 inches) with 12 rings, designed for serological flocculation tests, are used.§ Prepare a series of 2-fold dilutions of serum

---

* Atlas Powder Co., Wilmington, Delaware. Sold also as Difco's Bacto-Tween 80, item 3118-15. This detergent is recommended for globulin-coated bentonite by H. C. Goodman and J. Bozicevich, *in* "Immunological Methods" (J. F. Ackroyd, ed.), pp. 93–109. Blackwell, Oxford, 1964.

† Armour Labs., Chicago, Illinois.

‡ General Aniline Film Corp.

§ Glass test slides with 13 mm × 2 mm wells, provided with outer moats, are available as Thomas-Boerner Micro Test Slides (A. H. Thomas Co., Philadelphia).

in saline. Within each ring, place 0.1 ml of one of the serum dilutions, and add one drop of sensitized bentonite suspension thoroughly shaken, from a Pasteur-type capillary pipette. The drop is of such size that the capillary pipette should dispense about 40 drops per milliliter. The slide is then placed on a horizontal plate arranged to provide a circular rotatory motion over 0.75 inch in diameter* and rotated 100 to 120 times per minute for 20 minutes and read immediately—to avoid drying—at low power magnification ($\times 60$).

The reaction is graded 4-plus when all the bentonite particles are clumped in separate masses, either as a few large clumps or a number of small clumps, depending upon the titer of the serum. In both cases, the areas between the masses are essentially devoid of bentonite. A reaction is graded 3-plus when approximately three-fourths of the sensitized particles have clumped. In a 2-plus reaction, half of the particles are clumped and half are still in colloidal suspension. When only one-fourth of the bentonite particles are clumped, the reaction is scored as 1-plus. When all the sensitized bentonite particles are in colloidal suspension, the reaction is negative. Note that a negative serum usually causes no clumping in dilutions up to about 1:1000, but occasionally dilutions $\geq 1:1000$ can cause a 1- or 2-plus flocculation. False clumping can be avoided by the presence of protective colloid. For example, addition of 1 mg of polyvinylpyrrolidone (PVP) to 5 ml of sensitized particles after two washes with distilled water may inhibit nonspecific agglutination. If diluted serum (e.g., 1:1000) is used as protective colloid, the sensitivity of the test is reduced.

In each test, controls are run with a known positive and a known negative serum, diluted serially. When the test is positive, the particles are flocculated yet distributed evenly in the microscopic field, without "hyaline-like" material or other debris. If the sensitized bentonite preparation contains debris, nonspecific clumping may occur and give a false-positive reaction, readily seen with the negative control serum. As one gains experience, spurious aggregates can be distinguished readily from true flocculation.

Note that inhibition tests can be performed by adding inhibitor to the wells before adding the drop of sensitized bentonite particles.

e. Preparation of Antibody-Sensitized Bentonite Particles

A γ-globulin fraction is prepared from a high-titered antiserum in any of the usual ways—DEAE-cellulose chromatography, block electrophore-

---

* Several horizontal rotators (as Fisher, Eberbach) are available, introduced for venereal flocculation tests. A 9-place slide carrier for 3 $\times$ 2 inch slides, a useful accessory, is available for the Eberbach rotator.

sis, neutral salt precipitation, and so on. A 1% solution of the globulin is made in the barbital pH 8.6 buffer described in Section 16.F.2.b.i if a trial test shows clumping of the bentonite when pH 7.5 PBS is used. The bentonite particles are coated as in Section 16.F.2.c, and the test is conducted as described for antigen-coated particles, but now antigen dilutions are employed instead. When the test is performed with an excess of antigen, a prozone effect may occur. It is essential to use serial dilutions of antigen to get beyond the prozone effect.

CHAPTER 17

Complement*

A. Introduction†

1. THE CLASSICAL PATHWAY OF COMPLEMENT UTILIZATION

The term complement was given, historically, to ostensibly heat-labile factor(s) of normal serum which were necessary to allow hemolysis of sheep erythrocytes by heated (56°) anti-erythrocyte serum. Surveys of the history of development are given by Rapp and Borsos (1970)[1] and Mayer (1970).[2] Other extensive accounts of research on the complement system are available.[3-6]

Studies over many years, both with guinea pig and human complement, have shown that "complement" consists of more than 12 plasma proteins, which become activated in a sequential "cascade"; only a few of these are heat labile, but their deletion by heat interferes with the sequence of reaction steps. During the "cascade" (Fig. 1A), enzymes are generated (Table I; Figs. 1A,1B) that cleave precursors into products required for the next step in the chain, leading to sequential binding of the complement proteins to the surface of the cell under attack. In addition, soluble by-products arise during cleavage; some of these are biologically active, producing inflammation and promoting coagulation.

The enzymes are present in plasma in precursor form; they require

---

* The editors express their gratitude to the contributors of the various sections of Chapter 17 for permission to exercise wide editorial judgment in the arrangement of contributions within the chapter.

† Sections 17.A1–3 were contributed by Hans J. Müller-Eberhard, Louis G. Hoffmann, Manfred M. Mayer, and the Editors.

[1] H. J. Rapp and T. Borsos, "Molecular Basis of Complement Action." Appleton-Century-Crofts (Meredith), New York, 1970.

[2] M. M. Mayer, *Immunochemistry* **7**, 485 (1970).

[3] D. R. Schultz, "The Complement System," *Monogr. Allergy* **6** (1971).

[4] H. J. Müller-Eberhard, *Advan. Immunol.* **8**, 2 (1967).

[5] H. J. Müller-Eberhard, *in* "Progress in Immunology" (B. Amos, ed.), pp. 553–565. Academic Press, New York, 1971.

[6] R. A. Nelson, Jr., *in* "The Inflammatory Process" (B. W. Zweifach, L. Grant, and R. T. McCluskey, eds.), Chapter 25. Academic Press, New York, 1965.

TABLE I
NOMENCLATURE OF COMPLEMENT

1968 WHO system[a]		
Recognized constituents	Trivial names	1966 La Jolla system[b]
Components		
C1 (C1q, C1r, C1s)[c]		C'1
2		C'2
3		C'3
4		C'4
5		C'5
6		C'6
7		C'7
8		C'8
9		C'9
Intermediates		
EAC1		EAC'1a
EAC1,4		EAC'1a,4
EAC1,4,2	EAC 1-2	EAC'1a,4,2a
EAC1,4,2,3	EAC 1-3	EAC'1a,4,2a,3
EAC1,4,2,3,5	EAC 1-5	EAC'1a,4,2a,3,5
EAC1,4,2,3,5,6	EAC 1-6	EAC'1a,4,2a,3,5,6
EAC1,4,2,3,5,6,7	EAC 1-7	EAC'1a,4,2a,3,5,6,7
EAC1,4,2,3,5,6,7,8	EAC 1-8	EAC'1a,4,2a,3,5,6,7,8
EAC1,4,2,3,5,6,7,8,9	EAC 1-9	EAC'1a,4,2a,3,5,6,7,8,9
Enzymes[d]		
$\text{C}\overline{1\text{s}}$[c]	C1 with esterase activity	C'1a
$\text{C}\overline{4,2}$	C3 convertase	C'(4,2)a
$\text{C}\overline{4,2,3}$	C3 dependent peptidase	C'(4,2)a,3
Fragments		
C2a		—
C2b		—
C3a	Anaphylatoxin I; Chemotactic Factor I	FaC'3
C3b		—
C5a	Anaphylatoxin II; Chemotactic Factor II	FaC'5
C5b		—

[a] W.H.O. Committee on Complement Nomenclature [see Appendix I, reproduced with permission from *Bull. W.H.O.* **39**, 935 (1968)]. Bars over numbers indicate complexes possessing enzyme activity.

[b] Complement Workshop, La Jolla, 1966, see H. J. Müller-Eberhard, *Advan. Immunol.* **8**, 1(1968). Symbol a indicates "activation" to functional enzyme.

[c] The macromolecular complex represented by C1 is stabilized by serum calcium; it is dissociable into its three constituents by removing Ca^{2+} (Section 17.D.2). C1 activated as enzyme is designated by $\text{C}\overline{1}$; this activated complex is dissociable into C1q, C1r, and $\text{C}\overline{1\text{s}}$. $\text{C}\overline{1\text{s}}$ is the component carrying esterase activity.

[d] Enzymes associated with the "C3 shunt" or "alternative pathway," not recognized in 1968, are C3 proactivator-convertase (C3PA*ase* or factor $\overline{\text{D}}$) and C3 activator (C3A or Factor $\overline{\text{B}}$).

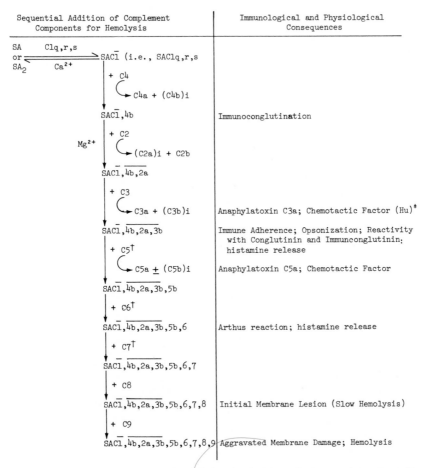

Sequential Addition of Complement Components for Hemolysis	Immunological and Physiological Consequences
SACl,4b	Immunoconglutination
SACl,4b,2a,3b	Anaphylatoxin C3a; Chemotactic Factor (Hu)[‡]
	Immune Adherence; Opsonization; Reactivity with Conglutinin and Immunconglutinin; histamine release
	Anaphylatoxin C5a; Chemotactic Factor
SACl,4b,2a,3b,5b,6	Arthus reaction; histamine release
SACl,4b,2a,3b,5b,6,7,8	Initial Membrane Lesion (Slow Hemolysis)
SACl,4b,2a,3b,5b,6,7,8,9	Aggravated Membrane Damage; Hemolysis

FIG. 1A. Schematic representation of the classical hemolytic complement reaction, applicable to human and guinea pig systems, based on data of H. J. Müller-Eberhard [*Annu. Rev. Biochem.* **38**, 389 (1969)] and of Manfred M. Mayer [*Immunochemistry* **7**, 485 (1970)].

S represents an antigenic site on the membrane surface of an erythrocyte. A single IgM antibody molecule (A) or two adjacent molecules of IgG antibody (A$_2$) will establish a complement-fixing site. The curved arrows connect individual substrates and products formed from them by enzymatic action. Enzymes that become activated are indicated by overbars (C$\overline{1}$, C$\overline{4b,2a}$, C$\overline{4b,2a,3b}$). The cleavage reactions are more or less wasteful, some fragments entering the fluid phase rather than fixing on the cell. Fragments that become hemolytically inactive are indicated by i.

† In the human complement system, components C5, C6, and C7 are reported to react most efficiently when present together, rather than when added sequentially *in vitro.*

‡ In the human system, an "activated complex" of C5, C6, and C7 appears to have chemotactic activity as well as the split products C3a and C3b.

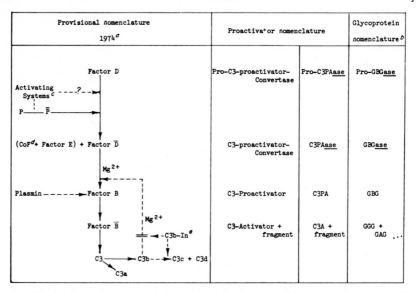

Provisional nomenclature 1974[a]		Proactivator nomenclature		Glycoprotein nomenclature[b]
Factor D		Pro–C3-proactivator-Convertase	Pro–C3PAase	Pro–GBGase
Activating ----?--→ Systems[c]				
P —¦— P̄ ——————→				
(CoF[d]+ Factor E) + Factor D̄		C3-proactivator-Convertase	C3PAase	GBGase
Mg²⁺				
Plasmin -----→Factor B		C3-Proactivator	C3PA	GBG
Factor B̄	Mg²⁺	C3-Activator + fragment	C3A + fragment	GGG + GAG ...
	-◄- -C3b-In[e]			
C3 ——→C3b- - -→C3c + C3d				
C3a				

FIG. 1B. A schematic representation of the C3 shunt, or "alternative," or properdin pathway of complement activation.

[a] The scheme shown here portrays current concepts in a rapidly expanding area of research and is designed to provide a guide to terminologies found in the literature. The reaction sequence is under intense investigation. According to provisional nomenclature, the active enzymes D̄ and B̄ are designated by overbars, their respective precursors being D and B. Factor B̄ acts on C3 with a specificity equivalent to C4̄,2̄ in Fig. 1A. See text.

[b] It was found [see T. Boenisch and C. A. Alper, *Biochim. Biophys. Acta* **221**, 529 (1970)] that a β-lipoprotein was split to a γ- and an α-lipoprotein. The lipoprotein being rich in glycine, the name glycine-rich β-lipoprotein, or GBG, was assigned to it, and the split products became GGG and GAG. GBG is now recognized as being β₂-lipoprotein II.

[c] Activating systems, properdin pathway, are listed in the text. Properdin (P) is a proenzyme serum protein of 5 S size which becomes activated to (P̄). *Purified* P cannot act directly but requires C3b (formerly known as properdin factor A).

[d] Cobra venom factor (CoF, Section 17.E.3.a), in the presence of Factor D, acts on factor B (C3PA) to form a complex enzyme. Factor E is mentioned in Section 17.E.5.

[e] C3b-In (C3b-inactivator, or KAF, Section 17.E.4) is a heat-labile β-globulin in normal serum which inactivates C3b to C3c and C3d and blocks C3b feedback.

activation or assembly. The activated principal enzymes are C1s̄ and C4̄,2̄, the latter splitting C3 and catalyzing the binding of C3b to produce the third enzyme, C4b,2a,3b. Different steps in the cascade require Mg²⁺ and/or Ca²⁺. Also present in plasma are C1-inhibitor, C3-inhibitor, and C6-inhibitor, which restrict the effective duration of enzymatic activity. Indeed the "cascade" is a transient albeit biologically effective event.

As seen in Fig. 1A, the cell surface (S) binds with antibody (A) and combines with C1, the only complement component which possesses an active immunoglobulin-combining site in its subunit C1q. C1 constitutes a Ca^{2+}-dependent complex of at least three different proteins, C1q, C1r, and C1s. After combination of C1 with antibody through C1q, subunit C1r (an enzyme) is enabled to activate the proenzyme subunit C1s to the actual enzyme $\overline{C1s}$. The activated $\overline{C1s}$, within the activated $\overline{C1}$, causes the $\overline{C4,2}$ enzyme to be assembled in a two-step reaction (Fig. 1A), namely, (a) binding of activated C4 to membrane or antibody receptors and (b) binding of activated C2 to cell-bound C4. Second, $\overline{C4,2}$ catalyzes binding of C3 to the cell surface and formation of the $\overline{C4,2,3}$ enzyme. This enzyme, in both the human and guinea pig complement systems, enables C5, C6, and C7 to interact with the cell surface in a complex manner[7]: the reaction is by far more efficient when the three proteins are allowed to act together rather than in sequence. Subsequent binding of C8 initiates the process of membrane damage. The lytic reaction becomes sharply accelerated by addition of C9. Membrane damage has been studied ultrastructurally.[8-10] Molecular aggregations of complement components on the surface of the cell are shown graphically by Kolb et al.[7] Mayer favors the concept of a rigid doughnutlike lesion passing through the phospholipid bilayer of the cell membrane, presenting a channel through which solutes of low molecular weight and water can exchange between the intracellular milieu and the extracellular fluid.[11]

The activation of complement proteins C2, C3, C4, and C5 is accompanied by cleavage (Fig. 1A). Cleavage of a complement molecule is believed to uncover its combining region for a short period of time, whereas secondary conformational changes are supposed to confine the combining region to the interior of the molecule. The activated combining site is lost rapidly (Fig. 1A, fragments designated by i). This loss perhaps constitutes a regulatory mechanism to prevent spreading of the cytolytic effect from the site of complement activation. The transient activation is partly responsible for the marked hemolytic inefficiency of some of these proteins, a circumstance of importance if one proposes to quantitate a complement protein by measurement of hemolytic activity.

Cleavage results also in liberation of smaller fragments, of which two,

[7] W. P. Kolb, J. A. Haxby, C. M. Arroyave, and H. J. Müller-Eberhard, *J. Exp. Med.* 135, 549 (1972).

[8] J. H. Humphrey and R. R. Dourmashkin, *Advan. Immunol.* 11, 75 (1969).

[9] M. J. Polley, *in* "Progress in Immunology" (B. Amos, ed.), pp. 597–608. Academic Press, New York, 1971.

[10] M. J. Polley, H. J. Müller-Eberhard, and J. D. Feldman, *J. Exp. Med.* 133, 53 (1971).

[11] M. M. Mayer, *Proc. Nat. Acad. Sci. U.S.* 69, 2954 (1972).

C3a and C5a arising, respectively, from C3 and C5, possess biological activity. Both serve as inflammatory mediators (anaphylatoxins) but are distinct: contraction of smooth muscle induced *in vitro* by either one does not desensitize the muscle toward the other anaphylatoxin (absence of tachyphylaxis). Both human C3a and C5a function as *chemotactic factors*, as does guinea pig C5a. Human C5a also liberates lysosomal enzymes from polymorphonuclear cells. As *anaphylatoxins*, C3a and C5a of both species release histamine, contract smooth muscle, and increase capillary permeability. As chemotactic factors, the active components attract polymorphonuclear and mononuclear leukocytes. Yet these double properties of the human C3a and C5a are dissociable, since cleavage of C3 by trypsin causes an immediate but transient appearance of anaphylatoxin and a slower formation of chemotactic factor. Also, natural plasma inhibitors of C3a and C5a are different proteins.

2. ALTERNATIVE PATHWAY FOR C3 ACTIVATION

The classical pathway to enzymatic attack on C3 involves the several discrete steps that lead to formation of the enzyme $C\overline{4,2}$ (Table I, Fig. 1A). Another mechanism for activation of complement, bypassing C1, C4, and C2, was suggested in early studies of Pillemer on the "properdin system,"[12, 13] but the existence of properdin as a special serum protein was doubted. Much later, an artificial system—a complex consisting of cobra venom factor (CoF), cofactors, and a special serum protein, which was later isolated as C3 proactivator—was shown to attack and activate C3.[14] (Indeed, purified CoF injected into animals would deplete their complement systems.[15, 16]) It was soon found that simple immune precipitates, made with guinea pig IgG_1-antibodies, would consume C3–9 in fresh serum, bypassing C1, C4, C2.[17, 18] The authors attributed their finding to IgG_1 aggregation and activation of an enzyme. Eventually, it was recognized that complement activation, described by Pillemer when

[12] L. Pillemer, L. Blum, I. H. Lepow, L. Wurz, and E. W. Todd, *J. Exp. Med.* **103**, 1 (1956).
[13] I. H. Lepow, *in* "Immunochemical Approaches to Problems in Microbiology" (M. Heidelberger and O. J. Plescia, eds.), pp. 280–294. Rutgers Univ. Press, New Brunswick, New Jersey, 1961.
[14] O. Götze and H. J. Müller-Eberhard, *J. Exp. Med.* **132**, 898 (1970).
[15] J. L. Maillard and R. M. Zarco, *Ann. Inst. Pasteur Paris* **114**, 766 (1968).
[16] C. G. Cochrane, H. J. Müller-Eberhard, and B. S. Aiken, *J. Immunol.* **105**, 55 (1970).
[17] B. Oliveira, A. G. Osler, R. P. Siraganian, and A. L. Sandberg, *J. Immunol.* **104**, 320 (1970).
[18] A. L. Sandberg, A. G. Osler, H. S. Shin, and B. Oliveira, *J. Immunol.* **104**, 329 (1970).

fresh serum was treated with zymosan (yeast cell walls), inulin, dextran, or agar, had opened the same pathway of attack on C3. Aggregated serum globulins and bacterial polysaccharides also engage this pathway. Interestingly, guinea pig IgG_2 antibody, which ordinarily fixes complement by the classical pathway, was found to use the alternative (properdin) pathway after peptic digestion: IgG accordingly possesses two sites of interaction with complement.[19]

A long, continuing study of the "alternative pathway" leading to utilization of the components of complement is summarized in Fig. 1B. The "C3 shunt" or "alternative pathway" to involvement of the late complement components (C5 through C9), bypassing C1, C4, and C2, is schematized in Fig. 1B.

The sequence involves two proenzymes and two enzymes. Two "languages" are in use, shown in the right half of Fig. 1B. Here, we adopt the provisional nomenclature of 1974, in which $D \rightarrow \overline{D}$ and $B \rightarrow \overline{B}$. When proenzyme D becomes activated to $\overline{D}$, this enzyme activates proenzyme B to $\overline{B}$, which in turn cleaves C3 to C3a and C3b.[20] The pathway requires Mg^{2+}. (C3b participates also, as shown in Fig. 1A, in forming the enzyme $\overline{C4b},2a3b$.)

The initiation of these events appears to occur when the properdin (P) in fresh plasma is activated to enzyme $\overline{P}$. Activating substances include zymosan (yeast cell walls), inulin, dextran, lipopolysaccharide or *Escherichia coli* cells, agar, aggregated IgG (G_1,G_2,G_3,G_4), aggregated IgA (A_1,A_2), aggregated IgE, antigen, and guinea pig IgG_1 antibody. The activation of $P \rightarrow \overline{P}$ may constitute a second step in the sequence of activation, since purified P cannot act directly; it requires C3b (formerly known as properdin factor A).

Activation can occur also by an isolated complex consisting of cobra venom factor (CoF) with properdin factors E and $\overline{D}$; also plasmin, if present, can act directly on factor B.

The effectiveness of the system is amplified by feedback of the cleavage product C3b into the $\overline{D} \rightarrow B$ pathway; but the amplifying system is restrained by C3b-inactivator (C3b-In), which interrupts the feedback by cleaving C3b into fragments C3c and C3d.

The C3b-inhibitor was first detected as a special heat-stable β-globulin exhibiting the property of a conglutinogen-activating factor, for which KAF became the symbol[21] (Section 17.E.3).

EDTA, binding Ca^{2+} and Mg^{2+}, blocks both the classical $\overline{C1,4,2}$ pathway and the alternative (properdin) pathway. Because the properdin

[19] A. L. Sandberg, B. Oliveira, and A. G. Osler, *J. Immunol.* **106**, 282 (1971).
[20] S. Ruddy and K. F. Austen, *J. Immunol.* **107**, 742 (1971).
[21] P. A. E. Noel and P. J. Lachmann, *Immunology* **24**, 259 (1973).

pathway requires only Mg^{2+}, the properdin pathway will function in the presence of 10 mM ethyleneglycoltetraacetic acid (EGTA), which chelates Ca^{2+} preferentially.[22] Thus analysis of the pathways utilized can be made.

There is evidence that the alternative pathway plays a special role in the body's defenses against bacterial and some viral infections after opsonization has occurred, apparently even by normal serum, and initiates a cascade of components C3—C9. The alternative pathway, when compared to the classical mechanism, has a low cytolytic capacity despite the consumption of complement components C3–9. Nevertheless, it can initiate cell lysis, provided the cells are particularly susceptible to complement attack, as are the erythrocytes from patients exhibiting paroxysmal nocturnal hemoglobinuria. Such cells lyse when serum is treated with inulin at pH 7.2.[23]

3. PRINCIPLES OF QUANTITATION OF COMPLEMENT COMPONENTS

The evolution of the molecular concept of complement function was entirely dependent on the development of methods allowing detection and isolation of complement proteins, isolation of intermediate reaction products, and precise quantitation of both complement activity and complement proteins.[5, 23-25]

All the complement components tested so far have yielded dose-response curves that are characteristic for a one-hit reaction. This principle states that a single cellular lesion (S*) produced by antibody and complement is sufficient for lysis of an erythrocyte.[23] Thus, it would seem that most, if not all, steps of the complement reaction require only a single molecule for progression of the reaction which eventuates in the manifestation of the membrane lesion E*. The one-hit concept therefore became the theoretical basis for quantitation of complement activity.[25] Although a single S* is sufficient, a cell can possess several S sites. Application of the Poisson distribution, assuming that sites S are randomly and independently distributed, yields an equation according to which the average number of molecular hits or lesions per cell (z) equals the nega-

[22] D. P. Fine, S. R. Marney, Jr., D. G. Colley, J. S. Sergent, and R. M. Des Prez, *J. Immunol.* **109**, 807 (1972).

[23] M. M. Mayer, *in* "Immunochemical Approaches to Problems in Microbiology" (M. Heidelberger and O. J. Plescia, eds.), pp. 268–279. Rutgers Univ. Press, New Brunswick, New Jersey, 1961.

[24] M. M. Mayer, *in* "Experimental Immunochemistry" (E. A. Kabat and M. M. Mayer, eds.), 2nd ed., pp. 133–240. Thomas, Springfield, Illinois, 1961.

[25] M. M. Mayer, *Complement, Ciba Found. Symp. 1964,* p. 4 (1965).

tive natural logarithm of the surviving cells. Lysed cells are represented by y, the surviving cells by $1 - y$. At 100% lysis, $y = 1$. Accordingly, $z = -\ln(1 - y)$. Since $y = 0.63$ when $z = 1$, i.e., at 63% lysis, the number of effective molecules of a complement protein which, under standard conditions, produces 63% lysis is equal to the number of cells used.

This method affords quantitation of *effective* molecules by hemolytic activity measurements, but does not detect those molecules that are potentially effective but do not register in the hemolytic titration owing to an inherent inefficiency of most hemolytic reaction steps. Quantitative molecular analysis of several reaction steps in the human complement system has revealed that the actual number of molecules of a complement protein that must be expended for a fruitful hemolytic reaction is a multiple of the theoretically postulated value of 1. For example, only 1 of 300 C4 molecules, or 1 of more than 1000 C2 molecules may be detected by effective molecular titration.[26] (On the other hand, the efficiency of guinea pig C2 is high, only 1.1 molecules being required for lysis of one cell; in the case of guinea pig C5, 10 molecules are required.) Inefficiency seriously limits the value of hemolytic titrations for quantitation of complement in absolute molecular terms unless correction factors are introduced. With the aid of such factors, the number of effective molecules measured may be converted to the absolute number of complement molecules initially present. When these efficiency factors are applied to the determination of a complement protein in human serum by hemolytic titration, then the corrected values are in excellent agreement with those obtained by independent immunochemical determination. It follows that for isolated complement components the ratio of effective molecules to protein molecules is considerably smaller than 1, with the exception of that of guinea pig C1 and C2. For each complement protein this ratio has a characteristic value, which may be used as a measure of purity and functional integrity.

Quantitation of components is assuming an increasing role in medicine in view of the findings of hereditary defects in the complement system and its inhibitors, with various clinical consequences. One of these is described in Section 17.E.2.a.ii. Hereditary defects in animals are known, such as C4-deficient guinea pigs, C6-deficient rabbits, and C5-deficient mice.[3, 27] Such animals are especially useful in testing for functional activity of the respective complement components. Reactions involving complement consumption which are given by C4-deficient guinea pigs implicate at once a utilization of the C3-shunt system (Section 17.A.2),

[26] H. J. Müller-Eberhard, *Ann. Rev. Biochem.* **38**, 389 (1969).
[27] "Biological Activities of Complement" (D. G. Ingram, ed.). Karger, Basel 1972.

e.g., the phagocytosis of pneumococci that have been opsonized by contact with *normal* guinea pig serum.[28]

4. COMPLEMENT FIXATION REACTIONS*

Methods for conducting complement fixation reactions are presented in Section 17.B. In principle, a carefully calibrated amount of fresh serum, usually guinea pig ("complement"), is mixed with some antigen and antibody of interest to allow binding of the complement components; then an indicator system is added, consisting of erythrocytes (commonly sheep in origin), coated with heat-inactivated, specific anti-red cell antibody. Lysis of the indicator system shows the presence of free complement, which usually is measured quantitatively. The use of 50% lysis of red cells by measurement of absorbancy was introduced by Maltaner (see Wadsworth *et al.*[29]).

The usual goals are these: detection of antibodies in low concentration; detection of antibodies to antigens in particulate or emulsion form; monitoring concentration steps with viral CF antigens (Vol. I, Chap. 1.D.1); miniaturization of antigen–antibody reactions in free solution (Vol. II, Chap. 12.D.1.c). In the classical Wassermann test for syphilis, an effective emulsified "antigen" extracted by alcohol from normal beef heart is used to detect the presence of syphilitic "reagins" in patients' sera.

5. TOPICAL PRESENTATION OF COMPLEMENT COMPONENTS†

The isolation of the hemolytic intermediates (Table I) is described in Section 17.C for both human and guinea pig complement. Preparations of complement components (Fig. 1A and Table I) are given in Section 17.D. Section 17.E details methods applicable to the several complement-related proteins: serum inhibitor of C$\bar{1}$; the C3-proactivator (C3PA or Factor B); properdin factor D; the C3b-inactivator previously known as conglutinogen-activating factor (KAF); and preparative procedures for C3a- and C3b-anaphylatoxins and for cobra venom factor (CoF). Section 17.F deals both with preparation of antisera to complement components and an immunological quantitation of these, and also with detection of complement in tissues by means of fluorescein-labeled antiserum to C3.

---

[28] J. A. Winkelstein, H. S. Shin, and W. B. Wood, Jr., *J. Immunol.* **108**, 1681 (1972).

* Section 17.A.4 was contributed by Merrill W. Chase.

[29] A. Wadsworth, F. Maltaner, and E. Maltaner, *J. Immunol.* **35**, 93 and 105 (1931).

† Sections 17.A.5–7 were contributed by the Editors.

6. KEY TO BUFFERS FOR THE COMPLEMENT SYSTEM

All buffers used with erythrocytes in hemolytic assays are isotonic, and reaction is at pH 7.4 unless specified otherwise. Sodium chloride solution is buffered with barbital (Veronal), and gelatin is added to 0.1%. Further, divalent cations are necessary in the hemolytic pathway (Figs. 1A, 1B), hence Ca^{2+} and Mg^{2+} are used in small, fixed amounts. This is the usual suspending medium for erythrocytes, designated simply as GVB^{2+} or GVB^{++} or GVB Me^{2+}. When gelatin is omitted, as in handling complement components prior to a hemolytic assay, the corresponding designations become simply VB or VB^{2+} according to omission or inclusion of the divalent metals. (Symbol Me^{2+} refers to the presence of *both* divalent metals.)

To reduce the ionicity, usually to 0.065, while retaining isotonicity, glucose or mannitol or sucrose are often added, the respective designations becoming $DGVB^{2+}$ (D for dextrose), $MGVB^{2+}$, or $SGVB^{2+}$ and so on.

To block the hemolytic pathway, the Ca^{2+} and Mg^{2+} of fresh serum can be chelated by adding EDTA. Thus EDTA–GVB (or EDTA–VB) becomes the diluent for serum prior to addition of erythrocytes.

7. COMPLEMENT IN SPECIES OTHER THAN MAN AND GUINEA PIG

It is outside the scope of this chapter to provide details. Review through 1970 is provided by Rapp and Borsos (p. 65).[1]

B. Immune Hemolysis and Complement Fixation*†

1. DILUENTS AND REAGENTS

The hemolytic action of complement varies with pH, ionic strength, and concentration of Ca^{2+} and Mg^{2+}.[1] Accordingly, an isotonic solution

* Section 17.B was contributed by Louis G. Hoffmann and Manfred M. Mayer.

† Section 17.B, dealing with technique of complement fixation tests, represents very largely the methods and procedures of Manfred M. Mayer, Louis G. Hoffmann, and their associates. Portions of this contribution were taken from the chapter on "Complement and Complement Fixation" by M. M. Mayer *in* "Experimental Immunochemistry" (E. A. Kabat and M. M. Mayer, eds.), 2nd ed. Thomas, Springfield, Illinois, 1961. The authors and editors express their appreciation to C. C. Thomas for permission to use this material.

[1] M. M. Mayer, "Complement and Complement Fixation," *in* "Experimental Immunochemistry" (E. A. Kabat and M. M. Mayer, eds.), 2nd ed., Chap. 4. Thomas, Springfield, Illinois 1961.

is used at pH 7.4, buffered either by barbital (Veronal) or triethanol-amine.[1a] $CaCl_2$ and $MgCl_2$ are added in optimal concentrations according to the intended procedure; e.g., the optimal divalent cation concentrations for the action of whole guinea pig complement are 0.15 mM Ca^{2+} and 0.5 mM Mg^{2+}, but the latter is raised to 1.0 mM for the C2 reaction. Human complement, however, requires 1.0 mM Mg^{2+}. In order to reduce spontaneous lysis of the red cells[2] as well as adsorption of complement protein or antibody to the glass surfaces of vessels, gelatin (0.1%, USP) is incorporated in the buffer. The pH of the final solution should be between 7.2 and 7.4. The conductivity of this buffer, measured at 0°, should not differ by more than 1% from a value of 8.17 mS. The appropriate concentrations of divalent cations will be indicated in each section.

The stock solutions of 0.03 M $CaCl_2$ and 0.1 M $MgCl_2$ should be checked for concentration by specific gravity, conductimetric titration with standard $AgNO_3$, or potentiometry with an ion-specific electrode. Volumetric glassware should be used.

In some of the procedures the optimal ionic strength of isotonic buffers is 0.065.[2a] An isotonic diluent of this ionic strength at pH 7.3–7.4 will be referred to as mannitol–gelatin–Veronal buffer (MGVB); its conductivity at 0° should not differ by more than 2% from 343 μS. Sucrose-gelatin-Veronal buffer (SGVB) can be used alternatively. Buffers are listed in Table I.

Procedures that require exclusion of divalent cations are carried out in a solution prepared with EDTA at pH 7.4, i.e., in the form $Na_3H \cdot EDTA$.

The working-strength isotonic buffer should not be kept longer than 1 day to avoid bacterial contamination.

a. BUFFERS AND SOLUTIONS

Composition of the principal reagents for handling erythrocytes, antibody, and complement are listed in Table I.

b. PREPARATION OF SHEEP ERYTHROCYTES (E)

Sheep blood is drawn aseptically into an equal volume of sterile Alsever's solution (Table I) or into commercial bleeding equipment [e.g., Fenwal Blood-Pack Unit No. JA-2C, containing ACD (acid–citrate–dextrose) solution, NIH Formula A]; when this is used, the blood is trans-

---

[1a] J. F. Kent, A. G. Otero, and R. E. Harrigan. *Amer. J. Clin. Pathol.* **27**, 539 (1957).
[2] P. Rous and J. T. Turner, *J. Exp. Med.* **23**, 219 (1916).
[2a] H. J. Rapp and T. Borsos, *J. Immunol.* **91**, 826 (1963).

TABLE I

COMPOSITION OF BUFFERS AND SOLUTIONS FOR ERYTHROCYTE AND COMPLEMENT[a]

1. ISOTONIC VERONAL (BARBITAL) BUFFER[b] WITH Ca^{2+}, Mg^{2+}, AND GELATIN, pH 7.3–7.4 (GVB and GVB^{2+}; VB if gelatin is omitted)

a. Prepare a 5× concentrate (stock VB) by dissolving to 1 liter: 5.095 gm of barbital sodium (Veronal), 41.5 gm of NaCl, and about 17.75 ml of 1.0 N HCl to pH 7.4, with stirring. At 4° stock VB is stable for a month.

b. $CaCl_2$, 0.03 M: dissolve 3.33 gm of anhydrous calcium chloride or 4.41 gm of the dihydrate in water to 100 ml.[c]

c. $MgCl_2$, 0.1 M: dissolve 20.33 gm of $MgCl_2 \cdot 6H_2O$ in water to 100 ml.[c]

d. *Working buffer* for use with guinea pig complement, to be prepared daily: blend 200 ml of a, 5 ml of b, and 5 ml of c and dilute to 1000 ml, including 1 gm of U.S.P. gelatin.[d] Added inorganic divalent ions supply 1.5×10^{-4} M Ca^{2+} and 5×10^{-4} M Mg^{2+}.

2. VERONAL (BARBITAL) BUFFER WITH DOUBLED MAGNESIUM: Blend solutions of buffer 1 above as in 1d, using 10 ml of 1c to supply 1.5×10^{-4} M Ca^{2+} and 1×10^{-3} M Mg^{2+}. This buffer is used for the C2 reaction with fractions of whole guinea pig complement. An alternative buffer with doubled Mg^{2+} can be prepared using buffer 5b. Buffer should be prepared daily.

3. VERONAL–MANNITOL BUFFER, WITH Ca^{2+}, Mg^{2+}, AND GELATIN, pH 7.3–7.4, $\Gamma/2 = 0.065$ ($MGVB^{2+}$)

a. Prepare an isotonic stock solution by dissolving to 500 ml: 1.019 gm of barbital sodium (Veronal) and 51.74 gm of reagent-grade D-mannitol; add approximately 3.55 ml N HCl to bring pH to 7.3–7.4; then add: 5.0 ml of 0.03 M $CaCl_2$ (solution 1b) and 10 ml of 0.1 M $MgCl_2$ (solution 1c), and bring to 1 liter; finally dissolve 1 gm of gelatin. The buffer should be prepared daily.

b. *Working buffer*: Mix 600 ml of above stock solution with 400 ml of solution 1d.

c. *Working buffer*: Prepare as in 3b but add, per liter, a further 5 ml of 0.1 M $MgCl_2$.

4. VERONAL–SUCROSE BUFFER, WITH Ca^{2+}, Mg^{2+}, AND GELATIN, pH 7.3–7.4, $\Gamma/2 = 0.065$ ($SGVB^{2+}$): Prepare as in 3a, but use 97.3 gm of sucrose in place of mannitol; dilute, as *working buffer*, as in 3b. This buffer can be prepared in 5 times the concentration given (stock VBS) and diluted to isotonicity as wanted.

(continued)

TABLE I (*Continued*)

5. TRIETHANOLAMINE BUFFER,[e,f] WITH Ca^{2+}, Mg^{2+}, AND GELATIN, pH 7.3–7.4 (GTB^{2+})

a. Prepare a 10× concentrate by dissolving to 1 liter: 28 ml of triethanolamine, 75 gm of NaCl, and ca 160 ml of 1.0 N HCl. Bring first to 975 ml, then check pH on an accurately prepared 1:10 dilution. Adjust stock as necessary with 1.0 N HCl or NaOH to bring pH of a 1:10 dilution to 7.4 ± 0.1, and bring volume to 1 liter. (It is recommended that 2 liters be prepared per batch.) Triethanolamine of Matheson, Coleman and Bell has given clear solutions; avoid any samples that give a slightly cloudy solution.

b. *Working buffer* for use with guinea pig complement: use 100 ml of 10× triethanolamine concentrate per liter in place of barbital sodium, but otherwise follow the procedure for preparing buffer 1d. Added inorganic divalent ions supply 1.5×10^{-4} M Ca^{2+} and 5×10^{-4} M Mg^{2+}.

6. TRIETHANOLAMINE BUFFER WITH GELATIN (GTB) BUT LACKING DIVALENT CATIONS, pH 7.3–7.4: Use 100 ml of 10× triethanolamine concentrate 5a per liter and add 1 gm of gelatin.

7. EDTA–VERONAL BUFFER LACKING DIVALENT CATIONS, pH 7.3 (EDTA–VB)

a. Prepare 0.1 M Na$_3$H·EDTA by dissolving 18.61 gm of disodium EDTA in 400 ml of water, titrating with 1.0 N NaOH to pH 7.3 and bringing to 500 ml. Alternatively, 19.0 gm of tetrasodium EDTA can be dissolved in 400 ml of water and titrated to pH 7.3 with 1.0 N HCl; the volume can be brought to 500 ml (0.1 M). At pH 7.4, trisodium EDTA is formed. Compare buffer 20, Appendix II, Vol. II.

b. Prepare *working buffer* by diluting 200 ml of solution 1a to 1 liter, including 50 ml of 0.1 M Na$_3$H·EDTA for a concentration of 5 mM, or:

c. Prepare *working buffer* by diluting 200 ml of solution 1a to 1 liter, including 100 ml of 0.1 M Na$_3$H·EDTA to provide 10 mmoles of the latter.

8. Na$_3$H·EDTA BUFFER WITH GELATIN, 0.09 M, pH 7.6, $\Gamma/2 = 0.15$ (EDTA–GVB): Dissolve 33.5 gm of Na$_2$H$_2$·EDTA in ca. 750 ml of water, adjust to pH 7.6 by adding 1 M NaOH. Bring to 1 liter and add 1 gm of USP gelatin. [After M. M. Frank, H. J. Rapp and T. Borsos, *J. Immunol.* **93**, 409 (1964).]

9. Na$_3$H·EDTA BUFFER CONCENTRATE, 0.2 M, pH 7.4: Dissolve 74.45 gm of Na$_2$H$_2$·EDTA in about 750 ml of distilled water and adjust to pH 7.4 by adding 1 M NaOH; bring to 1 liter. This stock buffer is diluted 1:25 in appropriate buffers of pH 7.4–7.6 to provide 8 mM Na$_3$H·EDTA, which chelates Ca^{2+} and Mg^{2+} and inactivates C1 and C2.

TABLE I (*Continued*)

10. ALSEVER'S SOLUTION, MODIFIED[g]: Dissolve in ca 750 ml of distilled
water: 8.0 gm of trisodium citrate dihydrate, 4.2 gm of NaCl, and 20.5 gm
of glucose. Add ca 5.5 ml of 10% citric acid to pH 6.1 and bring volume
to 1 liter. Filter if necessary to clarify. Sterilization may be effected by
autoclaving at 10 pounds pressure for 10 minutes or by membrane
filtration (Vol. I, Chap. 2.C.5). It is usual to dispense and store sterilely
in the containers that will receive the bleedings; keep at 4°, tightly
sealed. When 1 volume of sterile whole blood is added and immediately
mixed with 1.2 volumes of this solution, the storage concentrations per
milliliter are approximately 4.27 mg of citrate, 10.25 mg of glucose, and
2.1 mg of NaCl at constant pH. [From S. C. Bukantz, C. R. Rein, and
J. F. Kent, *J. Lab. Clin. Med.* **31**, 394 (1946).]

[a] Other buffers used in particular isolation procedures are listed in Section 17.D.1,
Tables I and III; Section 17.E, Table I.

[b] See buffer 6B, Appendix II, Vol. II.

[c] For use with whole guinea pig complement, it is convenient to dissolve the $CaCl_2$
and $MgCl_2$ together in 100 ml of water, adding 5 ml of the mixture to the working
buffer (buffer 1d).

[d] The gelatin should be allowed to swell in a small volume of water for about 10
minutes, then dissolved by mild heating on a steam bath or equivalent; foaming can be
avoided if the gelatin solution is pipetted beneath the surface of the buffer in the
volumetric flask, without blowing out. Alternatively, it can be allowed to swell in the
completed buffer and dissolved by mild heating.

[e] J. F. Kent, A. G. Otero, and R. E. Harrigan, *Amer. J. Clin. Pathol.* **27**, 539 (1957).

[f] See buffer 37A, Appendix II, Vol. II.

[g] The original blood preservatives of sodium citrate plus sugars were introduced by
P. Rous and J. T. Turner [*J. Exp. Med.* **23**, 219 (1916)], with differing formulations
for human, rabbit, sheep, and dog bloods. Alsever solution was introduced for human
blood by J. B. Alsever and R. B. Ainslie [*N. Y. State J. Med.* **11**, 126 (1941)]; the
amount of sodium citrate was reduced and NaCl was added (8.0 gm of trisodium
citrate dihydrate, 4.18 gm of NaCl, and 18.66 gm of glucose per liter). Modified
Alsever's solution listed above was introduced in 1946, with addition of citric acid to
form largely disodium citrate at pH 6.1. These laboratory devices employed one or
more volumes of diluent per volume of whole blood. More concentrated solutions
appropriate to human blood banks were needed to avoid dilution and to reduce the
sodium content of infused bloods. In 1943, J. F. Loutit and P. L. Mollison [*Brit. Med.
J.* **2**, 744 (1943)] had shown that 2 gm of *di*sodium citrate · H_2O and 3 gm of glucose
per 120 ml was an excellent preservative for 3.5 volumes of blood if initial mixing was
thorough; it remains the preservative used in Britain. The water can be reduced to
30 ml with effective preservation of 510 ml of blood. Other common formulations are
NIH formula A, NIH formula B, and citrate–phosphate–dextrose (CPD 5). NIH
formula A contains, per 100 ml, 2.2 gm of trisodium citrate · $2H_2O$, 0.8 gm of citric
acid, and 2.5 gm of dextrose · H_2O; 67.5 ml is mixed with 100 ml of blood although
15 ml is adequate (P. L. Mollison, "Blood Transfusion in Clinical Medicine," 4th ed.
F. A. Davis, Philadelphia, Pennsylvania, 1967). NIH formula B contains the same
chemicals: 1.32 gm of trisodium citrate · $2H_2O$, 0.48 gm of citric acid · H_2O, 1.47 gm
of dextrose, water to 100 ml, to be mixed with 400 ml of blood. CPD 5 [J. G. Gibson,
S. B. Rees, T. J. McManus, and W. A. Scheitlin, *Amer. J. Clin. Pathol.* **28**, 569 (1957)]
contains 25.8 gm of trisodium citrate · $2H_2O$, 3.2 gm of citric acid · H_2O, 2.18 gm of
$NaH_2PO_4 · H_2O$, 25 gm of dextrose in 1 liter at pH 5.63. Of this, 70 ml is mixed with
500 ml of blood, with final pH = 7.1.

ferred sterilely immediately on receipt in the laboratory to sterile screw-capped bottles or Erlenmeyer flasks with cemented rubber liners within the caps, the flasks being filled not more than half full. The blood is stored at 2° to 5°. Allow 3 to 7 days for stabilization of the cells. As long as sterility is maintained, the blood may be used for about 2 months, during which time the susceptibility of the erythrocytes to lysis by antibody and complement does not change much; however, blood is discarded when the first washing fluid shows excess hemoglobin or whenever the cell blank rises to more than 1 or 2% lysis.[3]

The lytic susceptibility of red cells from individual sheep may vary. Avoid pooling blood from several animals. Animals should not be bled more often than every 8 or 10 weeks; each bleeding may be as large as 500 ml.

To prepare the standardized sheep cell suspension, a volume of blood sufficient for the day's work is withdrawn aseptically from stock and centrifuged. The plasma and buffy coat are carefully aspirated and discarded; the sedimented cells are washed 3 times with 5 to 10 volumes of the isotonic diluent to be used in the experiment. (In procedures requiring rigorous exclusion of sheep C1, the cells are washed with 0.01 M EDTA buffer as in Table I, buffer 7c). The second and third wash fluids should be colorless. The sedimented, washed cells are resuspended in ca 18 volumes of diluent to an approximate 5% suspension and filtered through a small wad of glass wool in a funnel. Exactly 1.0 ml of the suspension is lysed with 14.0 ml of a 0.1% aqueous solution of anhydrous Na_2CO_3. The optical density ($OD_{541\,nm}^{1\,cm}$) of the clear lysate is measured in a spectrophotometer against a water blank. The desired standardization value is OD 0.704 $\pm$ 0.005, which corresponds approximately, in terms of hemoglobin concentration, to 1.0×10^9 erythrocytes per milliliter of cell suspension when the sheep blood is derived from healthy animals. A 5% cell suspension will yield a lysate of optical density slightly greater than the desired standardization value, and adjustment is made by diluting according to the following relationship:

$$V_t = V_i(OD/0.704)$$

where OD represents the desired optical density of the lysate of the 5% suspension, V_i is an accurately measured sample of the suspension, and V_t is the volume to which the sample should be diluted. Check the final OD after the calculated adjustment has been made. Washed erythrocytes can be added if the OD of the approximately 5% suspension is less than 0.704. The spectrophotometer should be checked with known

[3] M. M. Mayer, C. C. Croft, and M. M. Gray, *J. Exp. Med.* **88**, 427 (1948).

dilutions of a hemoglobin preparation* to verify that it follows Beer's Law in the relevant concentration range at 541 nm; if not, a calibration curve must be made to permit proper adjustment of the cell suspension.

After standardization in the manner just described, the cells are kept in a stoppered flask at refrigerator temperature until needed. It is advisable to make occasional checks of the standardization with a Coulter cell counter.

c. Hemolytic Antibody (A)

Antisera prepared by giving rabbits a single course of injections of boiled sheep erythrocyte stromata represents a convenient type of antibody since a constant level of hemolytic activity is approached when it is used in relatively large amounts with a constant, limited quantity of complement.[1]

i. Preparation of Boiled Sheep Erythrocyte Stromata

Collect 1 liter of sheep blood in 250 ml of 3.8% sodium citrate (dihydrate), with continuous mixing. After filtration of the blood through cheesecloth to remove any clumps, sediment the cells by centrifugation in the cold (fill the centrifuge bottles only one-third full), and wash once with one to two volumes of isotonic saline.

Add 4 ml of glacial acetic acid to 10 liters of ice-cold distilled water; then add the packed red cells slowly, with constant and vigorous mixing. Continue stirring for about 10 minutes to complete lysis; allow the red cell stromata to settle in the cold room overnight. Draw off as much of the supernatant fluid as possible. Transfer the stromata to at least six 250-ml centrifuge bottles, centrifuge for 15 minutes in the cold at 2000 rpm, or until the stromata are packed, and remove the supernatant fluid by suction.† Wash the stromata four to six times with cold 0.001 M acetate buffer, pH 5 (approximately 1.48 ml of 0.2 M acetic acid and 3.52 ml of 0.2 M sodium acetate trihydrate per liter). Use as much buffer as the centrifuge bottles will hold; after each wash, centrifuge in the cold for 15 minutes at 2000 rpm. (For large-scale preparations, washing with acetate buffer may be performed in 50-liter carboys; use two washes, each with 5 to 10 liters of acetate buffer for the stromata from 1 liter of blood, and let stromata settle overnight in the cold room.)

---

* Check-out for photometric linearity in the visible region (370 nm) is readily made by scanning different concentrations of alkaline K_2CrO_4. Two stock solutions are used: (a) 3.3 gm of KOH per liter (0.05 N) and (b) 20 mg of K_2CrO_4 per 500 ml of (a). Dilute to 50 ml with solution (b) 4 different volumes of (a), namely, 10 ml, 20 ml, 30 ml, and 40 ml. This test procedure is recommended by the National Bureau of Standards. Frequent checks of the spectrophotometer are advisable.
† A useful device for this purpose is shown in Vol. I, Chap. 2.A.2.b.

Suspend the stromata in an equal volume of cold 0.15 M NaCl and distribute among eight heavy-wall 100-ml centrifuge bottles. Spin in an angle head at 0° for 20 minutes at 4000 rpm, and make two similar further washings in cold 0.15 M NaCl. As the acetate is washed out, the stromata may settle less readily; if so, the time of centrifugation should be increased. Finally suspend the washed stromata in 0.15 M NaCl to a volume of about 300 to 400 ml.

Transfer the suspension to an Erlenmeyer flask containing a magnetic stirring bar; cap the flask and immerse it in a boiling water bath for 1 hour. Cool, then stir on a magnetic stirring apparatus until a smoothly dispersed suspension is obtained. Analyze a sample for nitrogen by micro-Kjeldahl analysis and then dilute with sterile saline to 1 mg of nitrogen per milliliter. Add Merthiolate to a final concentration of 1:10,000 (w/v) (1% of a 1% solution).

ii. Immunization of Rabbits

Rabbits are immunized with this suspension by 11 intravenous inoculations over a period of about 2 weeks according to the following sequence: make one intravenous injection of 0.1 ml, five injections of 1 ml, and five injections of 2 ml; do not skip more than two consecutive days.* Bleed the rabbits on the fourth and the fifth day after the last injection. Separate the sera (do not pool specimens from different rabbits) and heat for 30 minutes at 56° to inactivate complement. Store at −20°. For titration, make an initial 1:100 stock dilution; this dilution can be stored indefinitely at −20°.

d. Preparation of Sensitized Sheep Erythrocytes (EA)

On the basis of the determination of the optimal sensitization level (Section 17.B.2.a), an appropriate dilution of the antiserum is prepared, and this dilution is slowly pipetted *into* an equal volume of standardized cell suspension with constant swirling of the contents. Do not reverse the order of addition. The flask is stoppered and placed in a refrigerator until needed. Sensitized cells should be prepared daily as required.

The optimal sensitization level as determined by the procedure described in Section 17.B.2.a refers to use of whole complement of guinea pig serum. The complement of other species should be subjected to an experimental checking with use of the procedure described. Some of the procedures described below (e.g., Sections 17.B.3.a.iii; 17.C.2.a and b) require cells sensitized with larger amounts of antibody. The use of larger amounts of antibody requires modifications in the above procedure, as will be described where appropriate.

* It is advisable to dilute the suspension to 2 ml for each injection.

e. COLLECTION OF SERUM TO RETAIN ITS
   COMPLEMENT ACTIVITY

The hemolytic activity of complement deteriorates quickly unless precautions are taken during collection and storage of the serum. Pooled guinea pig blood is allowed to clot for 1 to 2 hours at room temperature. The serum is separated from the clot promptly, frozen immediately, and stored at −40° or lower in an electric deep freeze. If a Dry-ice storage box is used, the serum should be kept in sealed glass ampoules to avoid exposure to CO_2.

In studies of mouse complement by Borsos and Cooper,[4] the jugular veins were incised and the blood of about 45 mice was added, as obtained, to a large petri dish resting on crushed ice. Clotting was rapid; as soon as the last bleeding had clotted, the blood was transferred to plastic tubes and centrifuged at 8000 RCF for 30 minutes at 2° to 4°. The serum was removed by pipette and centrifuged again for 15 minutes at 2° to 4° at 1000 RCF. The clarified, pooled mouse serum was distributed in small tubes and stored at −50°. Serum obtained in this fashion contained 2 to 3 times more active complement than was yielded by mouse serum obtained from pooled blood that had been allowed to clot at room temperature. (The mouse serum collected in the cold did not clot on incubation at 37°.)

2. GENERAL PROCEDURES

a. DETERMINING THE CONCENTRATION OF ANTISERUM
   FOR OPTIMAL SENSITIZATION

i. Buffer

The diluent for this procedure with guinea pig complement is buffer containing 0.15 mM Ca^{2+} and 0.5 mM Mg^{2+} (GVB^{2+}, Table I, buffer 1d; or GTB^{2+}, Table I, buffer 5b).

ii. Hemolysin Required for Optimal Sensitization

To determine the dilution of antiserum needed for optimal sensitization, 5.0-ml portions of a series of antiserum dilutions (1:200, 1:400, 1:800, 1:1600, 1:3200, 1:6400) are added to 5.0-ml portions of a standardized sheep erythrocyte suspension (10^9 cells/ml) in 40-ml centrifuge tubes with constant swirling of the contents. One-milliliter portions of each of these cell suspensions are distributed among a series of 40-ml centrifuge tubes kept at 0°. Add 5.5 ml of ice-cold buffer to each, followed

[4] T. Borsos and M. Cooper, *Proc. Soc. Exp. Biol. Med.* **107**, 227 (1961).

by 1.0 ml of an appropriate dilution of complement also kept at 0°. The dilution is chosen so as to yield approximately 50% to 70% hemolysis (for optimally sensitized cells); a 1:200 dilution of fresh guinea pig serum should give this degree of hemolysis. The tubes are then incubated at 37° for 90 minutes with occasional agitation to suspend the cells. The cells are then centrifuged, and the supernatant fluid in each tube is examined for the extent of lysis by photometric analysis. Titration with each cell population should be performed in duplicate, and duplicate cell blanks should be set up for each cell suspension. In addition, for each of the cell suspensions a pair of tubes yielding complete lysis should be included. These "completes" are set up by lysing 1.0 ml of cell suspension with 6.5 ml of H_2O. A few milliliters of the complement dilution should be saved so that its optical density at 541 nm can be measured. This reading of the "complement color" is applied on a proportional basis as a correction to the optical density readings of the supernatant fluids from the analyses proper.

The extent of lysis is determined from the OD measurements made at 541 nm by the procedure described below for the titration of complement (Section 17.B.2.b.iv). It is then plotted arithmetically against the reciprocal antiserum dilution to identify the point at which the hemolytic response levels off and becomes virtually independent of further increases in antibody concentration. A dilution of the antiserum supplying roughly twice the amount of antibody present at this point is used for optimal sensitization of the sheep erythrocytes. In this way, the effect of small day-to-day variations in hemolysin dilution on complement titers will be minimized. Discard sera which do not show a plateau in the hemolytic response to within a few percent of lysis.

b. Measurement of Overall Hemolytic Activity of Complement

The hemolytic unit of guinea pig complement, CH_{50}, is defined as milliliters of undiluted serum sufficient to lyse 2.5×10^8 optimally sensitized sheep erythrocytes out of a total of 5×10^8 cells, in the presence of optimal concentrations of Ca^{2+} and Mg^{2+}, at pH 7.3 and ionic strength 0.149, in 1 hour of incubation at 37° in a total volume of 7.5 ml. All the aforementioned variables affect the hemolytic activity of complement and must be controlled.[1]

i. Incubation Time

Particular mention should be made of the incubation time, which represents an end point for the hemolytic action of guinea pig complement but not necessarily for that of complement from other species; e.g., it has been found that, with human complement, the cells lyse at a relatively rapid but declining rate during the first 90 minutes of incubation, and at a slower but nearly constant rate for hours thereafter, yielding ca 50% more lysis after 5 hours of incubation than after 90 minutes.[5] In titrations of human complement, accordingly, the incubation time represents an arbitrary factor that must be specified.

ii. Divalent Cations

It cannot be taken for granted that the concentrations of divalent cations which are optimal for guinea pig complement are also optimal for complement from other species; e.g., for human complement, the optimal divalent cation concentration is 1.0 mM Mg^{2+}.[5] As stated above, the diluent used in the titration of guinea pig complement is buffer containing 0.15 mM Ca^{2+} and 0.5 mM Mg^{2+}.

iii. Absorption of Guinea Pig Complement with Sheep Cells

Before titrating complement, natural hemolytic antibody must be removed from the guinea pig serum. This is done by absorbing 100 ml of ice-cold, undiluted serum three successive times with 3-ml portions of packed sheep erythrocytes previously washed with isotonic saline. The suspension is kept at 0° for 10 minutes for each absorption before being centrifuged at 0°. (The low temperature prevents hemolysis.)

iv. Procedure

In the titration procedure, the following sequence of adding reagents is recommended: (1) 1.0 ml of sensitized erythrocytes (Section 17.B.1.d); (2) buffer in a volume to make the *final* reaction volume 7.5 ml; (3) the desired volume of an appropriate dilution of complement delivered from a calibrated pipette, which is held to the inside wall of the tube above the surface of the liquid.

The hemolytic reaction is performed in wide-mouth 40- or 50-ml centrifuge tubes which permit mixing of the contents by rotary motion during addition of the complement. The tubes are stoppered or capped to prevent evaporation of water during incubation.

If experimental determination of the hemolytic response curve is desired, a series of closely spaced dilutions (approximately 1.1- or 1.2-fold steps) of complement is prepared with calibrated pipettes and volumetric flasks. In the reaction system described here, 1.0 ml of a 1:200 dilution of guinea pig serum will produce a degree of lysis ranging between 40% and 70%, hence 1.0-ml portions of a series of spaced dilutions from about

[5] L. G. Hoffmann, "Further Studies on the Terminal Transformation Reaction in Immune Hemolysis," Thesis, The Johns Hopkins University, School of Hygiene and Public Health (1958).

1:130 to about 1:300 or 1:350, should yield a series of points covering the entire range of the response curve. Instead of preparing such a series of dilutions with calibrated pipettes, it is simpler to prepare a 1:800 dilution of guinea pig complement and to add 2.50-, 3.00-, 3.50-, 4.00-, 5.00-, and 6.00-ml portions of this dilution with calibrated pipettes to the series of reaction tubes. The total reaction volume must be kept uniform, i.e., 7.5 ml, because of the "volume effect" in the hemolytic action of complement.[1]

It is advisable to hold the reagents at 0° and set up the reaction mixtures at 0° to retard the action of complement until all tubes are prepared. The entire set is then placed in the water bath at 37° for 60 minutes with occasional mixing of the contents to keep the cells in uniform suspension. Each set of titrations should include duplicate cell blanks, as well as duplicate "completes" for which 1 ml of a 1:40 dilution of guinea pig complement can be used.

At the end of the incubation period, the tubes are centrifuged to remove unlysed cells and the clear supernatant fluids are analyzed photometrically for oxyhemoglobin at 541 nm. In addition, an optical density reading is taken of a low dilution of the guinea pig complement (e.g., 1:40) in order to obtain the correction for complement color. The OD readings of the supernatant fluids from all the tubes, including the "completes," are corrected by subtraction of the absorbancy values of the cell blanks, which should not exceed 1 or 2% lysis, as well as by subtraction of the appropriate complement color values. In addition, it is advisable to apply corrections, positive or negative, for light absorption, if any, by the spectrophotometric cuvettes when filled with water. It is not uncommon to find that cuvettes differ in such blank readings by OD values of 0.002 or 0.003. The spectrophotometric cuvettes should be selected also for uniformity of light path; any appreciable deviation should be corrected factorially. After application of all these corrections, the fraction of cells lysed in each tube is calculated by dividing its corrected OD value by the corrected OD of the "complete."

The hemolytic dose-response curve of complement is described by the equation of von Krogh[6]:

$$x = K(y/1 - y)^{1/n}$$

or

$$\log x = \log K + (1/n)\log[y/(1 - y)]$$

where x = the amount of complement, in milliliters of diluted guinea pig serum; y = the fraction of cells lysed; $1/n$ is a number that depends on experimental conditions but equals 0.2 ± 0.02 under the standard

[6] M. von Krogh, J. Infect. Dis. **19**, 452 (1916).

conditions described above; and K is the CH_{50}, since $x = K$ when $y = 0.5$.

The experimental results are evaluated by plotting $\log[y/(1-y)]$ against $\log x$; the use of 2×3 cycle log-log graph paper is recommended. (Alternatively, the probit function can be used for evaluation of results.[7]) The values of $y/(1-y)$ corresponding to a range of y from 0.1 to 0.9 are given in Table II. Fit the best line to the experimental points and read the 50% lytic dose of complement from the graph. The complement titer is defined as the number of CH_{50} contained in 1 ml of undiluted serum. For example, if 4.0 ml of a 1:800 dilution of guinea pig serum is required for 50% hemolysis, the titer equals 200 CH_{50} per milliliter.

In addition to evaluating the results of a titration in terms of CH_{50}, the investigator should check the value of $1/n$ by measuring the slope of the line representing the logarithmic form of the von Krogh equation. Serious deviation of $1/n$ from the value 0.2 may indicate experimental error.

Sometimes it is not practicable to perform hemolytic analyses at several points within the range of partial lysis. If one point is available between 10 and 90% hemolysis, or better between 20 and 80%, the number of CH_{50} per milliliter can be calculated from the von Krogh equation by assuming that the value 0.2 for the exponent $1/n$ is applicable. The need for calculation can be avoided by use of the conversion factors given in Table III. This table shows the number of CH_{50} required to produce a given degree of lysis. The use of these conversion factors may be illustrated as follows: If 1.0 ml of a 1:250 dilution of complement produces 30% lysis ($y = 0.30$), the number of CH_{50} per milliliter of undiluted complement equals $250 \times 0.844 = 211$ CH_{50}. It should be emphasized that titrations based on a single point are valid only if there is sound basis for assuming a value of 0.2 for $1/n$.

The technique described here is recommended from the standpoint of accuracy of pipetting and photometric analysis, but when desired, titrations can be performed in smaller reaction volumes. Results will be the same, provided all reagents are scaled down proportionately. For example, with a sample of guinea pig complement containing 200 CH_{50} per milliliter, 0.2 ml of a 1:200 dilution added to 10^8 sensitized cells in a total reaction volume of 1.5 ml will yield 50% lysis.*

---

[7] B. H. Waksman, *J. Immunol.* **63**, 409 (1949).

* Such a procedure is approximately 5 times more sensitive than the one given above in detail. Where increased sensitivity is an important goal, and it is desired to avoid micromanipulation, the technique of J. F. Kent, S. C. Bukantz, and C. R. Rein [*J. Immunol.* **53**, 37 (1946)] is recommended.

TABLE II
$y/1 - y$ VALUES

	0	0.1	0.2	0.3	0.4	0.5	0.6	0.7	0.8	0.9	
10	0.111	0.112	0.114	0.115	0.116	0.117	0.119	0.120	0.121	0.122	10
11	0.124	0.125	0.126	0.127	0.129	0.130	0.131	0.133	0.134	0.135	11
12	0.136	0.138	0.139	0.140	0.142	0.143	0.144	0.145	0.147	0.148	12
13	0.149	0.151	0.152	0.153	0.155	0.156	0.157	0.159	0.160	0.161	13
14	0.163	0.164	0.166	0.167	0.168	0.170	0.171	0.172	0.174	0.175	14
15	0.176	0.178	0.179	0.181	0.182	0.183	0.185	0.186	0.188	0.189	15
16	0.190	0.192	0.193	0.195	0.196	0.198	0.199	0.200	0.202	0.203	16
17	0.205	0.206	0.208	0.209	0.211	0.212	0.214	0.215	0.217	0.218	17
18	0.220	0.221	0.222	0.224	0.225	0.227	0.229	0.230	0.232	0.233	18
19	0.235	0.236	0.238	0.239	0.241	0.242	0.244	0.245	0.247	0.248	19
20	0.250	0.252	0.253	0.255	0.256	0.258	0.259	0.261	0.263	0.264	20
21	0.266	0.267	0.269	0.271	0.272	0.274	0.276	0.277	0.279	0.280	21
22	0.282	0.284	0.285	0.287	0.289	0.290	0.292	0.294	0.295	0.297	22
23	0.299	0.300	0.302	0.304	0.305	0.307	0.309	0.311	0.312	0.314	23
24	0.316	0.318	0.319	0.321	0.323	0.325	0.326	0.328	0.330	0.332	24
25	0.333	0.335	0.337	0.339	0.340	0.342	0.344	0.346	0.348	0.350	25
26	0.351	0.353	0.355	0.357	0.359	0.361	0.362	0.364	0.366	0.368	26
27	0.370	0.372	0.374	0.376	0.377	0.379	0.381	0.383	0.385	0.387	27
28	0.389	0.391	0.393	0.395	0.397	0.399	0.401	0.403	0.404	0.406	28
29	0.408	0.410	0.412	0.414	0.416	0.418	0.420	0.422	0.425	0.427	29
30	0.429	0.431	0.433	0.435	0.437	0.439	0.441	0.443	0.445	0.447	30
31	0.449	0.451	0.453	0.456	0.458	0.460	0.462	0.464	0.466	0.468	31
32	0.471	0.473	0.475	0.477	0.479	0.481	0.484	0.486	0.488	0.490	32
33	0.493	0.495	0.497	0.499	0.502	0.504	0.506	0.508	0.511	0.513	33
34	0.515	0.517	0.520	0.522	0.524	0.527	0.529	0.531	0.534	0.536	34
35	0.538	0.541	0.543	0.546	0.548	0.550	0.553	0.555	0.558	0.560	35
36	0.563	0.565	0.567	0.570	0.572	0.575	0.577	0.580	0.582	0.585	36
37	0.587	0.590	0.592	0.595	0.597	0.600	0.603	0.605	0.608	0.610	37
38	0.613	0.616	0.618	0.621	0.623	0.626	0.629	0.631	0.634	0.637	38
39	0.639	0.642	0.645	0.647	0.650	0.653	0.656	0.658	0.661	0.664	39
40	0.667	0.669	0.672	0.675	0.678	0.681	0.684	0.686	0.689	0.692	40
41	0.695	0.698	0.701	0.704	0.706	0.709	0.712	0.715	0.718	0.721	41
42	0.724	0.727	0.730	0.733	0.736	0.739	0.742	0.745	0.748	0.751	42
43	0.754	0.757	0.761	0.764	0.767	0.770	0.773	0.776	0.779	0.783	43
44	0.786	0.789	0.792	0.795	0.799	0.802	0.805	0.808	0.812	0.815	44
45	0.818	0.822	0.825	0.828	0.832	0.835	0.838	0.842	0.845	0.848	45
46	0.852	0.855	0.859	0.862	0.866	0.869	0.873	0.876	0.880	0.883	46
47	0.887	0.890	0.894	0.898	0.901	0.905	0.908	0.912	0.916	0.919	47
48	0.923	0.927	0.931	0.934	0.938	0.942	0.946	0.949	0.953	0.957	48
49	0.961	0.965	0.969	0.972	0.976	0.980	0.984	0.988	0.992	0.996	49

TABLE II—(Continued)

	0	0.1	0.2	0.3	0.4	0.5	0.6	0.7	0.8	0.9	
50	1.000	1.004	1.008	1.012	1.016	1.020	1.024	1.028	1.033	1.037	50
51	1.041	1.045	1.049	1.053	1.058	1.062	1.066	1.070	1.075	1.079	51
52	1.083	1.088	1.092	1.096	1.101	1.105	1.110	1.114	1.119	1.123	52
53	1.128	1.132	1.137	1.141	1.146	1.151	1.155	1.160	1.165	1.169	53
54	1.174	1.179	1.183	1.188	1.193	1.198	1.203	1.208	1.212	1.217	54
55	1.222	1.227	1.232	1.237	1.242	1.247	1.252	1.257	1.262	1.268	55
56	1.273	1.278	1.283	1.288	1.294	1.299	1.304	1.309	1.315	1.320	56
57	1.326	1.331	1.336	1.342	1.348	1.353	1.358	1.364	1.370	1.375	57
58	1.381	1.387	1.392	1.398	1.404	1.410	1.415	1.421	1.427	1.433	58
59	1.439	1.445	1.451	1.457	1.463	1.469	1.475	1.481	1.488	1.494	59
60	1.500	1.506	1.513	1.519	1.525	1.532	1.538	1.545	1.551	1.558	60
61	1.564	1.571	1.577	1.584	1.591	1.597	1.604	1.611	1.618	1.625	61
62	1.632	1.639	1.646	1.653	1.660	1.667	1.674	1.681	1.688	1.695	62
63	1.703	1.710	1.717	1.725	1.732	1.740	1.747	1.755	1.762	1.770	63
64	1.778	1.786	1.793	1.801	1.809	1.817	1.825	1.833	1.841	1.849	64
65	1.857	1.865	1.874	1.882	1.890	1.899	1.907	1.915	1.924	1.933	65
66	1.941	1.950	1.959	1.967	1.976	1.985	1.994	2.003	2.012	2.021	66
67	2.030	2.040	2.049	2.058	2.067	2.077	2.086	2.096	2.106	2.115	67
68	2.125	2.135	2.145	2.155	2.165	2.175	2.185	2.195	2.205	2.215	68
69	2.226	2.236	2.247	2.257	2.268	2.279	2.289	2.300	2.311	2.322	69
70	2.333	2.344	2.356	2.367	2.378	2.390	2.401	2.413	2.425	2.436	70
71	2.448	2.460	2.472	2.484	2.497	2.509	2.521	2.534	2.546	2.559	71
72	2.571	2.584	2.597	2.610	2.623	2.636	2.650	2.663	2.676	2.690	72
73	2.704	2.717	2.731	2.745	2.759	2.774	2.788	2.802	2.817	2.831	73
74	2.846	2.861	2.876	2.891	2.906	2.922	2.937	2.953	2.968	2.984	74
75	3.000	3.016	3.032	3.049	3.065	3.082	3.098	3.115	3.132	3.149	75
76	3.167	3.184	3.202	3.219	3.237	3.255	3.274	3.292	3.310	3.329	76
77	3.348	3.367	3.386	3.405	3.425	3.444	3.464	3.484	3.505	3.525	77
78	3.545	3.566	3.587	3.608	3.630	3.651	3.673	3.695	3.717	3.739	78
79	3.762	3.785	3.808	3.831	3.854	3.878	3.902	3.926	3.950	3.975	79
80	4.000	4.025	4.050	4.076	4.102	4.128	4.155	4.181	4.208	4.236	80
81	4.263	4.291	4.319	4.348	4.376	4.405	4.435	4.464	4.495	4.525	81
82	4.556	4.587	4.618	4.650	4.682	4.714	4.747	4.780	4.814	4.848	82
83	4.882	4.917	4.952	4.988	5.024	5.061	5.098	5.135	5.173	5.211	83
84	5.250	5.289	5.329	5.369	5.410	5.452	5.494	5.536	5.579	5.623	84
85	5.667	5.711	5.757	5.803	5.849	5.897	5.944	5.993	6.042	6.092	85
86	6.143	6.194	6.246	6.299	6.353	6.407	6.463	6.519	6.576	6.634	86
87	6.692	6.752	6.813	6.874	6.937	7.000	7.065	7.130	7.197	7.264	87
88	7.333	7.403	7.475	7.547	7.621	7.696	7.772	7.850	7.929	8.009	88
89	8.091	8.174	8.259	8.346	8.434	8.524	8.615	8.709	8.804	8.901	89
90	9.000	9.101	9.204	9.309	9.417	9.526	9.638	9.753	9.870	9.989	90

TABLE III
Units of CH_{50} Required to Produce Given Degrees of Lysis[a]

Degree of lysis	CH_{50}	Degree of lysis	CH_{50}
0.10	0.644	0.55	1.041
0.12	0.671	0.60	1.084
0.14	0.696	0.65	1.132
0.16	0.718	0.70	1.185
0.18	0.738	0.75	1.246
0.20	0.758	0.80	1.320
0.25	0.803	0.82	1.354
0.30	0.844	0.84	1.393
0.35	0.884	0.86	1.438
0.40	0.922	0.88	1.490
0.45	0.961	0.90	1.552
0.50	1.000		

[a] Conversion factors calculated from the von Krogh equation for $1/n = 0.2$.

c. Titration of Hemolytic Antibody

The unit of hemolytic antibody, AbH_{50}, is defined as the amount of antiserum, in milliliters, that will lyse 5×10^8 sheep erythrocytes out of a total of 10^9 cells in the presence of 12 CH_{50} units of complement in exactly 15 minutes at 37° in a total reaction volume of 5.0 ml, at pH 7.3, ionic strength 0.149, and in the presence of optimal concentrations of Ca^{2+} and Mg^{2+}.

The following reagents are used: (1) buffer containing 0.15 mM Ca^{2+} and 0.5 mM Mg^{2+} and gelatin, either GVB^{2+} or GTB^{2+} of Table I; (2) standardized erythrocyte suspension containing 5×10^8 cells (not sensitized) per milliliter; (3) a series of accurately prepared dilutions of the hemolytic antiserum, spaced by a factor of ca 1.2; (4) a dilution of guinea pig complement containing 6 CH_{50} per milliliter; usually a dilution of ca. 1:30 or 1:40 is required. The natural hemolysin of the guinea pig serum must be removed (cf. Section 17.B.2.b). (5) Isotonic citrate–saline solution chilled to 0°: 1 part of aqueous 0.075 M sodium citrate (22.06 gm of sodium citrate dihydrate per liter) is mixed with 4 parts of aqueous 0.15 M NaCl; this solution serves to stop the lytic reaction. The procedure for the titration is as follows: Measure out a series of 2.0-ml portions of the cell suspension into 40- or 50-ml centrifuge tubes. Add 1.0 ml each of the appropriate dilutions of hemolytic antiserum slowly and with constant mixing to ensure uniform distribution of the hemolytic antibody upon the cells. Incubate 15 minutes at 37°. Add 2.0

ml of the diluted guinea pig complement (12 CH_{50}) and incubate at 37° with occasional mixing to maintain the cells in uniform suspension. After exactly 15 minutes, add 10.0 ml of ice-cold citrate–saline solution, mix, centrifuge, remove the clear supernatant fluid, and determine oxyhemoglobin photometrically as in complement titration (Section 17.B.2.a).

The incubation time for the lytic reaction is 15 minutes, which must be timed precisely. This is done conveniently by spacing the addition of complement to individual reaction tubes at intervals of exactly 0.5 or 1 minute. At the end of the 15-minute reaction period, the citrate–saline solution is added to the tubes in the same sequence at intervals of exactly 0.5 or 1 minute.

A less accurate, but more convenient, scaled-down procedure is as follows: Use 0.5-ml portions of red cell suspension, 0.5 ml of antiserum dilution, 0.25 ml of a dilution of guinea pig complement containing 12 CH_{50} per milliliter (ca. 1:15 or 1:20) and finally 2.5 ml of citrate–saline. In essence, this modified procedure represents an analysis with 1:4 the quantities of all the reagents, except for two alterations, i.e., doubling the volume of antiserum for the sake of greater precision of measurement and making a corresponding decrease in the volume of complement from 0.5 to 0.25 ml to maintain the total reaction volume at the proper volume (1.25 ml). In this procedure, the dilution of the guinea pig complement is altered by a factor of 0.5. Since twice the volume of antiserum is used, its dilutions should be double those employed in the large-scale titration.

Use the von Krogh equation (or probit function) to evaluate the data as in the titration of complement. In the large-scale assay, the titer of the hemolytic antiserum equals the reciprocal of the dilution yielding 50% hemolysis. In the small-scale titration, the reciprocal of the dilution yielding 50% lysis is divided by 2 to obtain the titer.

3. COMPLEMENT FIXATION TESTS

The many versions of the complement fixation test in use may be divided into two categories: the serologic type, used primarily for diagnostic work,* and the quantitative type, used for detailed studies of antigen–antibody reactions. Each type will be discussed separately.

* Other methodologies for diagnostic complement fixation, particularly for antiviral or antirickettsial antibodies, are given by E. H. Lennette and N. J. Schmidt, "Diagnostic Procedures for Viral and Rickettsial Infections," 4th ed., pp. 52–58, American Public Health Ass., Inc. (1969); and by the Public Health Service, U.S. Department of Health, Education, and Welfare [*Pub. Health Monogr.* No. 74, Standardized Diagnostic Complement Fixation Method and Adaptation to Micro Test (1965)] and A Guide to the Performance of the Standardized Diagnostic Complement Fixation Method and Adaptation to Micro Test (National Communicable Disease Center, Atlanta, Georgia, 1969). In the Public Health Monograph,

The diluent for all C-fixation procedures using guinea pig complement is buffer containing 0.15 mM and Ca^{2+} and 0.5 mM Mg^{2+} and gelatin (GVB^{2+} or GTB^{2+}; Table I).

a. Serologic Complement Fixation Test

i. Standard Procedure

This is the method originally described in Kabat and Mayer.[1] Pooled guinea pig serum, distributed in test tubes or glass ampoules after absorption of natural hemolysin with packed sheep erythrocytes (cf. Section 17.B.2.b.iii) and stored at −40°, serves as complement. The hemolytic activity of each pool is determined by titration (Section 17.B.2.c) of the contents of one or two ampoules. If all test tubes or ampoules containing the same pool of guinea pig serum have been treated uniformly, it can be assumed that their contents have the same titer of hemolytic complement. Hence it is not necessary to titrate the complement before each complement fixation test, yet a simple and approximate control titration is included with each complement fixation test, as explained below.

While a spectrophotometric titration of complement is performed in a total reaction volume of 7.5 ml (Section 17.B.2.a.ii), serologic complement fixation tests are set up on one-fifth this scale, i.e., with a final hemolytic reaction volume of 1.5 ml, and results are read by visual inspection. The unit of complement is also scaled down by a factor of 5. For example, with a sample of guinea pig complement that contains 200 CH$_{50}$ per milliliter (determined in the photometric titration with 5×10^8 optimally sensitized cells in a total reaction volume of 7.5 ml), 0.2 ml of a 1:200 dilution added to 1×10^8 sensitized cells in a total reaction volume of 1.5 ml will yield 50% lysis.

Appropriate dilutions of antiserum and antigen are prepared for the complement fixation test so that 0.4 ml of each will contain the desired quantity. Make a dilution of guinea pig serum so that 0.5 ml will contain 5 CH$_{50}$ (this statement applies to the one-fifth scale system). Since guinea pig serum usually contains about 200–250 CH$_{50}$ per 0.2 ml (one-fifth scale system), 0.5 ml of a 1:100 or 1:125 dilution will usually furnish approximately 5 CH$_{50}$ units. The actual dilution of guinea pig serum needed should be calculated from the hemolytic titer. The complement

---

popularly termed the Laboratory Branch CF Method, 11 hemoglobin color standards are prepared daily, to represent degrees of hemolysis (in percent, 0, 10, 20, 30, 40, 50, 60, 70, 80, 90, 100), as visual standards for recording results of complement-fixation tests.

fixation test is set up by mixing 0.4 ml of antiserum dilution, 0.5 ml of diluted guinea pig serum as a source of complement, and 0.4 ml of antigen dilution. This reaction mixture may be kept either for 90 minutes at 37° or for about 20 hours at 2 to 4°. Overnight incubation in the cold has been found to be the more sensitive procedure. At the end of the incubation period, 0.2 ml of a suspension of sensitized erythrocytes (5×10^8 cells per milliliter as in Section 17.B.1.d) is added, the contents are mixed, and the tubes are incubated at 37° for 60 minutes in a water bath with occasional agitation in order to maintain the cells in uniform suspension.

Several types of controls must be included; these are readily apparent in Table IV. The test proper appears as Part A, panel 1. Since antiserum or antigen, or both, may "fix" or inactivate complement alone, i.e., nonspecifically, it is necessary to include control tubes that contain antigen and complement without antiserum (Part A, panel 2) and antiserum and complement without antigen (Part A, panels 3a and 3b). In order to rule out nonspecific reactions reliably, it is advisable to run these "anticomplementary" controls in a dual fashion, viz., both with 5 CH_{50} (panel 3a) and with 3 CH_{50} (panel 3b). For 3 CH_{50} units, use 0.3 ml of the diluted guinea pig serum instead of 0.5 ml, and make up the difference in volume with 0.2 ml of diluent panel 3 b). It is essential to maintain constant volume, since the hemolytic activity of complement depends on concentration. Controls on the stability of complement during primary incubation are shown in Table IV, Part B.

It is also necessary to ascertain whether either antigen or antiserum contains any substance that hemolyses erythrocytes nonspecifically, i.e., without the benefit of complement (compare Table IV, Part C). This difficulty does not arise frequently, but the highest concentration of antiserum and the highest concentration of antigen should be checked for direct hemolytic activity on sheep erythrocytes in the *absence* of complement.

The antiserum to be tested for ability to fix complement should be heated for 30 minutes at 56° to inactivate its complement. Usually it is not advisable to work with dilutions less than 1:5, although in some routine diagnostic tests, in which patient's sera are tested within 1 or 2 days after collection, dilutions as low as 1:2 are used. In *titrations* of sera from patients or experimental animals the optimal quantity of antigen must be determined experimentally by testing a series of different dilutions as shown in Table IV, Part A.

The degrees of lysis in the test and in the control tubes are read visually; color standards for purposes of comparison may be prepared by mixing a standardized suspension of red cells and a solution of hemoglobin in such proportions as to simulate 0%, 25%, 50%, 75%, and 100%

TABLE IV

PROTOCOL FOR SEROLOGIC COMPLEMENT FIXATION[a]

Part A: Test for Complement Fixation

Antigen (volume and dilution)	Volume and dilution of antiserum					Control	
	0.4 ml 1:10	0.4 ml 1:20	0.4 ml 1:40	0.4 ml 1:80	0.4 ml 1:160	0.4 ml diluent	0.6 ml diluent
0.4 ml 1:1000 0.4 ml 1:2000 0.4 ml 1:4000 0.4 ml 1:8000 0.4 ml 1:16,000	(1) Complement (0.5 ml of a dilution containing 5 CH_{50}) is added to all tubes					(2) 0.3 ml of same dilution of complement	
0.4 ml diluent	(3a)						
0.6 ml diluent	(3b) 0.3 ml of same dilution of complement						

Part B: Test for Deterioration of Complement

Reagents	Tube number				
	1	2	3	4	5
Dilution of complement containing 5 CH_{50} per 0.5 ml (ml to be added)	0.1	0.2	0.3	0.4	0.5
Barbital–saline buffer (GVB) (ml to be added)	1.2	1.1	1.0	0.9	0.8
Dilution of complement containing 3 CH_{50} per 0.5 ml (ml to be added)	0.1	0.2	0.3	0.4	0.5
Barbital–saline buffer (GVB) (ml to be added)	1.2	1.1	1.0	0.9	0.8

Part C: Tests for Lytic Effects of Reagents

0.4 ml 1:10 antiserum + 0.9 ml of diluent
0.4 ml 1:1000 antigen + 0.9 ml of diluent

[a] Heat-inactivated (56° for 30 minutes in a water bath) antiserum is tested. The meaning of the various controls is explained in the text. After all tubes have been incubated at 37° for 90 minutes or at 2 to 4° for 20 hours, 0.2 ml of GVB or GTB diluent containing 2.5×10^8 sensitized erythrocytes is added to each tube. The final incubation is carried out at 37° for 60 minutes prior to reading the degree of lysis. Record as follows: 0 = no lysis; 1 = ca 25% lysis; 2 = ca 50% lysis; 3 = ca 75% lysis; 4 = approximately 100% lysis. Note that triethanolamine buffer (GTB) can be used instead of GVB.

lysis. Tubes showing 50% lysis or less are read best by comparing the clear supernatants after the unlysed cells have settled, while those above 50% lysis can be read readily when the unlysed cells are kept in suspension.

With human and rabbit antisera, the highest dilution of antibody fixing C (i.e., the apparent "antibody titer") will generally vary in a systematic fashion with the dilution of antigen, i.e., the apparent antibody titer will increase with increasing dilutions of antigen up to a point beyond which a higher dilution of antigen will not fix complement with any dilution of antibody. A representative example is shown in Table V. The amount of complement fixed depends on both the amount and composition of immune aggregates present. No fixation is observed below a minimum amount of immune aggregate, hence the failure of very high dilutions of antigen to fix complement with any dilution of antibody. On the other hand, complement fixation is inhibited by excess antigen, a condition that will occur at a high antibody dilution if a low antigen dilution is used. The complement-fixing titer of an antiserum is therefore expressed as

TABLE V

TWO-DIMENSIONAL COMPLEMENT-FIXATION TEST WITH BOVINE SERUM ALBUMIN AND HOMOLOGOUS RABBIT ANTIBODY (SECOND COURSE ANTISERUM)[a,b]

Bovine serum albumin N per test mixture (μg)	Antibody nitrogen per test mixture (μg)									
	4	2	1	0.5	0.25	0.125	0.063	0.031	0.016	0
1	0	0	1	1	4	4	4	4	4	4
0.5	0	0	0	0	4	4	4	4	4	4
0.25	0	0	0	0	4	4	4	4	4	4
0.125	0	0	0	0	1	4	4	4	4	4
0.063	0	0	0	0	0	3	4	4	4	4
0.031	0	0	0	0	0	1	4	4	4	4
0.016	0	0	0	0	0	0	4	4	4	4
0.008	0	0	0	0	0	0	2	4	4	4
0.004	0	0	0	0	0	0	1	4	4	4
0.002	0	0	0	0	0	0	3	3.5	4	4
0.001	3	3	3	3	3	3	3	3.5	4	4
0	4	4	4	4	4	4	4	4	4	4

[a] From A. L. Wallace, A. G. Osler, and M. M. Mayer, *J. Immunol.* **65**, 661 (1950).
[b] Five CH_{50} units of guinea pig complement were used; total fixation volume = 1.3 ml; 0.2 ml of sensitized red cells standardized as described in experimental part; fixation for 20 hours at 2 to 4°; hemolytic reaction 60 minutes at 37°. Readings are given as degree of hemolysis, with 0 representing no lysis, 4 representing complete lysis.

the highest dilution which fixes complement (i.e., produces 0–50% lysis) with the optimal dilution of antigen. Thus, in the example shown in Table V the optimal amount of antigen is 0.004 μg of nitrogen and the antibody titer corresponds to 0.06 μg antibody nitrogen.

Unfortunately, the optimal dilution of antigen is not constant for a given antigen–antibody system but depends on the quality of the antiserum. Thus, Wallace et al.[8] described two rabbit antisera to bovine serum albumin (BSA), one of which gave optimal complement fixation with 0.063–0.5 μg of BSA nitrogen in the test system, the other with 0.002–008 μg. Accordingly, it is not possible to accept an optimal antigen dilution for a given antigen–antibody system, observed with one serum, as a standard that will allow measuring the antibody content of other sera with the same antigen dilution. Instead, a number of antigen dilutions must be tested with each antiserum.

ii. Microtechnique

A micro modification of the serologic complement-fixation test, which is performed on spot plates made of transparent plastic, has been developed by Fulton and Dumbell.[9] This technique conserves both time and materials, although suitable controls are more difficult to establish.*

In each well in the plastic or lucite depression plate, a microdrop (0.02 ml) of an antiserum dilution is mixed with equal amounts of complement and antigen. The plate is placed in a vapor-tight box containing some water in the bottom. The container is kept in a cold room overnight. The next morning, a large drop (0.04 ml) of sensitized sheep erythrocyte suspension is added to each well, and the plate is incubated for 2 hours in a similar box kept at 37°. Precautions must be taken against evaporation of water since such loss of water will have a double effect on complement activity, viz., reduction of the reaction volume and increase in ionic strength. All additions to the spot plates are performed with calibrated dropping pipettes to minimize variations, particularly in the amounts of complement and EA added, since the actual amount of added complement

[8] A. L. Wallace, A. G. Osler, and M. M. Mayer, J. Immunol. 65, 661 (1950).
[9] F. Fulton and K. R. Dumbell, J. Gen. Microbiol. 3, 97 (1949).
* An even more convenient complement-fixation technique makes use of the Takatsy spiral loops (0.05- and 0.025-ml sizes) and "microtiter" equipment [G. Takatsy, Kiserletes Orvostudomany 2, 393 (1950)] according to J. L. Sever [J. Immunol. 88, 320 (1962)]. Presently, the Cooke Microtiter System with calibrated slotted metal heads is available from Microbiological Associates, Bethesda, Maryland. Diagnostic microtests are described in detail by the Public Health Service, U.S. Department of Health, Education, and Welfare, Public Health Monograph No. 74 (1965) (see footnote, Section 17.B.3).

will determine how much is left after fixation, while the complement titer reflects the cell concentration sensitively.[1]

iii. Indirect Complement Fixation

Heat-inactivated antisera from a number of species (Aves, Bovidae), although known to contain antibody on the basis of other immunologic tests, fail to fix guinea pig complement in the presence of homologous antigen. Such sera have, in fact, been shown to inhibit the fixation of guinea pig complement by homologous antigen and rabbit antibody.[10-13] These observations formed the basis of the development of the indirect complement-fixation test,[14] which is essentially an antigen-binding test.

Procedure. In the indirect complement-fixation test, the antiserum to be analyzed is heat-inactivated and is first allowed to react with its antigen and complement for 2 hours at $0°$; then, a known rabbit antiserum to the antigen is added in sufficient quantity to achieve equivalence between the rabbit antibody and the total amount of antigen present; next, the standard procedure for complement fixation (Section 17.B.3.a.i) is followed. The volumes of reagents added should be adjusted so that the final volume of the test, comprising test serum, antigen, complement, and rabbit antiserum, is 1.3 ml; addition of 0.2 ml of sensitized erythrocyte suspension will bring the volume to the standard 1.5 ml. The results are interpreted in a manner opposite to the one applicable to direct complement fixation: Hemolysis, indicating absence of complement fixation upon addition of rabbit antibody, denotes a positive result, viz., binding of antigen by the test serum. The indirect complement-fixation titer of the test serum is the highest dilution giving 50–100% lysis.

Controls should include: (1) a series of dilutions of the test serum + complement + diluent, to check for inactivation of complement by the test serum alone; (2) a parallel series of dilutions of the test serum with complement, antigen, and diluent, to check for *direct* complement fixation by the test serum; (3) a few dilutions of the standard rabbit antiserum, both higher and lower than that used in the test, with antigen and complement and diluent, to make certain that the dilution of standard antiserum employed is near equivalence; and (4) a similar test with several dilutions of antigen with complement and standard rabbit antiserum and diluent, to ascertain that the amount of antigen used is the minimum

[10] K. Goodner and F. L. Horsfall, Jr., *J. Exp. Med.* **64**, 201 (1936).
[11] C. E. Rice, *Can. J. Comp. Med. Vet. Sci.* **11**, 236 (1947).
[12] C. E. Rice, *J. Immunol.* **59**, 365 (1948).
[13] C. E. Rice and J. B. Brooksby, *J. Immunol.* **71**, 300 (1953).
[14] C. E. Rice, *J. Immunol.* **60**, 11 (1948).

required for complement fixation in the absence of test serum. Additional controls for complement activity, complement inactivation by antigen alone, and hemolysis by the test serum alone, should be included as in the direct complement-fixation test (cf. Table IV).

The dilutions of antigen and standard rabbit antiserum should be chosen on the basis of a preliminary direct complement-fixation test, so that the antigen dilution provides the minimum amount of antigen required for complete fixation; the standard antiserum dilution should contain enough antibody to place the system in the equivalence zone or in slight antibody excess with respect to the amount of antigen used.

The conditions for the primary interaction between the test serum and antigen may have to be altered to suit the requirements of the system under study; complement should be omitted at this point and added later with the standard rabbit antiserum if incubation for prolonged periods or at temperatures above 2° is necessary. The specificity of the antigen and standard rabbit antiserum is of obvious importance: If several antigens and antibodies are present, a test serum containing antibody to only some of the antigens will produce negative results because the remaining antigen(s) will be left to fix complement with the corresponding rabbit antibodies.

iv. Problems Encountered with Avian and Cattle Antisera

The failure of heated antisera of several species to fix guinea pig complement may be circumvented in a number of ways other than indirect complement fixation. The simplest of these is omitting heat inactivation. It has been found that avian antisera which fail to fix guinea pig complement after being heated do so when fresh.[15, 16] Unfortunately, this immediately leads to the problem that various amounts of a presumably heat-labile factor are introduced into the test with the various antiserum dilutions, and it is no longer possible to tell whether the test is measuring antibody or this heat-labile factor. Brumfield and Pomeroy[17] showed that this difficulty can be avoided by introducing fresh normal chicken serum into the test to replace the factor that is lost from the test serum by heat inactivation. The amount used is the maximum that will not inactivate guinea pig complement in the absence of antigen and antibody. Benson et al.[18] concluded, from the solubility properties and Ca^{2+} requirement of the heat-labile factor in question, that it is chicken C1. They

[15] L. D. Bushnell and C. B. Hudson, *J. Infec. Dis.* **41**, 388 (1927).
[16] H. P. Brumfield and B. S. Pomeroy, *Proc. Soc. Exp. Biol. Med.* **94**, 146 (1957).
[17] H. P. Brumfield and B. S. Pomeroy, *Proc. Soc. Exp. Biol. Med.* **102**, 278 (1959).
[18] H. N. Benson, H. P. Brumfield, and B. S. Pomeroy, *J. Immunol.* **87**, 616 (1961).

showed that chicken midpiece and guinea pig endpiece* could replace fresh chicken serum and guinea pig complement in a direct complement-fixation test with heat inactivated fowl antisera.

Likewise, Marucci[19, 20] showed that antibody could be detected by complement fixation in heat-inactivated sera from cattle infected or vaccinated with foot-and-mouth disease virus if vesicular fluid was used as the antigen, but not if a suspension of ground, infected tongue epithelium or a filtrate of ground, infected tissue culture material was used. It has been suggested[1] that the vesicular fluid supplies a heat-labile factor similar to the one discussed above; this might explain the anomalous results obtained with high antigen dilutions, which fix complement only with low antiserum dilutions, in contrast to the usual finding that the highest antigen dilution which fixes complement at all produces the highest antiserum dilution titer (cf. Table V, Section 17.B.3.a.i).

One reason for failure to observe fixation of guinea pig complement by heated antisera may be the low sensitivity of the serologic complement-fixation test; thus, Osler et al.[21] showed that horse antiserum to pneumococcal polysaccharide fixes guinea pig complement in the quantitative complement-fixation test, but not in the serologic test. Nevertheless, differences between the behavior of antibodies of different species can be pronounced.

b. QUANTITATIVE COMPLEMENT FIXATION

i. Standard Procedure

As described by Mayer et al.[22] these analyses are performed by allowing the desired quantities of antigen and antibody to react with a rather large quantity of complement (50, 100, or 200 or more CH_{50} units) either for 90 minutes at 37° or 20 hours at 2° to 4°. At the end of the fixation period, accurately measured samples of the reaction mixture are diluted appropriately and quantitative hemolytic complement titrations are performed (Section 17.B.2.c) in order to determine the number of residual CH_{50}.

---

* Complement components were shown in 1907 to 1910 to be split into two fractions which separately displayed no activity. "Midpiece" is the fraction precipitated with serum globulin; it fixes directly to sensitized erythrocytes. "Endpiece" is serum deprived of midpiece; it attaches to and allows hemolysis of the midpiece-sensitized cell complex. See Section 17.D.1.a.

[19] A. A. Marucci, Amer. J. Vet. Res. 18, 785 (1957).
[20] A. A. Marucci, Amer. J. Vet. Res. 19, 979 (1958).
[21] A. G. Osler, M. M. Hawrisiak, Z. Ovary, M. Siqueira, and O. G. Bier, J. Exp. Med. 106, 811 (1957).
[22] M. M. Mayer, A. G. Osler, O. G. Bier, and M. Heidelberger, J. Immunol. 59, 195 (1948).

In most studies in which this procedure has been employed, a total volume of 10 ml has been used for the fixation reaction. Thus, 2.5 ml of an appropriate dilution of antiserum are mixed in the cold in 40-ml wide-mouth Pyrex centrifuge tubes, with 5.0 ml of a dilution of guinea pig serum containing the number of CH_{50} desired. Large tubes are used in order to facilitate mixing of reagents. After addition of complement, 2.5 ml of an appropriate dilution of the antigen are added with thorough mixing. The tubes are capped and incubated in a water bath at 37° or kept in a refrigerator at 2° to 4° overnight. (In cross-reacting systems it is advisable to maintain accurate control of temperature; for fixation in the cold, the tubes should be kept in an insulated container of crushed ice placed in a refrigerator.) After the indicated period of fixation, the tubes are chilled in ice-water in order to retard any further fixation of complement. A portion of the contents of each tube is diluted with chilled isotonic barbital buffer (GVB^{2+}) to yield a dilution suitable for the estimation of the residual activity of complement in terms of CH_{50}. For example, if it is anticipated that of 50 CH_{50} added, 20 will have been fixed, the 10-ml fixation mixture would then contain 30 CH_{50}, or 1 CH_{50} in 0.33 ml. Hence, hemolytic activity in the range of partial lysis would then be determined by testing 3.0-, 3.5-, and 4.0-ml portions of a 10-fold dilution of the reaction mixture with 1.0 ml of sensitized cells (5×10^8 cells) and sufficient chilled isotonic buffer (in this instance 3.5, 3.0, and 2.5 ml) to make a final volume of 7.5 ml. The contents of the tubes are mixed, and the tubes are capped and incubated at 37° for 60 minutes. After centrifugation the supernatant fluids are analyzed photometrically for hemoglobin to determine the degree of lysis. The activity, in terms of CH_{50}, is obtained by graphic evaluation of von Krogh plots or by calculation with the conversion factors given in Table III (Section 17.B.2.b).

Controls should include two tubes each of complement and diluent, complement and antiserum, complement and antigen. If there are no significant differences among the spectrophotometric readings found in these controls, they are averaged to provide the base line from which the number of CH_{50} fixed in the experimental tubes is calculated. If either the antigen or the antiserum has inactivated some complement, the amount of complement remaining in that control is used as the base line. If both show inactivation, it becomes difficult to choose the correct base line; the best guess is that the amounts of complement inactivated by antigen and antiserum alone are additive, but this cannot be taken for granted.

The range of application of quantitative complement fixation is almost as broad as that of the quantitative precipitin method (described in Vol. III, Chap. 13). A conspicuous exception to this statement is the estimation of the antibody content of an immune serum. This is so, because quantitative complement fixation measures a biological activity of anti-bodies, and the antibodies in different sera, and even in a single serum, are heterogeneous. Thus, the amount of complement fixed under standard conditions per microgram of antibody nitrogen with an equivalent amount of antigen varies over a rather broad range, as can be shown by simultaneous application of the quantitative precipitin and comple-ment-fixation methods.[8] Hill and Osler[23] established a correlation between the aggregation capacity of antibody and its complement-fixing potency.

In other respects, quantitative complement fixation serves as well as the quantitative precipitin method but requires less material and time. By using a constant amount of antibody and varying amounts of antigen, a quantitative complement-fixation curve may be constructed; this curve is similar in appearance to the quantitative precipitin curve, except that complement fixation appears to be less sensitive to excess antigen than precipitation. Once the quantitative complement-fixation curve of an antiserum is established, it can be used for the estimation of antigens with a precision approaching that of the quantitative precipitin method. Quantitative complement fixation has also been used successfully for the study of cross-reactions and inhibition phenomena.

To study the inhibitory action of antigenic fragments on the antigen-antibody reaction by quantitative complement fixation, various amounts of the material to be examined for inhibitory effect are added to a mixture of complement, sufficient antibody to fix ca 80% of the complement, and antigen in equivalent proportion or in slight antigen excess, as established by a quantitative complement-fixation curve. The inhibitor should be added before the antigen; according to Wasserman and Levine,[24] incuba-tion of inhibitor and antibody prior to addition of complement and anti-gen does not affect the results, at least in the pneumococcal system studied by quantitative micro-complement fixation. However, this obser-vation might not be valid generally. All reaction mixtures should be set up in identical volumes. The results are expressed as percent of inhibition; e.g., if the antigen and antibody fix 80 out of 100 CH_{50} in the absence of inhibitor and 60 CH_{50} in the presence of a certain amount of inhibitor, the percentage of inhibition is $100 \times (80 - 60)/80 = 25\%$.

ii. Micromethod

A modification of the quantitative complement-fixation method, capa-ble of detecting nanogram (10^{-9} gm) amounts of antigen and antibody,

[23] B. M. Hill and A. G. Osler, *J. Immunol.* **75**, 146 (1955).
[24] E. Wasserman and L. Levine, *J. Immunol.* **87**, 290 (1961).

has been developed.[24] This method is based on reducing the reaction volume, cell concentration, and complement concentration. The amount of complement used is chosen so as to yield ca 70% lysis with hemolysin and erythrocytes in the absence of antigen and antibody under the conditions of the test. The 10-fold reduction in cell concentration, compared to the standard system, produces a steeper complement dose-response curve, with the result that the fixation of minute amounts of complement results in a detectable reduction in the degree of lysis. The total volume of the test is 0.7 ml, and the reactants are delivered from micropipettes. Hemoglobin concentrations are measured at 413 nm in microcuvettes.

The amount of complement to be used is determined by titration under the conditions of the test. Sensitized sheep erythrocytes are prepared as described in Section 17.B.1.d and diluted to 5×10^7 EA/ml. Samples of zero, 100, 200, 300, 400, 500, and 600 μl of complement, diluted 1:1000, are held for 18 hours at 2° to 4° in a reaction volume of 600 μl in 13×100 mm test tubes, and 100-μl portions of EA are added. The mixtures are incubated for 1 hour at 37°, and the tubes are centrifuged, and the supernatant fluids are collected for hemoglobin measurement. The incubation of the complement samples at 2° to 4° is important because, at the high dilution employed, 25–30% of the complement activity is lost by inactivation. Failure to observe the 2° to 4° temperature step would therefore result in a wrong choice of complement concentration.

The degree of lysis in each tube is calculated in the usual manner (cf. Section 17.B.1.b) and the amount of complement required for 50% lysis is determined by interpolation from a plot of the data. The quantity of complement to be used in the test is 1.1–1.2 times that required for 50% lysis.

The test is set up with 300 μl of buffer, 100 μl of diluted antiserum, 100 μl of complement diluted to the required concentration, and 100 μl each of various dilutions of antigen. Each point is set up in triplicate. Controls include a set of tubes containing complement alone, another set containing antiserum and complement, another set containing the highest concentration of antigen with complement, and a set containing buffer only. The procedure described above for the titration of complement is repeated. Since evaporation of water will give rise to serious errors, the tubes should be capped for all incubations.

The absorbancy values obtained for the antiserum + complement controls are averaged and used as the base line from which complement fixation is reckoned. The difference, ΔOD, between these controls and the tubes containing antigen is taken as a measure of complement fixation and is plotted against the amount of antigen added. A curve similar to the quantitative complement-fixation and precipitin curves is obtained.

The microtechnique may be employed for inhibition studies by incorporating the inhibitor in the diluent. The choice of conditions is the same as for the standard quantitative complement-fixation procedure. The precentage of inhibition is expressed simply as

$$(1 - \Delta OD_{(+inhibitor)})/\Delta OD_{control} \times 100$$

A curious observation has been made in comparing the standard procedure with the microtechnique of quantitative complement fixation for the study of cross-reactions. Murakami et al.[25] reported that a certain rabbit antiserum to denatured T6 phage-DNA showed 40% and 50% cross-reaction with T2 and T4 phage DNA, respectively, with the standard procedure, but no cross-reaction with the micromethod. This phenomenon, which seems to be a general one, has been subjected to detailed investigation by Reichlin et al.[26] and appears to be due, at least in part, to the steeper dose-response curve for immune hemolysis in the microsystem. The practical result is that in the study of cross-reactions, the objective should dictate the choice of complement-fixation method to be used: The micromethod offers maximal sensitivity to small *differences* in antigenic specificity, whereas the standard procedure provides maximal sensitivity to slight *similarities*.

A more extensive discussion of complement fixation, including other modifications, is given by Mayer.[1*]

4. PASSIVE IMMUNE HEMOLYSIS

Sheep erythrocytes may be lysed by complement and antibody directed against a nonerythrocyte antigen if the antigen is first adsorbed on the erythrocytes.[27] A method for performing experiments of this nature has been described by Bloch et al.[28]

Sheep erythrocytes carrying adsorbed antigen are prepared in the same manner as for passive hemagglutination (Section 16.B.1). With protein antigens, several hundred micrograms of antigen are used per billion tanned erythrocytes. An 0.5% suspension of the antigen-coated erythrocytes is prepared in buffer containing 0.15 mM Ca^{2+} and 0.5 mM Mg^{2+},

---

* A modification of the complement-fixation test capable of detecting antigens in the range of 1 to 10 pg (1 to 10×10^{-12} gm) is described by B. W. Moore and V. J. Perez, *J. Immunol.* 96, 1000 (1966).

[25] W. T. Murakami, H. Van Vunakis, H. I. Lehrer, and L. Levine, *J. Immunol.* 89, 116 (1962).

[26] M. Reichlin, M. Hay, and L. Levine, *Immunochemistry* 1, 21 (1964).

[27] G. Middlebrook, *Bull. N.Y. Acad. Med.* 28, 474 (1952).

[28] K. J. Bloch, F. M. Kourilsky, Z. Ovary, and B. Benacerraf, *J. Exp. Med.* 117, 965 (1963).

which is used as the diluent throughout. The antiserum to be examined is heated 30 minutes at 56° to inactivate complement, and absorbed twice with packed sheep erythrocytes to remove natural hemolysin before use. Serial dilutions of the antiserum are prepared, and 0.5 ml of each dilution is added to 0.1 ml of cell suspension. The mixtures are kept at 5° for 18 hours, and then 0.1 ml of guinea pig complement, diluted to 12 CH_{50} per milliliter, is added to each tube, the contents are mixed, and the tubes are incubated 15 minutes at 37°. The degree of lysis is estimated visually as in Section 17.B.3.a.*i*, and the dilution yielding 50% hemolysis is taken as the end point. A control substituting erythrocytes not coated with antigen should always be included.

This technique may be applied to the study of two kinds of inhibition: Antigen in solution may inhibit the lysis of antigen-coated erythrocytes by binding the antibody, and nonhemolytic antibody may inhibit lysis by competing with the lytic antibody for antigen sites on the erythrocytes.

C. Preparation of Hemolytic Intermediates

1. INTRODUCTION*

The complexity of events leading to hemolysis of erythrocytes by complement was approachable only because "erythrocyte reagents" were prepared—erythrocytes coated by specific antibody and then by some of the complement factors, thereby allowing the testing of serum fractions for completion of the hemolytic event. Early reagents were R1, R2, and R3, i.e., serum deprived of $C\overline{1}$ (R1) or of C2 (R2) or of C3-9 (R3); these were found to be inadequate as the complexity of the "complement cascade" (Section 17.A, Fig. 1A) was appreciated. Preparation of these reagents, described as "hemolytic intermediates," requires the availability of separated complement components, presented in Section 17.D.

The reagents used by research workers to titrate components C1 through C9 include the following. To test for C1, there are needed EAC4 and functionally pure C2; for C2, EAC1,4; for C3, EAC1,4,2 + C5–9; for C4, EAC1 and C2; for C5, EAC1,4,2 + C3, C6, C7, C8, C9; for C6, EAC1,4,2 + C3, C5, C7, C8, C9, or use of C6-deficient rabbit serum; for C7, EAC1,4,2,3 + C5, C6, C8, C9; for C8, EAC1–7 plus C9; for C9, EAC1–7 plus C8. (The reaction sequence in testing for C1, C2, or C4 is completed in each instance by adding C-EDTA. EAC1,4,2 can be replaced by EAC1,4 + C2.) EAC4,3 and EAC1q are additional reagents.

An alternative scheme of titration demands monospecific antisera for

* Section 17.C.1 was contributed by the Editors.

each complement component, by means of which one can prepare agar plates containing component-specific antibody and quantitate an unknown *vs* dilutions of the standardized, functionally separated component, by radial immunodiffusion; this test, introduced by Feinberg,[1] is popularly called the "Mancini" test (Vol. III, Chap. 14.C.6.a). Tests that can be arranged to hinge on conversion of C3 to C3a and C3b can be followed by immunoelectrophoretic analysis *vs* anti-C3, since C3 (a β_2-globulin) and its principal fragment (a β-globulin) cross-react: the extent of conversion is shown by shift in electrophoretic migration of the antigen–antibody arc (Section 17.F.2.b, Fig. 1).

By comparison of immunochemical with hemolytic analyses, it was first learned that CĪ-inhibitor could be present in some patients as an immunochemically intact, yet functionally inactive material.[2]

2. PREPARATION OF HEMOLYTIC INTERMEDIATES FROM GUINEA PIG COMPLEMENT*

a. EAC1 (GUINEA PIG)

This labile intermediate is used to measure C4 with use of separated C2 and C-EDTA, and to form other intermediates.

i. Formation

Erythrocytes are sensitized with four times the amount of antibody required for "optimal" sensitization (cf. Section 17.B.2.a), which is nearly the maximal antibody-binding capacity of the cells. Because this entails use of relatively high concentrations of rabbit antiserum (usually about 1:200), precautions must be taken to avoid absorption of rabbit C components and to eliminate rabbit serum proteins from the cell preparation. The erythrocyte suspension and antibody dilution are therefore both made up in 0.01 M EDTA—Veronal buffer (buffer 7c, Section 17.B, Table I), and allowed to react for 15 minutes at 37°. The cells are separated by centrifugation, resuspended in low ionic strength Veronal-mannitol buffer (buffer 3, Section 17.B, Table I) and then standardized to a concentration of 2 × 10⁹ cells/ml.

The sensitized and standardized cells are mixed with guinea pig CĪ (Section 17.D.3.a), in a concentration to supply 200 or more molecules of CĪ per cell. The tube is incubated 10 minutes at 37°. The EACĪ cells are sedimented and resuspended in an appropriate volume of mannitol buffer and standardized to the desired cell concentration, without washing, since washing leads to loss of CĪ.

---

* Sections 17.C.2.a—e were contributed by Louis G. Hoffmann and Manfred M. Mayer.

[1] J. G. Feinberg, *Int. Arch. Allergy Appl. Immunol.* **11**, 129 (1957).

[2] F. S. Rosen, P. Charache, J. Pensky, and V. Donaldson, *Science* **148**, 957 (1965).

$\text{EAC}\overline{1}$ prepared according to this procedure have been found in our laboratory to carry ca 1450 site-forming units (SFU) per cell (see Section 17.D.3.a.iii for the definition of SFU) in an assay in which the $\text{C}\overline{1}$ is transferred to EAC4 (see below). This number of SFU must be regarded as a minimum estimate.

ii. Stability

$\text{EAC}\overline{1}$ should be used on the day of preparation.

b. EAC$\overline{1}$,4 (GUINEA PIG)

This intermediate is used to measure C2 with use of C-EDTA. The rate of formation of the intermediate provides an assay for $\text{EAC}\overline{1}$.

i. Formation of the Intermediate

The transfer of $\text{C}\overline{1}$ to EAC4 is measured in terms of the number of sites bearing antibody and C4 (SAC4) which become converted to $\text{SAC}\overline{1}$,4. Preparations of $\text{EAC}\overline{1}$,4 are characterized in terms of their t_{max}, i.e., the time at which SAC1,4,2 formation reaches a maximum in a kinetic experiment with a limited amount of C2.[3] The value of t_{max} is inversely related to the effective number of $\text{SAC}\overline{1}$,4 per cell at a given cell concentration. In our laboratory, the procedure described below has consistently yielded $\text{EAC}\overline{1}$,4 preparations with t_{max} values between 4 and 7 minutes. The procedure for measuring t_{max} is described in Section 17.D.3.b.iv(a).

Ten milliliters of sensitized erythrocytes at a concentration of 10^9 cells/ml (usually, 2 to 4 times optimal sensitization level of antibody under conditions described in Section 17.C.1.a) in buffer containing 1 mM Ca^{2+} (buffer 3c, Section 17.B, Table I) are treated in one of the following ways.

Method A. The C4 erythrocyte suspension is cooled to 0° and mixed with 0.25 to 2.0 ml of ice-cold C which has *not* been absorbed with packed erythrocytes. The mixture is kept at exactly 0°, usually for 5 to 10 minutes. The level of sensitization of the cells, the amount of C to be used, and the length of time required may vary for different lots of antiserum and C and have to be worked out by trial and error. The addition of more than 1 ml of C usually does not enhance SAC14 formation and may even be inhibitory. The time of treatment should be adjusted so that the extent of E* formation is less than 5%. Nishioka and Linscott[4] limit reaction time to 7.5 minutes so as to avoid fixation of C3.*

---

[3] T. Borsos, H. J. Rapp, and M. M. Mayer, *J. Immunol.* 87, 310 (1961).

[4] K. Nishioka and W. D. Linscott, *J. Exp. Med.* 118, 767 (1963).

* To avoid the presence of C3 on the EAC1,4 (the presence of C3 can be detected by immune adherence), E. Becker and co-workers add phlorizin to the guinea

The complement treatment is terminated by centrifugation; the cells are washed twice with ice-cold buffer, resuspended in 20 ml of the same buffer, and incubated for 90 minutes at 37°. This incubation allows lysis of any E* that have formed; furthermore, any SAC1,4,2 that may have formed will decay to SAC1,4. The suspension is then centrifuged and the supernatant fluid is removed for absorbancy measurement; the percentage of E* formation is determined from this reading.

Method B. The C4 erythrocyte suspension is treated with partially purified guinea pig $C\bar{1}$ to supply 200 to 400 molecules of $C\bar{1}$ per cell: after 10 minutes at 20°, the cells are sedimented and washed several times in the suspending buffer, then resuspended to a concentration of 10^9 cells/ml in buffer containing the usual concentration of 0.15 mM Ca^{2+} and doubled Mg^{2+} (buffer 2, Section 17.B, Table I).

ii. Stability

Washed $EAC\bar{1},4$ are stable for several weeks when stored at 0° and may be used until the cells become so fragile that the cell blank exceeds 1% lysis. It should be noted that frequent washing of $EAC\bar{1},4$ should be avoided since it leads to loss of $C\bar{1}$ by dissociation and hence to an increase in t_{max}.

iii. C2 Titrations with $C\bar{1},4$

For use in titrations of C2, cells are centrifuged and resuspended in buffer containing 0.15 mM Ca^{2+} and 1.0 mM Mg^{2+}, and standardized at a concentration of 1.5×10^8 cells/ml. (A 1:15 dilution of a cell suspension at this concentration in distilled water has an OD = 0.932 at 412 nm.)

c. EAC4 (GUINEA PIG)

This intermediate is used to measure $C\bar{1}$ with the aid of C2 and EDTA-C.

---

pig complement in the proportion of 1.5 volumes of 0.01 M phlorizin (4.4 mg/ml) to 1 volume of guinea pig serum. Weigh out 4.4 mg/ml for the desired volume of 0.01 M phlorizin and add two-thirds of the final desired volume of buffer containing 1 mM Ca^{2+}. Warm the phlorizin gently over a bunsen burner until it dissolves. It should not get too warm to hold in the hand. Cool to room temperature and bring to pH 7 to 8 (pH paper) with 0.1 N NaOH. Add buffer with Ca^{2+} to the desired final volume. The same amount of complement in the phlorizin–complement mixture is added to EA as is called for in the text. The other conditions, such as time and temperature of incubation, are also the same as given in the text.

i. Formation of the Intermediate

EAC$\overline{1}$,4 is a complex prepared from EAC$\overline{1}$ and whole guinea pig serum. Removal of C$\overline{1}$ by EDTA leaves EAC4. Alternatively, an excellent preparation results if EAC$\overline{1}$ is prepared with partially purified C$\overline{1}$ and treated at 0° after the addition of C-EDTA. Both methods are given.

(a) *Modification of the Method of Becker.*[5] Ten milliliters of EAC1,4 (Section 17.C.1.b) are centrifuged, the cells resuspended in 10 ml of 0.01 M EDTA–Veronal buffer (buffer 7c, Section 17.B, Table I) and incubated 5 minutes at 37°. The cells are washed twice with 10 ml of the same EDTA buffer and then three times with 10 ml of buffer containing 0.15 mM Ca^{2+} and 1.0 mM Mg^{2+} (buffer 2, Section 17.B, Table I), and resuspended in 10 ml of the latter buffer.

(b) *Method of Borsos and Rapp.*[6] Sedimented sheep erythrocytes are suspended in gelatin–EDTA–VBS and held at 37° for 10 minutes, sedimented, washed once with the same buffer and three times with gelatin–VBS^{2+}. The final suspension (1 × 10^9/ml) in gelatin–VBS^{2+} is sensitized with rabbit hemolysin, enough being used to supply 200 molecules of IgM antibody per cell; 20 ml (5 × 10^8 cells/ml) at 0° is treated with 2 ml of C$\overline{1}$ to provide ca 400 molecules per cell. After being stirred, the suspension is held at 0° for about 20 minutes (tube should stand in a small thermos jar with floating ice); then add rapidly, at 0°, 50 ml of 1:10 guinea pig complement in gelatin–EDTA–VBS which has been heated at 37° for 15 minutes before being chilled to 0°. After 15 minutes at 0°, sediment the cells, wash twice with the same buffer and then three times with gelatin–VBS^{2+}, and suspend in this buffer. The cold EDTA treatment removes the C$\overline{1}$, leaving C4.

ii. Stability

Washed EAC4, like EAC$\overline{1}$,4, are stable for several weeks at 0° and may be used until the cell blank exceeds 1% lysis.

iii. C$\overline{1}$ Titrations with EAC4

For use in the titration of C$\overline{1}$, a portion of EAC4 is centrifuged and the cells are resuspended in low ionic strength Veronal–mannitol buffer (buffer 3b, Section 17.B, Table I) to a concentration of 1.5 × 10^8 cells/ml, and standardized.

d. EAC$\overline{1}$,4,2

This labile intermediate is used directly to titrate C3 when C5 to C9 are supplied and to form EAC1,4,2,3 for titrating C5, C6, C7, C8, C9.

[5] E. L. Becker, *J. Immunol.* **84**, 299 (1960).
[6] T. Borsos and H. J. Rapp, *J. Immunol.* **99**, 263 (1967).

i. Formation of the Intermediate

$EAC\overline{1},4,2$ are prepared by exposing $EAC\overline{1},4$ (Section 17.C.2.b) in Veronal–mannitol buffer to purified C2 (Section 17.D.3.b). Ten milliliters of $EAC\overline{1},4$ (10^9 cells/ml) are mixed with 10 ml of purified C2 diluted so as to obtain the desired number of SFU of C2 per cell (usually 100–300) and incubated at 30°. The incubation time should be determined by preliminary experiment so as to obtain maximal formation of $SAC\overline{1},4,2$. If t_{max} (Section 17.D.3.b.iv.(a)) is known, use about one-half to three-fifths of this interval. (A comparison of the effects of cell density and C2 concentration at 30° on t_{max} is given in Table I.)

At the end of the incubation period, 60 to 80 ml of ice-cold buffer are added and the tube is chilled to 0°. The suspension is centrifuged im-

TABLE I
Conversion of EAC1,4 to SAC1,4,2[a]

No. of SFU[b] (C2/cell)	Cell concentration	t_{max} (min)
2.5	7.5×10^7	6
255	7.5×10^7	7–8
2.5	5×10^8	2
255	5×10^8	3–4

[a] A single preparation of EAC1,4 was used throughout.
[b] SFU, site-forming unit.

mediately at 0°, and the cells are resuspended to the desired concentration in ice-cold EDTA buffer (buffer 7b, Section 17.B, Table I), and standardized.

ii. Stability

The suspension is stored at 0° until needed and should be used promptly since $SAC\overline{1},4,2$ decay with a half-life of 10 hours at 0°. ($EAC\overline{1},4^{oxy}2$, as prepared with human components, is rather stable owing to oxidation of C2.)

iii. Assay. See Section 17.C.3.a.

e. $EAC\overline{1,4,2,3},5,6,7$ (Guinea Pig)[7]

This stabilized intermediate serves for assay of C8 and C9. Its counterpart in the human system is given in Section 17.C.4.c.

[7] F. A. Rommel and R. Stolfi, *Immunology* **15**, 469 (1968).

i. Two-Step Preparation of C2 + C4 + C7 and C3 + C5 + C6

Step 1. Removal of Euglobulins. Five milliliters of guinea pig serum at 4° was adjusted to pH 7.5 with acetic acid and diluted with distilled water to a conductance equivalent to 0.04 M NaCl. The precipitate was removed after 30 minutes. The supernatant was adjusted to 0.16 M NaCl and pH 5.0 (using 0.1 N HCl).

Step 2. Chromatography on CM-Cellulose. The yield from step 1 (26 ml) was applied to a 2.6 × 30 cm column of CM-cellulose equilibrated with 0.16 M NaCl + acetate, pH 5.0, at an initial rate of 15 ml per hour. The proteins in the first effluent include C2, C4, and C7. A linear NaCl gradient was then started in acetate buffer, pH 5.0. at a rate of 30 ml per hour, proceeding to 0.24 M NaCl. Fractions of about 4.2 ml were collected into tubes containing 0.8 ml of a solution of Tris base to bring the pH to 7.0. C8 and C9 are excluded since they elute after C3, C5, C6, which were harvested approximately between 190 and 380 ml of effluent under conditions where total effluent was 715 ml. The activity of each complement component was determined by the microtiter plate technique of Nelson *et al.*[8] Six out of 10 trials yielded C3, C5, and C6 without contamination with C8.

ii. EAC1-7 Reagent

(a) *Preparation.* The two pools from step 2 were mixed to provide C4,2,3,5,6,7, and additional functionally purified C5[8] was added to increase its concentration. Gelatin was added to 1%, and small aliquots were frozen at −75°.

(b) *Use.* The buffer was gelatin–DVB^{2+}, used at 0°. 1.0 ml of an appropriate dilution (between 1:3 and 1:25) of the C2 through C7 mixture was mixed with 1.0 ml of a moderate excess of either C9 or C8 to allow assay of C8 or C9. Then 0.5 ml (0.5 × 10^8) EAC1-7 at 0° was added. The tubes were incubated in a 37° bath, with mechanical shaker, for 90 minutes. The reaction was stopped by adding 5 ml of 0.086 M EDTA at 0°. Absorbancy of the supernatants was read at 415 nm.

(c) *Stability.* The half-life of EAC1-7 containing more than a limited number of C7 sites per cell was stable at 0° during at least 2 weeks when stored in gelatin–DVB with penicillin and streptomycin.

---

[8] R. A. Nelson, Jr., J. Jensen, I. Gigli, and N. Tamura, *Immunochemistry* **3**, 111 (1966).

3. MEASUREMENT OF HEMOLYTIC INTERMEDIATES
OF GUINEA PIG COMPLEMENT*

a. ASSAY OF SAC1,4,2 AND SAC4,2

The intermediate, SAC4.2, may be converted to S* by whole complement diluted in 5 mM EDTA buffer (buffer 7b, Section 17.B, Table I) which blocks the action of C1, C2, and C4. The solution is termed C-EDTA. SAC1,4,2 (Section 17.C.2.d) is automatically converted to SAC4,2 by EDTA.[4] and therefore cannot be distinguished from SAC4,2 in terms of the procedure described here.

Conversion to S* is accompanied by decay of some of the SAC4,2 to SAC4.[3] This decay can be overcome by increasing the C-EDTA concentration to a very high level,[3] but this procedure frequently leads to high blanks for cells that do not contain C2, and in this range some specimens of C have proved to be inhibitory. As a compromise, a final dilution of 1:62.5 is used; the conversion of SAC4,2 to S* which is attained with this dilution at 37° is 70% of that attained asymptotically at final dilutions of 1:16 to 1:8.

In a typical procedure, 2.0 ml of C-EDTA, diluted 1:25, are added to 3.0 ml of EAC1,4,2 (Section 17.C.2.d) in EDTA buffer (5×10^7 cells/ml) in 40-ml centrifuge tubes at 0°. The tubes are mixed, stoppered, and incubated at 37° for 90 minutes, the cells being resuspended at intervals of 10 to 20 minutes. Exactly 10-ml portions of isotonic NaCl solution are added to each tube, and the tubes are centrifuged. The supernatant fluids are collected for measurement of OD at 412 nm.

Controls include a cell blank (CB) in which EDTA buffer is substituted for C-EDTA, another control in which cells that have not reacted with C2 are exposed to C-EDTA (CBC), a complete lysis control (OD_{100}) in which 3.0 ml of cell suspension are lysed with 12.0 ml of distilled water after incubation at 37°, and a C color blank consisting of 3.0 ml of EDTA buffer + 2.0 ml of C-EDTA.

The optical densities of all samples are corrected by subtraction of the values obtained for CB and C color, except for the complete lysis control which is corrected only for CB:

$$OD' = OD - OD_{CB} - OD_{C\text{-}Col}$$

except

$$OD'_{100} = OD_{100} - OD_{CB}$$

* Section 17.C.3 was contributed by Louis G. Hoffmann and Manfred M. Mayer.

The degree of lysis, y, is computed by dividing the corrected optical density value of each sample by that of the complete lysis control:

$$y = OD'/OD'_{100}$$

The average number of S^* per cell, z, is obtained from y by applying the Poisson distribution; corrected for the number of S^* per cell found in the CBC control; and converted to the average number of SAC4,2 per cell, z', by multiplying by 1.4 to correct for decay:

$$z = -\ln(1 - y); z' = 1.4(z - z_{CBC})$$

Experiments in which the CB or CBC controls exceed 1% lysis should be regarded as suspect.

It should be noted that the correctness of the factor 1.4 depends on the homogeneity of the SAC4,2 population being examined. Appreciable contamination of SAC4,2 with later and more stable intermediates in the hemolytic sequence[4, 9] means that the true correction factor should be less than 1.4. When in doubt, the investigator should check the homogeneity of the SAC4,2 preparation directly by studying its decay, which should follow first-order kinetics for its entire course.[10]

Another fact to be noted is that the conversion of SAC4,2 to S^* and the lysis of E^* are sensitive to deviations in ionic strength from that of EDTA buffer.[11, 12] Arbitrary changes, therefore, cannot be made in this parameter without first examining their effect.

The procedure described above is limited to EAC4,2 preparations containing no more than three SAC4,2 per cell because at higher multiplicities, close to 100% lysis is attained. Such cell preparations may be analyzed by extrapolating decay curves to zero time as described by Borsos et al.[3]

b. ASSAY OF SAC4

A method for the measurement of SAC4, based on the establishment of a steady state between the formation and decay of SAC1,4,2 in the presence of excess $C\bar{1}$ and C2, has been developed by Hoffmann et al.[13]

[9] U. Nilsson and H. J. Müller-Eberhard, Fed. Proc., Fed. Amer. Soc. Exp. Biol. **23**, 506 (1964).
[10] M. M. Mayer, Complement and Complement Fixation, in "Experimental Immunochemistry" (E. A. Kabat and M. M. Mayer, eds.), 2nd ed., Chap. 4. Thomas, Springfield, Illinois, 1961.
[11] H. J. Rapp and T. Borsos, J. Immunol. **91**, 826 (1963).
[12] L. G. Hoffmann and A. T. McKenzie, Proc. Soc. Exp. Biol. Med. **115**, 977 (1964).
[13] L. G. Hoffmann, A. T. McKenzie, and M. M. Mayer, Immunochemistry **2**, 13 (1965).

The reaction system is affected by the concentrations of $C\bar{1}$, C2, and cells, and by ionic strength and temperature. The procedure described below results in the conversion of ca 95% of the SAC4 to SAC1,4,2 or SAC4,2. It is applicable to cells that have been sensitized with four times the "optimal" amount of antibody; if less antibody is used, the extent of conversion of SAC4 to SAC1,4,2 + SAC4,2 can be expected to be somewhat higher. The reaction medium is low ionic strength Veronal–mannitol buffer (GVM, buffer 3, Section 17.B, Table I).

One milliliter of EAC4 containing 3.13×10^7 cells is mixed at 0° with 1.0 ml each of C2 (Section 17.D.3.b) containing 90 units/ml and of $C\bar{1}$ (Section 17.D.3.a) containing 6×10^9 SFU/ml (Section 17.D.3.a.iii); alternatively, the ice-cold $C\bar{1}$ and C2 solutions may be mixed immediately beforehand and 2.0 ml of the mixture be used. The reaction mixtures are incubated at 30° for 30 minutes and centrifuged in the cold. The supernatant fluids are quickly decanted, the tubes drained for a few seconds and wiped with absorbent tissue, and the cells are resuspended at 0° in 4.0 ml of C-EDTA 1:62.5 for determination of the number of SAC4,2 per cell (cf. Section 17.C.3.a).

Controls should include a sample of EA or EAC4 that is allowed to react with $C\bar{1}$ + C2 and then resuspended in EDTA buffer instead of C-EDTA (cell blank), a sample of EA exposed successively to $C\bar{1}$ + C2 and C-EDTA (CBC), several complete lysis controls of EAC4 exposed to $C\bar{1}$ + C2 and then resuspended in 4.0 ml of water, and a C color control.

The supernatant fluids obtained after incubation at 37° and centrifugation are subjected to OD measurement at 412 nm without further dilution. To avoid subtracting the high C color value that is obtained with this procedure (OD = 0.15), the C color control is placed in the reference cuvette and all samples except the complete lysis controls are compared to it directly; the latter are read against water at the same slit width but with reduced electrical sensitivity. The results are calculated as described in the preceding section, except that the proper correction factor to convert S* to SAC4 is 1.47.

The procedure described above was developed for EAC4 preparations with less than 3 SAC4 per cell and is applicable only to such preparations since it is subject to the same limitation as the SAC1,4,2 assay described in the preceding section. However, since the conversion efficiency of SAC4 to SAC1,4,2 + SAC4,2 depends in a known fashion on the concentrations of C1 and C2,[13] it should be possible to extend the method to EAC4 preparations with larger numbers of SAC4 per cell by using lower concentrations of $C\bar{1}$ and C2.

4. PREPARATION OF HEMOLYTIC INTERMEDIATES FROM HUMAN COMPLEMENT*†[14,15]

a. HUMAN EAC$\overline{1}$; EAC$\overline{1}$,4; EAC$\overline{1}$,4,^{oxy}2 (HUMAN)

The EAC$\overline{1}$,4,^{oxy}2 cells may be used to assay C3 activity (Section 17.A, Fig. 1). Unlike the unstable EAC1,4,2 as prepared with untreated C2, the reagent EAC$\overline{1}$,4,^{oxy}2 is relatively stable, having a half-life at 37° of 150 to 200 minutes. Further, since ^{oxy}C2 (iodine-oxidized C2) is approximately 13 times as active as native C2, its use for the preparation of intermediate complexes is very economical.

In the steps detailed below, it is necessary to have available human C4 (Section 17.D.2.c) and human ^{oxy}C2 (Section 17.D.2.b.v) as well as antibody-coated erythrocytes (EA) described in Section 17.B.1.d.

Step 1. Preparation of Euglobulin (Source of Crude C1). Fresh human serum is adjusted to pH 7.5 and diluted 1:3 with distilled water. After 1 hour at 4° the finely dispersed precipitate is collected by centrifugation for 30 minutes at 1000 g. The precipitate is washed with Veronal buffer containing 0.05 M NaCl and 7.5 × 10^{-4} M CaCl$_2$. It is dissolved in one-half the original serum volume with twice isotonic barbital-NaCl, containing 7.5 × 10^{-4} M CaCl$_2$. Floatable lipids are removed by brief ultracentrifugation, and the material is frozen in liquid nitrogen and stored at −70°.[8,14]

Step 2. Preparation of EAC$\overline{1}$. Five milliliters of 1 × 10^9 cells/ml of antibody-coated erythrocytes (EA) in gelatin–Veronal–sucrose buffer (SGVB, buffer 4, Section 17.B, Table I) are mixed with 0.5 ml of crude fraction containing C1 (prepared as above) and the mixture is incubated for 15 minutes at 37°. The cells are washed once in gelatin–VB and finally resuspended in 5 ml of the same buffer.

Step 3. Preparation of EAC$\overline{1}$,4.‡ The cells are then allowed to react for 30 minutes at 37° with 100 μg of purified human C4 (see Section 17.D.2.c),

* Section 17.C.4 was contributed by Hans J. Müller-Eberhard.

† Sections 17.C,4, 17.D.2.a.iii, 17.D.2.b-g, 17.E.3.a,b, 17.E.4, 17.F.2.a,b as well as portions of 17.A and 17.D.1, constitute publication No. 177 from the Department of Experimental Pathology, Scripps Clinic and Research Foundation. Acknowledgment is made of support by U.S. Public Health Service Grant AI-07007, United States Atomic Energy Commission Contract AT (04-3)-730 and American Heart Association, Inc., Grant 68-666.

[14] N. R. Cooper, and H. J. Müller-Eberhard, *Immunochemistry* **5**, 155 (1968).

[15] N. R. Cooper, M. J. Polley, and H. J. Müller-Eberhard, *Immunochemistry* **7**, 341 (1970).

‡ An alternative method of preparing human or guinea pig C1,4 is given by T. Borsos and H. R. Rapp, *J. Immunol.* **99**, 263 (1967).

corresponding to 1×10^{12} effective molecules; this results in specific binding of a minimum of 3000 C4 molecules per cell. The cells are washed twice in gelatin–barbital–saline (buffer 1, Section 17.B, Table I) and allowed to react again with 0.5 ml of human C1 for 15 minutes at 37° to replace the C1 that will dissociate during the formation of $EAC\overline{1},4$ and subsequent washing.

Step 4. Combination with $^{oxy}C2$. The cells are washed once in the same gelatin–VBS reagent and immediately treated with human $^{oxy}C2$ (see Section 17.D.2.b.v). Five milliliters of 1×10^9 cells per milliliter of $EAC\overline{1}, 4$ are incubated for 10 minutes at 30° with 5×10^{11} effective molecules of $^{oxy}C2$, which corresponds to approximately 30 μg of the purified, iodine-treated protein. The cells are washed once with ice-cold GVB and resuspended in the same buffer.

b. HUMAN $EAC\overline{1,4},^{oxy}2,\overline{3}$ [16]

This intermediate complex can be used to quantitate C5 activity. For accurate quantification, 500 μg of purified human C3 (see Section 17.D.2.d) is added to 5 ml of $EAC\overline{1,4},^{oxy}\overline{2}$ (see Section 17.C.4.a) containing 1×10^9 cells/ml in GVB (buffer 1, Section 17.B, Table I) After 20 minutes at 30° the cells are washed twice in ice-cold GVB. This intermediate complex contains a minimum of 25,000 specifically bound C3 molecules per cell. Owing to the $^{oxy}C2$, the complex is quite stable and may be stored at 4° for several days without loss of activity.

For semiquantitative assays, i.e., for screening fractions of separated serum, etc., a useful complex may be prepared without the use of purified complement proteins. In brief, serum diluted 1:2 with single-strength barbital–saline buffer (VB, buffer 1, Section 17.C, Table I, prepared without divalent ions or gelatin) is treated with zymosan (0.5 mg/ml) for 60 minutes at 37°, and the zymosan is removed by centrifugation. The supernatant diluted serum is then mixed with an equal volume of a carefully selected iodine solution containing a 50-fold molar excess of potassium iodide selected as described below. The mixture is kept for 5 minutes at room temperature and then is exhaustively dialyzed at 4° against barbital–saline buffer. Antibody-coated erythrocytes (EA) at a concentration of 2×10^8 cells/ml in GVBS with doubled Mg^{2+} is then treated for 50 minutes at 37° with the reagent in a final dilution of 1:100 with respect to the original serum.

The optimum concentration of the iodine solution is determined separately: small aliquots of the zymosan-treated serum are mixed with an equal volume of either 2, 4, 6, 8, or 10×10^{-4} M I_2 in 50-fold molar excess

[16] H. J. Müller-Eberhard, A. P. Dalmasso, and M. A. Calcott, *J. Exp. Med.* **123**, 33 (1966).

of KI (Section 17.D.2.b.v). After treatment as described above, the ability to convert EA to $EAC\overline{1,4,}^{oxy}2,3$ is tested and the optimal I_2 concentration is used for preparation of the $C\overline{1,4,}^{oxy}2,3$-reagent.

c. $EAC\overline{1,4,}^{oxy}2,3,5,6,7$

This intermediate complex is stable and may be stored for several days in the cold. The cells cannot by lysed by C9 alone, but they lyse completely within a few minutes on addition of C8 and C9. The complex is prepared either by treating $EAC\overline{1,4,}^{oxy}2$ (Section 17.C.4.a) or $EAC\overline{1,4,}^{oxy}2,3$ (17.C.4.b) with (a) isolated C5 (see Section 17.D.2.d.iii), C6 and partially purified C_7 (see Sections 17.D.2.e and f), or (b) more economically with a chromatographically obtained reagent containing C3, C5, C6, and C7.[17]

To prepare the (C3, C5, C6, C7) reagent, 60 ml of human serum, dialyzed overnight at 4° against phosphate buffer, pH 6.0, ionic strength 0.1 (buffer A, Section 17.D, Table I) is applied to a 4.5 × 60 cm column of carboxymethyl (CM) cellulose that has been equilibrated with this buffer. After 100 ml of this buffer have passed the column, a sodium chloride gradient in the same buffer is begun, the limiting buffer containing 1.8% NaCl. Fifteen-milliliter fractions are collected, conductance is measured, and all fractions with a conductance less than 10 mS are pooled, thus avoiding contamination of the pool with C8 which is eluted at higher salt concentration. The pool of C3–C7 reagent is concentrated to one-quarter its volume by ultrafiltration, such as by a UM-10 membrane (Amicon Corp., Cambridge, Massachusetts) and stored at −70°.

$EAC\overline{1,4,}^{oxy}2$ (Section 17.C.4.a) at a concentration of 1 × 10⁹ cells/ml in GVB containing 0.02 M $Na_3H \cdot EDTA^*$ is then incubated with an equal volume of C3–C7 reagent rendered isotonic by adding dextrose* and supplemented with 10 μg/ml of purified C5 (see Section 17.D.2.d.iii). After 45 minutes at 37° the cells are washed three times or more in the $Na_3H \cdot EDTA$–GVB reagent and resuspended in GVBS. They may be stored in the cold for several days.

d. $EAC\overline{1,4,}^{oxy}2,3,5,6,7,8$ (EAC1–8 Cells)

EAC1–7 (Section 17.C.4.c) in a concentration of 1 × 10⁹ cells/ml is allowed to react with an excess of purified human C8 (see Section 17.D.2.g) for 10 minutes at 37°, i.e., with 0.2 μg of C8 per milliliter of cells, which corresponds to approximately 5 × 10¹⁰ effective molecules. The cells are washed and stored in 0.09 M $Na_3H \cdot EDTA$ with gelatin pH 7.6 (buffer 8, Section 17.B, Table I), which prevents, to a large extent,

---

[17] J. A. Manni and H. J. Müller-Eberhard, *J. Exp. Med.* **130**, 1145 (1969).

* Note that 5.05% of anhydrous dextrose or 5.51% of the usual monohydrate are isotonic solutions.

the protracted spontaneous lysis that is characteristic for these EAC1–8 cells.

e. EAC4 (HUMAN)

This intermediate is used to titrate human C1q, C1r, C1s, and C1$\bar{s}$ [17.D.2.a, subsections ii(c), iii(c), v(d), vi(d) (2)].

Method A. EA in GVB with 0.01 M EDTA (buffer 7c, Section 17.B, Table I) is treated with 8 units of rabbit anti-E hemolysin which has been heated at 56° for 30 minutes to inactivate rabbit C1q. After 30 minutes at 37°, the cells are sedimented by centrifugation, resuspended in GVB (buffer 1d, Section 17.B, Table I) and adjusted to a concentration of 1.5×10^9 cells/ml. EA is treated with 400 μg of purified human C4 (Section 17.D.2c) and 40 μg of purified C1$\bar{s}$ (Section 17.D.2.a.vi) per milliliter of cells for 30 minutes at 37°. This circumvents the use of C1q-containing C1 complex and the necessity of its later complete removal, a task that has proved difficult. The cells are washed three times with GVB and resuspended in sufficient GVB to yield 0.75×10^8 cells/ml. Diisopropylfluorophosphate (DFP) (see footnote to Section 17.D.2.b) is added to a final concentration of 0.5×10^{-3} M, and the mixture is incubated for 30 minutes at 37° to inactivate residual C1$\bar{s}$. The flask must be securely stoppered during DFP treatment and cooled in an ice bath before opening. After three washes with GVB, the EAC4 cells are resuspended in low ionic strength sucrose–GVB (buffer 4, Section 17.B, Table I) to a concentration of 1.5×10^8 cells/ml.

Method B. The two-step method of Borsos and Rapp[6] may be used to obtain human C4 as well (see Section 17.C.2.c).

f. EAC43 (HUMAN)[18]

The intermediate EAC43 was prepared to assay properdin factors B and D (Sections 17.E.6.a–c and 5.a–c) as well as to test for the Cb3-inactivator (KAF) (Section 17.E.3.c).

i. Procedure

Step 1. The precursor was EAC$\overline{1}$4, prepared either by the method of Borsos and Rapp[6] or directly by allowing purified C4 to react with EAC$\overline{1}$; 1×10^8 EAC$\overline{1}$ were reacted with 100 U of purified C4.

Step 2. Preparation of EAC42. EAC$\overline{1}$4, 1×10^8 cells/ml in gelatin–DVB^{2+}, were treated at 30° with the same volume of C2 at 1000 U/ml for "t_{max} time" [Section 17.D.3.b.iv(a)]. The cells were sedimented and promptly washed in EDTA–GVB at 0°.

Step 3. Preparation of EAC43. EAC42, 1×10^8 cells/ml in

[18] D. T. Fearon, K. F. Austen, and S. Ruddy, *J. Exp. Med.* **138**, 1305 (1973).

EDTA–GVB, was mixed with the same volume of a solution of C3 at 8.3 μg/ml in the same buffer and incubated at 30° for 30 minutes. The cells were washed twice and suspended in EDTA–GVB, then held at 37° for 2 hours to allow decay of C2.

ii. Tests

C3–9 was supplied either by (a) 1:19 dilution of normal guinea pig serum in EDTA–GVB or (b) functionally pure C3–9.

EAC43, 0.5×10^8, + 0.3 μg of factor B + 0.4 μg of factor $\overline{D}$ and, each in 50 U quantities, C3, C5, C6, and C7, were mixed and held at 30° for 30 minutes; all reagents were supplied in DGVB^{2+}. Then 25 U each of C8 and C9 were added to yield a final volume of 2.5 ml, and incubation was allowed for 60 minutes at 37°. After dilution with 5 ml of saline, debris was sedimented and supernatant was read spectrophotometrically. The average number of Z—effective hemolytic sites per cell—was calculated. Variations in this pattern were made, using variable amounts of factor B or factor $\overline{D}$.

g. R1q (HUMAN)

This reagent, prepared as described in Section 17.D.2.a.iii(c), is serum deprived of C1q. Fresh human serum containing EDTA is absorbed with soluble human γ-globulin aggregates and fully clarified. The EDTA effect is reversed by addition of Ca^{2+} and Mg^{2+} to normal levels. The reagent should lack C1q, and at 1:50, should cause no hemolysis when incubated with EA.

D. Isolation and Assay of Complement Components

1. INTRODUCTION*

a. HISTORICAL SURVEY

The multiple component nature of complement was discovered in 1907 when it was found that either the euglobulin (midpiece) or the pseudoglobulin (endpiece) fractions of guinea pig serum, used alone, failed to lyse antibody-sensitized sheep erythrocytes (EA) but were hemolytically active when recombined.[1] This classical procedure served, in current nomenclature, to precipitate the first component of complement (C1)

---

* Section 17.D.1 was contributed by Irwin H. Lepow, Hans Müller-Eberhard and the Editors.

[1] A. Ferrata, *Berlin Klin. Wochenschr.* **44,** 366 (1907).

with other euglobulins of serum, separating it from the second component (C2), a pseudoglobulin. The remaining components of complement which were then unrecognized—C3 through C9 (see Section 17.A, Table I)— were distributed between the two fractions, making it possible to reconstitute hemolytic activity by mixing the two crude fractions.

At the present time, ten of the eleven proteins constituting the human complement system, and two in their enzymatic modes, have been obtained in a degree of purity approaching or exceeding 95% and in quantities permitting immunological and chemical characterization as discrete serum constituents. These are C1q, C1r, C1s, C1s̄, (C1), C2, C3, C4, C5, C6, C8, and C9. C7 has been purified so far as activities only; i.e., it has been separated from other complement components and from the bulk of the serum proteins. However, the degree of purification is still relatively low according to the rigid criteria of protein chemistry.

From guinea pig serum, C1̄, C2, C3, C5, C6, and C9 have been obtained in a high state of purity which is comparable to that of the isolated human proteins (Section 17.D.3).

b. LABILITY OF COMPLEMENT

In view of the lability of "complement," the bulk of the serum should be separated within 1 to 3 hours of the drawing of blood in order to preserve C3, C4, and C5, as described for guinea pig complement (Section 17.B.1.e). Human blood obtained from apparently healthy donors is collected by venipuncture without anticoagulant, allowed to clot at room temperature for 1 hour to several hours and held at 1° for several hours, and centrifuged at 1100 g for 30 minutes at 1°, after which the serum is siphoned off. A further collection may be taken after clots have been left overnight for maximal clot retraction. Sera from multiple donors may be pooled at 1°, as required, provided that the individual sera are cell-free. Results have been indistinguishable with individual or pooled sera if sera are used fresh, or prepared promptly and placed in storage at −70° for prolonged periods. An alternate method is described below.

Specimens of identical ABO group collected in acid–citrate–dextrose (ACD)* are pooled, and 10 ml of a 16 gm% solution of $CaCl_2 \cdot 2H_2O$ are added per liter of ACD blood. Clotting and clot retraction are allowed to proceed for 2 hours at 37° and for 15 hours at 4°. The serum is separated from the clot by filtration through nylon gauze. Maximal yield is obtained by applying manual pressure to the residual clot, the operator wearing sterile gloves. It is to be noted that outdated human blood (3 to 4 weeks old) can be used for isolation C1q, C1s, C2, C8, and C9.

---

* Acid–citrate–dextrose, NIH formula B, is described in Chap. 16.A.5.

c. METHODOLOGY

Purification of complement components involves the successive use of a series of specified procedures, such as column chromatography on DEAE- or TEAE-cellulose, gel filtration on Sephadex, preparative zone electrophoresis employing Pevikon C-870 as anticonvection medium, chromatography on hydroxylapatite, and sometimes gradient density centrifugation and polyacrylamide gel electrophoresis. The basic techniques are given as described in Volume II, but specific details accompany each step of isolation of complement components. It is to be noted that workers with complement have usually operated at temperatures of 0–4°, but have measured conductivity and pH of buffers and column effluents at 20°.

With identification of each component of complement, the methods for isolation will undergo elaboration or simplification; yet the rather detailed descriptions of the present methods should be a useful guide to immunologists in undertaking resolutions of other complex mixtures of proteins.

Because of the lability of most complement proteins, it is of paramount importance that isolation procedures be carried out in the shortest possible time, a minimum of 10 days usually being required. For rapidity of concentration of the rather large volumes handled, it is usual to achieve concentration by ultrafiltration using Amicon positive pressure filtration devices and the ultrafilter UM 10 (Amicon Corp., Cambridge, Massachusetts). Pressure dialysis through cellophane is also possible.

d. BACTERIOLOGICAL CONSIDERATIONS

Since most complement proteins are exceedingly susceptible to inactivation by proteolytic enzymes, it is essential for successful preparative work to prevent bacterial growth in buffers and protein solutions. Therefore, all preparative steps are performed strictly in the cold at 0° to 5° and it is well to start with sterile stock buffers and to check periodically for pH shifts and for bacteria by culturing (Vol. I, Chap. 17.2.C.5.e).

In the laboratory of one of us (H. J. M-E.), the stock concentrates of buffers are autoclaved before use and upon dilution antibiotics are added to all buffers, except that used for electrophoresis. Two different antibiotics are preferably added, e.g., chloramphenicol* (5×10^{-5} M) and kanamycin† (3×10^{-5} M), and the combination of antibiotics is planned to be changed periodically to prevent growth of resistant strains.

As a routine precaution, pools of column or block fractions are usefully

---

* Add 0.75 ml of 2% solution of chloramphenicol in 95% ethanol (w/v) per liter of buffer.

† Add 60 µl of 25% kanamycin (Bristol Laboratories, Syracuse, New York) per liter of buffer.

passed through a Millipore filter (pore size 0.45 μm)* several times in the course of the preparation of a protein, except in the case of C1q, which is retained by the filter and would thus be lost.

e. STORAGE

The final product should be stored in liquid nitrogen or transferred to a $-70°$ freezer until used. Before freezing, it is well to dialyze against phosphate buffer, pH 6.0, ionic strength 0.2 (buffer A in double strength, Table I) and divide into portions not exceeding a volume of 1 ml using siliconized glass tubes, preparatory to freezing in liquid nitrogen.

f. "FUNCTIONAL SEPARATION" OF COMPONENTS

As purified components and monospecific sera became available, successful attempts were made to effect "functional separation" of complement components; i.e., serum fractions were accepted that contained high reactivity and low content of other proteins, so that, in proper dilution, they functioned as single components. The first functional separation of 9 components was made from guinea pig serum (Nelson et al.[2] and elaborated by Zarco et al.[3]). Parallel schemes for use with human serum were developed by Vroon et al.[4] to functionally isolate 9 components and 2 inhibitors, and by Lachmann et al.[5]

2. COMPLEMENT COMPONENTS FROM HUMAN SERUM

a. HUMAN C1 AND ISOLATION OF SUBCOMPONENTS

i. Concepts and the Development of Procedures†‡

Early attempts at further purification of C1 took advantage of the euglobulin nature of this component and its limited solubility in ammo-

---

* Handling of Millipore filters is described in Vol. I, Chap. 2.C.5, as is equipment for larger and smaller volumes.

[2] R. A. Nelson, J. Jensen, I. Gigli, and N. Tamura, *Immunochemistry* 3, 11 (1966).

[3] R. M. Zarco, R. A. Cort, and D. R. Schultz, Cordis Corporation, under contract with NIAID and NCI, scheme reproduced in H. J. Rapp and T. Borsos, "Molecular Basis of Complement Action," p. 98. Appleton-Century-Crofts, New York, 1970.

[4] D. H. Vroon, D. R. Schultz, and R. M. Zarco, *Immunochemistry* 7, 43 (1970).

[5] P. J. Lachmann, M. J. Hobart, and W. P. Aston, *in* "Handbook of Experimental Immunology" (D. M. Weir, ed.), 2nd ed., pp. 5.1–5.17. Karger, Basel, 1972.

† Section 17.D.2.a.i was contributed by Irwin H. Lepow.

‡ This work, represented by subsections i, ii, and iv, was supported by U.S. Public Health Service Grant AI-01255 and was performed in part during tenure of a Research Career Award of the National Institutes of Health (GM-K6-15,307).

nium sulfate solutions.[6, 7] The possibility that C1 was a proenzyme was inferred from experiments on factors required for inactivation of complement by plasmin and by antigen–antibody complexes.[8] Finally, direct evidence was obtained for the proenzymatic nature of this component and activation to an enzyme that could hydrolyze certain amino acid esters and attack C4 and C2.[9] Also, an apparently identical enzyme was eluted from antigen–antibody complexes which had been exposed to serum reagents containing C1.[10] The active enzyme, presently termed $\overline{C1}$ (Section 17.A, Table I), was previously designated C'1a, converted C'1, activated C'1, or C'1 esterase. The enzymological properties of $\overline{C1}$ were characterized and a normal serum inhibitor of the active enzyme[9, 11] was identified (Section 17.E.2.a). The kinetics of the activation process[12] was established as well as the role of $\overline{C1}$ in several complement-dependent immunological reactions.[13–15] Levine[16] and Becker[17, 18] working with guinea pig complement also concluded that C1 contains a proenzyme that can be activated by certain immune complexes.

With the advent of column chromatography, attempts were initiated to isolate both the proenzymatic (C1) and active forms ($\overline{C1}$). A euglobulin fraction of normal serum was applied to columns of DEAE-cellulose at pH 7.4 and eluted with a salt gradient. For separation of $\overline{C1}$, the euglobulin was first incubated at 37° to convert C1 to active enzyme,[9, 11, 12] assayed as the capacity to hydrolyze N-acetyl-L-tyrosine ethyl ester. Later, by chromatography on TEAE-cellulose, a highly purified preparation of $\overline{C1}$($C1\bar{s}$) was secured.[19]

The isolation of C1 in proenzymatic form posed more formidable technical problems because of the propensity of partially purified frac-

[6] L. Pillemer, E. E. Ecker, J. L. Oncley, and E. J. Cohn, *J. Exp. Med.* **74**, 297 (1941).

[7] L. Pillemer, S. Seifter, C. L. San Clemente, and E. E. Ecker, *J. Immunol.* **47**, 205 (1943).

[8] I. H. Lepow, L. Wurz, O. D. Ratnoff, and L. Pillemer, *J. Immunol.* **73**, 146 (1954).

[9] I. H. Lepow, O. D. Ratnoff, F. S. Rosen, and L. Pillemer, *Proc. Soc. Exp. Biol. Med.* **92**, 32 (1956).

[10] I. H. Lepow, O. D. Ratnoff, and L. Pillemer, *Proc. Soc. Exp. Biol. Med.* **92**, 111 (1956).

[11] O. D. Ratnoff and I. H. Lepow, *J. Exp. Med.* **106**, 327 (1957).

[12] I. H. Lepow, O. D. Ratnoff, and L. R. Levy, *J. Exp. Med.* **107**, 451 (1958).

[13] I. H. Lepow and A. Ross, *J. Exp. Med.* **112**, 1107 (1960).

[14] C. F. Hinz, M. E. Picken, and I. H. Lepow, *J. Exp. Med.* **113**, 193 (1961).

[15] I. H. Lepow and M. A. Leon, *Immunology* **5**, 22 (1962).

[16] L. Levine, *Biochim. Biophys. Acta* **18**, 283 (1955).

[17] E. L. Becker, *Nature (London)* **176**, 1073 (1955).

[18] E. L. Becker, *J. Immunol.* **77**, 462, 469 (1956); **82**, 43 (1959); **84**, 299 (1960).

[19] A. L. Haines and I. H. Lepow, *J. Immunol.* **92**, 456 (1964).

tions to convert to $C\overline{1}$.[9, 12] The euglobulin fraction was therefore prepared in the presence of $Na_3H \cdot EDTA$, a chelating agent for Ca^{2+} which was known to inhibit activation of C1, and manipulations were performed at temperatures of 0° to 5°. When euglobulin so treated was chromatographed on columns of DEAE-cellulose under the same conditions used for isolation of $C\overline{1}$, an essentially identical chromatogram was observed.[20] However, hemolytic $C\overline{1}$ activity could not be detected in any individual fraction. Fortunately, by recombination experiments it was found that fractions from three discrete areas of the chromatogram would, upon mixing, reconstitute the hemolytic $C\overline{1}$ activity if Ca^{2+} were present, measured as formation of the intermediate complex $EAC\overline{1}$ from EA, or of $EAC\overline{1},4$ from EAC4. The three fractions were arbitrarily designated C1q, C1r, and C1s, in the order of their elution from DEAE-cellulose. C1q was identical with a previously described serum protein, referred to as the "11 S factor"[21, 22]; C1r (7 S) appeared to be a new component; and C1s (4 S) could be identified as the proenzymatic form of $C1\overline{s}$ esterase.

Interaction of the three components in free solution in the presence of Ca^{2+} resulted in a macromolecular complex (18 S)[23] that was the functional unit of hemolytic $C\overline{1}$ activity; C1q supplied binding sites for the antigen–antibody complex, C1r was somehow involved in the mechanism of enzyme activation, and C1s possessed the structure necessary for developing the catalytic site of C1 esterase. Well purified C1 esterase ($C\overline{1}$) proved to be derived[24] from only the C1s portion of the C1 macromolecule. Although highly active in hydrolyzing N-acetyl-L-tyrosine ethyl ester and inactivating the hemolytic activity of C4 and C2 in free solution, purified $C1\overline{s}$ was nonfunctional in hemolytic systems.[4–18, 25] Yet, in the presence of C1q, C1r, and Ca^{2+}, a complex was formed that could attach to antigen–antibody complexes and so initiate the further action of complement in immune hemolysis.[20]

Isolation of C1q, C1r, and C1s provides fractions for further purification of these subcomponents and for studies on the mechanism of activation of C1 to $C\overline{1}$.[26, 27]

[20] I. H. Lepow, G. B. Naff, E. W. Todd, J. Pensky, and C. F. Hinz, *J. Exp. Med.* **117**, 983 (1963).
[21] H. J. Müller-Eberhard and H. G. Kunkel, *Proc. Soc. Exp. Biol. Med.* **106**, 291 (1961).
[22] A. Taranta, H. S. Weiss, and E. C. Franklin, *Nature (London)* **189**, 239 (1961).
[23] G. B. Naff, J. Pensky, and I. H. Lepow, *J. Exp. Med.* **119**, 593 (1964).
[24] A. L. Haines and I. H. Lepow, *J. Immunol.* **92**, 468 (1964).
[25] A. L. Haines and I. H. Lepow, *J. Immunol.* **92**, 479 (1964).
[26] O. D. Ratnoff and G. B. Naff, *J. Exp. Med.* **125**, 337 (1967).
[27] G. B. Naff and O. D. Ratnoff, *Proc. Cent. Soc. Clin. Res.* **40**, 22 (1967).

Since the function of C1q is to provide sites of attachment of C1 to the antigen–antibody complex and C1r is involved in the activation of C1s to C1s̄, C1s̄ by itself can serve as the enzymatic initiator of subsequent steps of the complement sequence *in free solution*. This principle makes possible analysis of reaction mechanisms in simpler systems uncomplicated by the presence of a solid-phase reactant (e.g., EA) to which complement components or their reaction products can bind. This approach has contributed significantly to understanding the mechanism of the earlier steps of complement function.[27, 28]

ii. Preparation of Human C1q, C1r, and C1s[20]*

(a) *Characteristics.* C1q, C1r, and C1s behave electrophoretically as γ_2-, β-, and α_2-globulins, respectively. In the isolated state or upon dissociation of the C1 complex in human serum by binding Ca^{2+} with $Na_3H \cdot EDTA$, the three components exhibit respective sedimentation constants of 11 S, 7 S, and 4 S. In the presence of Ca^{2+}, the three subunits reassociate to form an 18 S macromolecular complex. In normal human serum, C1q is present at a concentration of 100 to 200 $\mu g/ml$,[29] C1s at a concentration of about 20 $\mu g/ml$,[20] but the normal concentration of C1r has not been determined. C1r loses activity during incubation at 45° for 30 minutes, C1q during incubation at 56° for 30 minutes, and C1s resists complete inactivation under these conditions.

(b) *Functional Separation.* Serum euglobulins are precipitated (step 1) at final pH 6.1 to 7.3, final ionic strength 0.034, serum dilution of 1 in 9 to yield a partially purified fraction of C1 fully separated from the *serum C1̄-inhibitor* described in Section 17.E.2. The euglobulin is dissolved and brought to pH 7.4, ionic strength 0.15 at low temperature in the presence of 10^{-3} M $Na_3H \cdot EDTA$, thereby dissociating C1 into its subunits and preventing activation of C1 to C1̄. The dissociated subunits of C1 are chromatographically separated on DEAE-cellulose (step 2) in the presence of 10^{-3} M $Na_3H \cdot EDTA$. In common with other γ-globulins, C1q is not adsorbed on the column at pH 7.4, ionic strength 0.15. With increasing salt concentration, the β-globulins emerge early. These include C3–C5, C1r, and small amounts of C4, successively. Finally, at higher salt concentration C1s, an α_2-globulin, is displaced from the column.

Step 1. Concentration of Euglobulin. Euglobulin fractions of human serum may be prepared under various conditions of pH and ionic strength. The variables of greatest importance are (a) maintenance of temperature

[28] H. J. Müller-Eberhard and I. H. Lepow, *J. Exp. Med.* **121**, 819 (1965).

* Section 17.D.2.a.ii was contributed by Irwin H. Lepow.

[29] H. J. Müller-Eberhard, *Advn. Immunol.* **8**, 1 (1968).

close to the freezing point and (b) presence of $Na_3H \cdot EDTA$ when the separated euglobulin fraction is adjusted to physiological values of pH and ionic strength. Otherwise, activation of C1 to C$\overline{1}$ will occur and the C1s subunit will be obtained as the active enzyme C1$\overline{s}$.

One volume of undeteriorated human serum is added slowly with constant stirring at 1° to 8 volumes of acetate buffer, pH 5.5, ionic strength 0.02 (10 ml of 2 M sodium acetate and 2.9 ml of 1 N acetic acid diluted to 1 liter with distilled water). After the preparation has stood undisturbed overnight at 1°, the supernatant fluid is withdrawn by siphon. The precipitate is centrifuged at 4000 rpm for 30 minutes at 1° and washed with the same acetate buffer with a volume equal to the original serum volume. The washed precipitate is suspended at 1° in 0.5 M NaCl containing 10^{-3} M EDTA, to one-tenth the original volume of serum and centrifuged cold at 30,000 rpm for 60 minutes in a No. 30 rotor in the Spinco preparative ultracentrifuge. The supernatant fluid is poured through a filter of glass wool to exclude particles of lipid, and the filtrate is dialyzed at 1° vs 50 volumes of pH 7.4 phosphate buffer, ionic strength 0.15 (buffer D, Table I), containing 10.0 ml of 0.1 M $Na_3H \cdot EDTA$ per liter. After overnight dialysis, the fraction is centrifuged at 4000 rpm for 30 minutes at 1°. The resulting opalescent crude euglobulin, concentrated 10-fold with respect to serum, is the starting material for step 2. The preparation is a potent source of C1 in forming the intermediate complex EAC1 from EA, or EAC1,4 from EAC4 and in completing the cold phase of the Donath–Landsteiner reaction (leading to lysis of erythrocytes of patients exhibiting paroxysmal nocturnal hemoglobinuria); it is enzymatically inactive on synthetic substrates such as N-acetyl-L-tyrosine ethyl ester unless the solution is recalcified and incubated at 37°.[24]

*Step 2. Chromatography on DEAE-Cellulose.** Diethylaminoethyl-(DEAE)-cellulose (type 20, exchange capacity 1.05 mEq/gm, Schleicher and Schuell Co., Keene, New Hampshire) is suspended in 30 times its weight of water, stirred vigorously, and allowed to settle for several hours. The supernatant fluid, containing fine particles, is decanted, and resuspension is repeated until the supernatant fluid is clear after 30 minutes of settling. Washing is continued on a coarse sintered-glass funnel with a solution of 0.125 M NaOH and 0.125 M NaCl, followed by water until washings are alkali-free. The washed adsorbent is suspended in starting buffer (pH 7.4 phosphate, ionic strength 0.15, 10^{-3} M $Na_3H \cdot EDTA$) for packing into chromatography columns.

A magnetically stirred slurry of DEAE-cellulose (10 to 20 gm/liter) is forced into a chromatography column (2.5 cm diameter) under 5 psi

* See also Vol. II, Chap. 9.C.2.

of air pressure to a packed height of 25 cm. The column is placed at 5° and washed with several liters of cold starting buffer.

Twenty milliliters of euglobulin fraction, concentrated 10-fold with respect to serum, is allowed to drain into the head of the equilibrated column and flushed from the walls with several 2-ml aliquots of cold starting buffer. The head of the column is layered carefully with cold starting buffer, which is then allowed to percolate through the column at about 30 ml per hour under gravity flow, the effluent being collected in 10-ml aliquots on a volumetric fraction collector. A sharp peak of unadsorbed proteins, including C1q, emerges with the void volume of the column and trails on the descending side, requiring several hundred milliliters of additional starting buffer to reach values approaching zero as read at OD 280 nm. This peak contains most of the γ-globulins in the euglobulin starting material. C1q activity is maximal in the protein front but falls off somewhat less sharply than the protein content of subsequent fractions.

A linearly increasing gradient of salt concentration at constant pH is then run into the column at a flow rate of about 30 ml per hour. The gradient is produced by allowing 1 liter of 0.5 M NaCl in starting buffer in a 1-liter Erlenmeyer flask to flow through a capillary tube into an *identical* mixing flask containing starting buffer in hydrostatic equilibrium with the contents of the first flask, and thence into the column. The mixing flask is stirred magnetically, and the effluent is again collected in 10-ml aliquots. Elution of the column is discontinued after 125 additional aliquots of 10 ml have been obtained. At this point, a total of about 80% of the applied protein has left the column.

The salt gradient elutes a series of protein peaks which are monitored by absorbancy at 280 nm. The first eluted peak emerges at ionic strength 0.21 (0.06 M NaCl in starting buffer) and is incompletely resolved from a second, much larger peak emerging at ionic strength 0.23. The latter is highly enriched in C3 and C5 and may be successfully employed for further purification of these components (Section 17.D.2.d). A third group of proteins peaks at ionic strength 0.30. The ascending side of this peak may be either asymmetrical or show discrete resolution into a smaller peak. In either case, C1r activity is found in this area of the chromatogram at ionic strength 0.27, i.e., conductance equal to 0.27 M NaCl. A fourth group of proteins emerges as a very small peak at ionic strength 0.37; C1s activity is found in these fractions. An inconstant finding is the presence of very small protein peaks just before and after the peak which is associated with C1s.

Aside from the variabilities noted above, the elution pattern described has been sufficiently constant in our hands so that identification of the activity areas of C1q, C3–C5, C1r, and C1s can be made by inspection of the absorbancy patterns and then confirmed by appropriate assays. It must be emphasized, however, that this situation holds only under these given empirical conditions. Different batches of DEAE-cellulose show variable behavior, and slightly different ionic strengths may correspond with the peaks.*

Larger volumes of euglobulin concentrate (100 ml, equivalent to 1 liter of serum) may be chromatographed in entirely analogous fashion, using 4.4 × 40 cm columns and increasing the volume of starting and limit buffers in gradient elution to 2 liters each.

Column fractions containing C1q, C1r, and C1s are stable at 1° for at least 1 week and at −70° for at least one year. They are best kept at the ionic strength and concentration of $Na_3H \cdot EDTA$ at which they emerge from the column, being adjusted to other desired conditions just before use.

(c) *Yield of Product and Activity Assays.* Because the individual activities of C1q, C1r, and C1s cannot be measured in whole serum, it is not possible to calculate the yields of each of the separated subunits. Since almost all the C$\bar{\text{I}}$ activity of serum is present in the euglobulin fraction and approximately 50% of this can be accounted for by appropriate recombinations of pools of fractions of C1q, C1r, and C1s, it may be inferred that yields of the subunits are ca 50%.

All the various possible hemolytic assays for the activity of C1q, C1r, and C1s are based on the requirement for all three subunits to reconstitute the hemolytic activity of C$\bar{\text{I}}$. The most satisfactory system is formation of the intermediate complex EAC$\bar{\text{I}}$,4 from EAC4. The latter complex may be prepared as described in reference 16 or by other methods (Section 17.C.2.c for guinea pig complement and Section 17.C.4.e for human complement).

Centrifuged sediments of the complex EAC4 containing 5×10^8 cells are suspended in 0.5 ml each of 1:200 dilutions of the recalcified (5×10^{-4} *M* excess Ca^{2+}) pools of C1q and C1r and 0.5 ml of 1:400 dilutions of the recalcified fractions to be tested for C1s activity. The buffer diluent is pH 7.4 barbital (buffer 1d, Section 17.B, Table I) or triethanolamine-buffered saline (Section 17.B, buffer 5b, Table I), but with gelatin reduced to 0.05%. The suspensions are incubated at 37° for 10 minutes and centrifuged warm. The pellets are then suspended in 3 ml of buffer diluent at 37° and centrifuged again. The washed pellets are then tested for reactivity as EAC$\bar{\text{I}}$,4 by attempted lysis in the presence of the re-

---

* High-capacity lots of DEAE-cellulose (e.g., 1.05 mEq/gm) appear to have given much more satisfactory resolution of these components than preparations of lower exchange capacity.

maining components of complement, as below. In entirely analogous fashion, fractions to be tested for C1q or C1r activity are diluted 1:400 and added to EAC4 in the presence of 1:200 dilutions of C1r and C1s, or C1q and C1s, respectively.

In the screening assays, a satisfactory reagent is human serum diluted 1:100 in buffer diluent containing 16×10^{-3} M $Na_2Mg \cdot EDTA$. $Na_2Mg \cdot EDTA$ chelates Ca^{2+}, thereby preventing $C\overline{1}$ in serum from reacting but permitting subsequent components requiring Mg^{2+} to react. Accordingly incubation of $EAC\overline{1},4$ with $Na_2Mg \cdot EDTA$-serum at 32° for 60-minute results in hemolysis which can be quantitated by measurement of released hemoglobin in the supernatant measured at 541 nm. For greater precision, $EAC\overline{1},4$ can be converted to $EAC\overline{1},4,2$ with purified C2 (Section 17.D.2.b), and the erythrocytes will then lyse upon incubation with $Na_3H \cdot EDTA$-treated normal serum. Regardless of the developing reagents selected, hemolysis should not occur if only two rather than all of the three subunits are incubated with EAC4 in the first step of the assay.

In addition to hemolytic assays, the activity of C1q, C1r, and C1s may be estimated by taking advantage of the requirement for all three subunits to generate esterolytic activity for N-acetyl-L-tyrosine ethyl ester (ATE). Fractions or pools to be tested are recalcified, adjusted to ionic strength 0.15, and incubated together at 37° for 30 minutes. The resulting solutions are then assayed for esterolysis of ATE (see below). If C1q, C1r, and C1s are present in sufficient concentration, enzymatic activity is demonstrable. By maintaining constant concentrations of two of the subunits and diluting the third to limiting concentration, an estimate of subunit activities can be made independently of a hemolytic system. The enzymatic assay is, however, several orders of magnitude less sensitive than the hemolytic assay.

iii. Isolation of Human C1q[*][30]

(a) Characteristics. C1q occurs in serum as a calcium-dependent macromolecular complex with C1r and C1s (18 S) resembling, in chemical composition, collagen. C1q possesses specific affinity for the Fc region of immunoglobulins, a property that has been exploited to great advantage, as in detection of circulating antigen–antibody complex in certain types of patients. C1q is present in human serum at an average concentration of 200 μg/ml. It has an $s^o_{20,w}$ of 11.1 S corresponding to a molecular weight

---

[*] Section 17.D.2.a.iii, Method A, was contributed by Hans J. Müller-Eberhard. Methods B, C, and D were contributed by the Editors.

[30] M. A. Calcott and H. J. Müller-Eberhard, *Biochemistry* 11, 3443 (1972).

of approximately 388,000. It cannot pass a Millipore 0.45 μm membrane. For gel diffusion studies, it is necessary to use 0.6% agarose, not agar. The complex structure, with 6 subunits, can be visualized in the electron microscope[31,32]; subunits of 220,000 and 150,000 daltons have been described,[33] but upon treatment with urea and iodoacetamide smaller units are found (70,000 and 50,000 daltons). It is a highly basic protein. It behaves as a slow γ-globulin upon Pevikon block electrophoresis at pH 6.0, 7.0, and 8.6, but immunochemically it is distinct from γ-globulin. C1q is inactivated when serum or the isolated protein is heated at 56° for 30 minutes.

(b) *Procedures.* Several schemes have been used in isolating the highly basic, high molecular weight C1q. Calcott and Müller-Eberhard[30] prepare euglobulin and fractionate on CM-cellulose, Sephadex G-200, and Pevikon block electrophoresis (Method A). Agnello *et al.*[34] precipitate C1q with DNA, digest the DNA, and pass the digest through Sephadex G-200; this product was subjected to a further useful step by Knobel *et al.*[35]—passage through CM-cellulose (Method B). Or C1q can be chelated with EGTA at low ionic strength, the precipitate being then subjected to preparative polyacrylamide fractionation,[36] a procedure suitable for obtaining monospecific antibody (Method C). C1q can also be prepared by affinity chromatography, a C1q–IgG complex being dissociated in high ionic strength solution, low pH, by diaminoalkyl compounds[37] (Method D).

Method A. Column Chromatography and Block Electrophoresis[30]

The rationale of the given procedure is as follows. Precipitation of the euglobulins from serum achieves an approximately 100-fold purification of C1q and concentrates C1r, C1s, C3, C5, and C4 also (step 1). Since C1q is highly cationic—one of the most basic proteins of human serum, it is possible to separate it (step 2) from most of the other euglobulins, excepting for γM-globulin and electrophoretically slow γG-globulin. Utilizing the molecular size difference existing between C1q and γG-globulin, γG-globulin is eliminated (step 3). Step 4 affords the complete separation of C1q from γM-globulin, because of the distinctly different electrophoretic mobility of the two proteins. To minimize interaction be-

[31] E. Shelton, K. Yonemasu, and R. M. Stroud, *J. Immunol.* **107**, 310 (1971).

[32] M. J. Polley, *J. Immunol.* **107**, 322 (1971) (Abstract).

[33] K. Yonemasu and R. M. Stroud, *J. Immunol.* **107**, 309 (1971).

[34] V. Agnello, R. J. Winchester, and H. G. Kunkel, *Immunology* **19**, 909 (1970).

[35] H. R. Knobel, C. Heusser, M. L. Rodrick, and H. Isliker, *J. Immunol.* **112**, 2094 (1974).

[36] K. Yonemasu and R. M. Stroud, *J. Immunol.* **106**, 304 (1971).

[37] C. R. Sledge and D. H. Bing, *J. Immunol.* **111**, 661 (1973).

tween C1q and γG- or γM-globulin, the buffers utilized throughout the isolation procedure are of relatively low pH and high ionic strength. Note that all manipulations must be carried out as sterilely as possible since C1q cannot be sterilized by passage through a Millipore 0.45 μm membrane. Buffers for column chromatography as used in the authors' laboratory are given in Table I.

Step 1. Precipitation. The pH of 850 ml of fresh or outdated human serum is adjusted to 7.0 by addition of glacial acetic acid. Three volumes of cold distilled water are added, and after standing at 4° for 60 minutes the developing precipitate is sedimented by centrifugation at 1100 g and 4° for at least 30 minutes. The precipitate is washed with ice-cold phosphate buffer, pH 7.0, ionic strength 0.02 (1:5 dilution of buffer B, Table I). It is then dissolved in 8 ml of starting buffer for carboxymethyl (CM)-cellulose chromatography (buffer C, Table I) and subjected to ultracentrifugation for 45 minutes at 4° in a Spinco No. 40 rotor at 35,000 rpm. The cleared solution is recovered by puncturing the bottom of the centrifuge tube with a 20-gauge needle, leaving behind the layer of flotated lipids.

Step 2. Chromatography on CM-Cellulose. The material from step 1 is applied to a 4.5 × 60 cm column containing 700 ml of packed CM-cellulose equilibrated with phosphate buffer, pH 5.0, ionic strength 0.2 (buffer C, Table I). The protein is eluted stepwise, first with 1200 ml of the starting buffer containing 0.09 M NaCl and having a conductance of 19 mS. Then the buffer is removed from the top of the column and elution is continued with 1200 ml starting buffer containing 1.4 M NaCl and having a conductance of 100 mS. The protein diluted in this step is contained in approximately 100 ml and is concentrated by precipitation with ammonium sulfate (28 gm/100 ml, 4°, overnight). The precipitate is collected by centrifugation at 4° and 670 g for 30 minutes, and the supernatant is removed by siphon. It is then dialyzed against 2 liters of phosphate buffer, pH 5.3, ionic strength 0.3 (equivalent to 0.3 M NaCl) (buffer D, Table I), until the bulk of the protein is in solution.

Step 3. Filtration on Sephadex G-200. The material from step 2, contained in maximally 8 ml, is centrifuged at 670 g for 5 minutes to remove undissolved protein and applied to a 5 × 100 cm column containing 1300 ml of packed Sephadex G-200 equilibrated with buffer D. The protein solution, with its density raised by means of NaCl to a slightly greater value than that of the column buffer, is layered between the upper surface of the Sephadex column and the supernatant buffer through a thin polyethylene tubing fitted to a syringe. The flow rate is adjusted to 30 ml per hour, and 10-ml fractions are collected. The protein appearing in the exclusion volume is concentrated by precipitation with ammonium sulfate

TABLE I

BUFFERS FOR COLUMN CHROMATOGRAPHY[a,b]

A. Phosphate pH 6.0, $\Gamma/2 = 0.1$: 1050 ml of 1 M NaH$_2$PO$_4$ + 350 ml of 0.5 M Na$_2$HPO$_4$ + H$_2$O to 15 liters

B. Phosphate pH 7.0, $\Gamma/2 = 0.1$: 256 ml of 1 M NaH$_2$PO$_4$ + 896 ml of 0.5 M Na$_2$HPO$_4$ + H$_2$O to 16 liters

C. Phosphate pH 5.0, $\Gamma/2 = 0.2$: 2800 ml of 1 M NaH$_2$PO$_4$ + 132 ml of 0.5 M Na$_2$HPO$_4$ + H$_2$O to 15 liters

D. Phosphate pH 5.3, $\Gamma/2 = 0.3$: 910 ml of 0.3 M NaH$_2$PO$_4$ + 45 ml of 0.2 M Na$_2$HPO$_4$ + 45 ml of H$_2$O

E. Phosphate pH 6.0, $\Gamma/2 = 0.06$ containing EDTA; conductance 3.5 to 4.0 mS: 716 ml of 1 M NaH$_2$PO$_4$ + 165 ml of 0.5 M Na$_2$HPO$_4$ + 180 ml of 0.2 M Na$_3$EDTA + H$_2$O to 18 liters

F.a. Phosphate pH 5.8, conductance 3.3 mS: 4.12 gm of NaH$_2$PO$_4$ in 1000 ml of H$_2$O + 115 ml of a solution of 5.22 gm of K$_2$HPO$_4$ per 1000 ml of H$_2$O

F.b. Phosphate pH 5.8, conductance 12 mS: 24.89 gm of NaH$_2$PO$_4$ in 1000 ml of H$_2$O + 115 ml of a solution of 32.44 gm of K$_2$HPO$_4$/1000 ml of H$_2$O

F.c. Phosphate pH 5.8, conductance 13 mS: 27.6 gm NaH$_2$PO$_4$ in 1000 ml of H$_2$O + 115 ml of a solution of 34.84 gm of K$_2$HPO$_4$/1000 ml of H$_2$O

F.d. Phosphate pH 5.8, conductance 68 mS: 4000 ml of 0.65 M K$_2$HPO$_4$ + 200 ml of 0.65 M NaH$_2$PO$_4$

G. Veronal (Barbital) buffer pH 8.6, $\Gamma/2 = 0.05$: 143.7 gm of sodium barbital + 103.2 ml of 1 N HCl + H$_2$O to 16 liters

H. Tris pH 7.0, 0.0125 M: 125 ml of 1 M Tris + 106 ml of 1 N HCl; adjust to pH 7.0 with 1 N HCl, add H$_2$O to 10 liters

I. Phosphate pH 7.3, 0.02 M: 360 ml of 0.5 M Na$_2$HPO$_4$ + 75 ml of 1 M NaH$_2$PO$_4$ + H$_2$O to 15 liters.

J. Phosphate pH 8.1, 0.03 M: 22 ml of 1 M NaH$_2$PO$_4$ + 900 ml of 0.5 M Na$_2$HPO$_4$ + H$_2$O to 15 liters.

K. Phosphate pH 7.9, 0.02 M: 5000 ml of 0.2 M Na$_2$HPO$_4$ + 250 ml of 0.2 M NaH$_2$PO$_4$; the pH is adjusted to 7.9 by adding small increments of 0.2 M of NaH$_2$PO$_4$. The stock solution is diluted 1:10 with H$_2$O

L. Phosphate pH 7.9, 0.65 M: 4000 ml of 0.65 M K$_2$HPO$_4$ + 200 ml of 0.65 M NaH$_2$PO$_4$; the pH is adjusted to 7.9 with small increments of 0.65 M NaH$_2$PO$_4$

M. Phosphate pH 5.4, $\Gamma/2 = 0.02$: 352.5 ml of 1 M NaH$_2$PO$_4$ + 20 ml of 0.5 M Na$_2$HPO$_4$ + H$_2$O to 20 liters

N. Phosphate pH 5.1, $\Gamma/2 = 0.1$: 470 ml of 0.2 M NaH$_2$PO$_4$ + 10 ml of 0.2 M Na$_2$HPO$_4$ + H$_2$O to 1 liter

O. Tris pH 8.2, containing 1 M NaCl: 250 ml of 0.2 M Tris + 110 ml of 0.2 N HCl + 58.45 gm of NaCl + H$_2$O to 1 liter

P. EDTA, 0.008 M, pH 5.4: Dissolve 4.5 gm of Na$_4$·EDTA and 70.5 gm of Na$_2$ · EDTA to 1 liter as stock solution. Dilute 1:25 as working strength (conductance 1.25 mS)

Q. Oxidizing reagent, 0.01 M I$_2$ and 0.5 M KI: Dissolve 8.3 gm of KI and 0.25 gm of iodine crystals in 4 ml of phosphate buffer, pH 6.0, ionic strength 0.1 (buffer A), then bring volume to 100 ml with the same buffer. Store in a dark bottle at 4°. The solution is stable for 1 week. Working solutions are prepared by diluting this concentrate in the same buffer

---

[a] Readings of pH and conductance are made at 20°.

[b] Unless the work load of the laboratory will consume large quantities in a relatively short time, smaller volumes should be prepared. Unless antibiotics are added (Section 17.D.1), frequent replacement and cleaning of carboys is highly advisable (see Vol. II, Appendix II, Section 2). Pressure filtration through 142-mm or larger membranes is done speedily (Vol. I, Chap. 2.C.5). Periodic culturing of carboy contents can be a highly useful procedure (Vol. I, Chap. 2,C.4.f).

as described above and dissolved in 5 ml of phosphate buffer, pH 6.0, ionic strength 0.1 (buffer A, Table I), which is used for electrophoresis.

Step 4. Preparative Block Electrophoresis. After dialysis against electrophoresis buffer (buffer G, Table I), the material of step 3 is applied to a $1 \times 18 \times 50$ cm block of Pevikon C-870 with the application made 20 cm from the anodal end of the block. Electrophoresis is carried out for 40 hours at a potential gradient of 2.5 V/cm. The block is cut into 1.25 cm-wide segments, which are eluted with electrophoresis buffer; the protein content of each fraction, after dialysis, is determined by the Folin method. The well defined, narrowly distributed protein peak, which during electrophoresis moved from the origin toward the cathode and which corresponds exactly to the distribution of C1q activity, is recovered, and the protein is concentrated by precipitation with ammonium sulfate. The precipitate is dissolved and dialyzed using phosphate buffer B, Table I.

Method B[34]

Step 1. Precipitation with DNA.[34] Recalcified plasma or normal human serum is dialyzed *vs* barbital buffer (0.025 M), pH 8.6, containing 0.01 M Na$_4$·EDTA. Calf thymus DNA (Worthington Biochemical Corporation) is used to establish a precipitin curve with each batch of serum. The serum is treated with the optimal amount of DNA, 25 μg/ml usually, stirring being continued for 1 hour; then the solution is transferred to 4° for 24 hours. The precipitate is collected by centrifugation, washed 4 times with barbital buffer, and finally suspended in phosphate buffer 0.05 M, pH 6.9, with MgCl$_2$ 0.3 mM and NaCl 0.05 M. The suspension is adjusted to pH 6.9 with 1 N HCl.

Step 2. Digestion with DNase. DNase I (Worthington) is added, 100 μg/ml of suspension, and digestion is allowed to proceed with stirring for 3 hours in the room. The suspension is dialyzed *vs* the pH 6.9 phosphate buffer until the precipitate has largely dissolved. It is clarified by centrifugation at 100,000 g for 30 minutes.

Step 3. Gel Filtration on Sephadex G-200. The supernatant from step 2 is passed through G-200 in 0.3 M phosphate, pH 5.3, to remove DNA and DNase digestion products.

Step 4. Chromatography on CM-Cellulose.[35] The product from step 3, greater than 90% pure, is equilibrated with 0.02 M phosphate, pH 5.1, containing 0.01 M EDTA. The solution is passed through a column of CM-cellulose in the same buffer. After the column has been washed, a linear NaCl gradient is established (limit buffer, 1 M NaCl) to cover conductivity from 5 to 25 mS. After a minor peak, C1q is eluted at 8 mS.

Method C

A simple method for effective concentration of C1q was developed by Yonemasu and Stroud.[36] To obtain monospecific antisera, the product was then subjected to preparative polyacrylamide gel electrophoresis in two steps.

Step 1. Chelation of C1q. Whole human serum (125 ml) is dialyzed for 4 hours in the cold *vs* 1000 ml of 0.026 M ethylene glycol bis(amino-ethyl)tetraacetic acid (EGTA) at pH 7.5, conductance being equivalent to 0.03 M NaCl, and dialysis is continued for 11 hours with fresh buffer. The precipitate is collected and washed once with the same solution and then dissolved in 32 ml of 0.02 M acetate buffer, pH 5.0, containing 0.75 M NaCl and 0.01 M EDTA. The solution is freed of insoluble aggregates.

Step 2. Precipitation with EDTA. The clarified yield from step 1 is dialyzed in the cold for 4 hours *vs* 4 liters of 0.06 M EDTA, pH 5.0 (conductance that of 0.065 M NaCl), and the precipitate is secured and washed. It is dissolved in 32 ml of 0.005 M phosphate. pH 7.5, containing 0.75 M NaCl and 0.01 M EDTA and clarified by centrifugation.

Step 3. Reprecipitation with EDTA. The yield from step 2 is dialyzed in the cold for 5 hours against 0.035 M EDTA, pH 7.5, conductance equal to 0.069 M NaCl. The precipitate is collected and washed, then dissolved to 16 ml with 0.02 M phosphate buffer, pH 7.5, containing 0.75 M NaCl and 0.01 M EDTA.

Purity. The preparation did not contain detectable IgG, IgM, or IgA, and gave only one arc by IEA *vs* anti-human serum, and one major band in disc electrophoresis. For the preparation of monospecific anti-C1q, two successive runs in polyacrylamide gel were made. Details are given by the authors.

Method D[37]

The principle consists of adsorption of C1q from serum euglobulin to a column of human IgG-Sepharose, linked covalently, followed by elution with 1,4-diaminobutane. The yield is 3 to 4 mg of C1q from 100 ml of serum in about 2 days (about 25% of total C1q).

Step 1A. Preparation of Euglobulin as Source of C1q. Human serum was precipitated with acetate buffer, pH 5.5, $\Gamma/2 = 0.02$ (final pH 6.4, $\Gamma/2 = 0.03$). Precipitate was redissolved in 0.3 M NaCl to 0.1 volume of original serum. After dialysis for 18 hours *vs* excess Tris·HCl, pH 8.0, containing 0.01 M EDTA, $\Gamma/2 = 0.1$, the solution was clarified by centrifugation at 12,000 g for 30 minutes.

Step 1B. Preparation of Resin. Settled Sepharose, 40 ml, was linked covalently with human IgG,[38] about 370 mg of IgG becoming bound. The

[38] D. H. Bing, *J. Immunol.* **107**, 1243 (1971).

IgG was prepared by chromatography on DEAE-cellulose and showed, in IEA *vs* rabbit anti-human serum, only IgG immunoglobulin. The coupled Sepharose was packed into a 2.5 × 9 column and equilibrated at 4° with Tris·HCl, pH 8.1, containing 0.01 M EDTA, $\Gamma/2 = 0.075$.

Step 2. Affinity Chromatography. The column was charged with 6 ml of euglobulin concentrate from step 1A, and column buffer was passed to wash the column thoroughly; collections were 4 ml. Elution was conducted with 0.4 M NaCl and 0.01 M EDTA to remove some dissociable proteins. Specific elution was then made with 0.2 M 1,4-diaminobutane (Aldrich Chemical Co., Milwaukee, Wisconsin). Protein effluent was pooled and dialyzed vs Tris·HCl, pH 8.1, with 0.01 M Tris, $\Gamma/2 = 0.15$.

Step 3. Fractionation on Sucrose Gradient. Step 2 yields as secured from 30 ml of euglobulin concentrate were brought to 11 mg/ml and applied to a 10 to 40% sucrose gradient. Tubes having C1q activity (in the 10 S region) were pooled, rejecting 19 S material (IgM) in the lower part of the tube.

(c) C1q Activity Assay[30]

(i) Qualitative assay to detect C1q during the isolation procedure

(a) ASSAY. The assay can be carried out using a simple serum reagent called R1q[21] in conjunction with soluble γ-globulin aggregates. R1q lacks only C1q. This reagent precipitates when C1q is added; it is usual to leave the tubes at 4° for 15 to 20 hours.

Soluble γ-globulin aggregates. These are prepared by heating 1 gm of Cohn fraction II γG-globulin dissolved in 100 ml saline at exactly 63° for 15 minutes. The solution is cooled, and the aggregates are separated from unaggregated γ-globulin by precipitation with 7 gm of sodium sulfate. The precipitate is dissolved in 10 ml of distilled water and dialyzed against saline. After addition of 0.3 ml of a 10% solution of sodium azide, the aggregates are stored at room temperature, as they are less soluble in the cold.

Preparation of R1q. To 4 ml of fresh human serum containing 0.01 M Na$_3$H·EDTA (prepared from buffers 7 or 9, Section 17.B, Table I) is added 4 ml of a 35 mg/ml solution of soluble γ-globulin aggregates. The mixture is kept overnight in the cold and then subjected to ultracentrifugation for 90 minutes at 35,000 rpm in a Spinco No. 40 rotor. The aggregates are thus removed and the top four-fifths of the supernatant are recovered. Normal calcium and magnesium concentrations are established to overcome the added EDTA, and the R1q reagent is used at a final dilution of 1:50; at this concentration it should be totally nonlytic when tested with sensitized sheep erythrocytes (EA).

(b) AGGLUTINATION OF LATEX PARTICLES. The particles, coated with Cohn fraction II of human serum* can be used to monitor C1q by microtests in flat-bottomed wells of plastic trays. Glycine-saline buffer, pH 8.2, with added EDTA is used.

(ii) *Quantitative assay.*[30] This method is exact; it requires the use of purified human C4 (prepared as in Section 17.D.2.c), purified C1r (17.D.2.a.iv) and C1s̄ (17.D.2.a.vi), human ^{oxy}C2 (17.D.2.b.v) and di-isopropylfluorophosphate (DFP).[16] DFP must be handled with extreme care.†

Formation of C1 in the presence of C1r and C1s̄ is measured by quantitation of conversion of EAC4 to EAC1̄,4. The general plan of assay outlined in Section 17.D.2.a.ii(c) is followed.

Of C1q dilution (ranging from 1 to 100 ng), 0.2 ml is incubated with 0.4 ml of an optimal amount of C1r and C1s for 15 minutes at 37°, using GVB as diluent. Functionally C1r and C1s may be obtained as in Section 17.D.2.a.ii according to Lepow et al.,[20] and a concentration is selected which in the absence of C1q does not initiate hemolysis. Then 0.2 ml of EAC4 (1.5 × 10^8 cells/ml) (Section 17.C.4.e) is added and incubation is continued for 30 minutes at 37°. The cells are washed twice with GVB at room temperature, resuspended in 0.2 ml of GVB, and treated with 0.2 ml of ^{oxy}C2 (Section 17.D.2.b.v) containing approximately 3 × 10^{10} effective molecules. After 10 minutes at 32°, 2.4 ml of guinea pig serum diluted 1:100 in 0.04 M EDTA–GVB is added. Lysis is determined after 60 minutes at 37°, and the number of effective molecules is calculated from a plot of $-\ln(1 - y)$ vs dose, where y is the percentage of hemolysis.

(d) *Purity Criteria and Yield.* The maximal yield of C1q by Method A has been 6%, or approximately 10 mg of protein from 850 ml of serum. When examined in the analytical ultracentrifuge at a concentration of 5 mg/ml or more, C1q yields a well defined, self-sharpening boundary due to the asymmetry of the molecule. No other boundary should be de-

---

* The coated latex particles and basal buffer are available commercially (Hyland Laboratories, Los Angeles, California).

† Diisopropylfluorophosphate [(CH₃)₂CH·O]₂PFO, MW 208.17, is hazardous to handle. It is stable as the anhydrous compound or in solution in dry, triglyceride oils in sealed glass containers. A 1-ml portion of anhydrous DFP (Boots, Nottingham, England) is diluted with 1 ml of anhydrous isopropyl alcohol to reduce the volatility of the reagent. By means of a disposable micropipette, add 20 μl of this dilution (equivalent to 2.5 M concentration) to 100 ml of the cell suspension to secure a final concentration of 0.5×10^{-3} M. DFP forms an unstable solution in water (solubility 1.54%, pH 2.5). HF and oxides of phosphorus arise. Avoid inhaling vapors or contact with skin or eyes. Respiratory, laryngeal, and visual disturbances may be produced. Disposable pipettes must be flushed with isopropyl alcohol before discarding.

tectable. When tested with a potent antiserum to whole serum, using the Ouchterlony double-diffusion technique and agar concentrations of 2% and 0.7%, no precipitin line should be detectable with 2% agar since C1q does not enter the gel, but with the agar concentration of 0.7%, C1q can be detected. Agnello et al.[54] strongly recommended the use of agarose, not agar, and described the optimal conditions for gel diffusion of C1q (400,000 daltons) to be 0.6% agarose; pH 7.2 buffer of ionic strength 0.09 containing 0.01 M EDTA; use of macro-Ouchterlony plates containing a 5 mm depth of agar, with wells of 9 mm and center-to-center spacing of 12 mm; and a developmental period of 5 days, the first for 2 days at 22°, followed by 3 days at 0°. C1q may be quantitated with use of a specific antiserum. C1q does not enter starch gel or 4% polyacrylamide gel.

Method B yields a product more than 90% pure, functionally useful in gel-diffusion studies to detect soluble immune complexes in certain disease states (normal γ-globulin does not precipitate). The extent of purity was estimated by radial immunodiffusion vs rabbit anti-human C1q, prepared by injection of C1q in incomplete Freund's adjuvant. After step 4,[35] only 1 arc was seen in IEA vs anti-normal human serum.

Method C, after step 2, yielded a product negative for C1s and C1r when tested for esterolysis on synthetic substrates. After step 3, one weak precipitin arc was found by IEA against rabbit anti-human serum, and a single arc vs rabbit anti-human euglobulin; human IgM was absent.

iv. Isolation of C1r Proenzyme*

(a) *Procedure.* C1r proenzyme was purified by de Bracco and Stroud in 1971[39] from a crude euglobulin preparation by sequential steps of DEAE- and CM-chromatography followed by preparative polyacrylamide gel electrophoresis. The account given here follows the 4-step procedure of Valet and Cooper.[40] Information from both sources on properties of the proenzyme are complementary.

Step 1. Separation of Euglobulin. Human serum, 120 ml at 0°, was brought to pH 6.0 and dialyzed against 8 volumes of 0.013 M phosphate buffer, pH 6.0, conductivity 1.8 mS. After 14 hours, the precipitate was collected and washed twice with this buffer. Yield was dissolved in 250 ml of a solution containing 0.047 M phosphate, 0.04 M NaCl, and 0.001 M EDTA (pH 7.5, conductance 9.3 mS) and dialyzed overnight against 8 volumes of the same solution.

---

* Section 17.D.2.a.iv was compiled by the Editors.

[39] M. M. E. de Bracco and R. M. Stroud, *J. Clin. Invest.* **50,** 838 (1971).
[40] G. Valet and N. R. Cooper, *J. Immunol.* **112,** 1667 (1974).

Step 2. Chromatography on DEAE-Cellulose. The yield from step 1 was applied to a 3×40 cm column of DE-32 in the same buffer (conductance 9.3 mS), followed by washing with 2 liters. Elution was carried out by a linear gradient of 0.18 M NaCl in the same buffer. Fractions containing the C1r proenzyme (ca 12 mS) were pooled and adjusted to pH 8.0 and diluted to a conductance of 8 mS.

Step 3. Chromatography on TEAE-Cellulose. The selected pool from step 2 was applied to a 2.5×35 cm column of TEAE-cellulose in 0.047 M phosphate, 0.04 M NaCl, 0.001 M EDTA buffer at pH 8.0, 8 mS. After the column was washed, elution was carried out by a linear NaCl gradient, limit buffer 0.2 M NaCl. Fractions with C1r activity (ca 12 mS) were pooled and concentrated on an Amicon membrane to 1.5 ml.

Step 4. Gel Filtration on Sephadex G-200. The yield from step 3 was applied to a 2×100 cm column of G-200 equilibrated with pH 7.5 buffer (0.047 M phosphate, 0.1 M NaCl, 0.001 M EDTA) with conductance of 15 mS. The central peak represented C1r proenzyme.

(b) *Hemolytic Assay.*[39] A 5-step procedure was developed, based on the Borsos and Rapp plan for measuring C1.[41] (1) The C1r unknown, diluted variously in DGVB^{2+}, is incubated at 30° for 45 minutes with constant, excess amounts of C1q (9.9 μg/ml) and C1$\bar{s}$ (0.4 μg/ml) to generate C$\bar{1}$. (2) The reaction mixture is diluted 1:600; EAC4 (1.5×10^8/ml) are added, incubating for 10 minutes at 30° (C$\bar{1}$ binds to the cells). (3) The cells are washed twice and (4) incubated for 10 minutes at 30° with 0.25 ml of C2 solution providing 50 site-forming units (SFU) per milliliter to form EAC$\overline{142}$. (5) Guinea pig serum treated with EDTA is added to supply C3–C9. Hemolysis is read after 90 minutes at 37°.

(c) *Purity.* In disc electrophoresis run under special conditions to avoid precipitation at low ionic strength, one band was visualized; it proved to contain the C1r activity. Necessary conditions were: preliminary washing of 6% gels with 0.1 M Tris·HCl with NaCl added to 8 mS, pH 8.3; running buffer then replaced with glycine-Tris at 0.2 mS; samples and gel overlay set at conductance of 8 mS (added NaCl).

(d) *Yield.* ~1.3 mg/1200 ml of serum. The product sedimented as 7.5 S; the molecular weight was calculated as 188,000 (168,000 according to de Bracco and Stroud[39]).

(e) *Properties.* C1r proenzyme required activation by trypsin in order to activate C1s to C1$\bar{s}$. C1r would associate reversibly with C1q, but it formed a firm complex with C1s: C1r added to C1q and C1s was unable to reconstitute C1. C1r is reported[39] to be labile at 37°, pH 7 to 8 and low ionic strength.

[41] T. Borsos and H. J. Rapp, *J. Immunol.* **91,** 851 (1963).

v. Purification of C1s (C1 Proesterase)*

The isolation here follows K. Sakai and R. M. Stroud.[42] An alternative procedure is given by Valet and Cooper,[43] who used successive columns of DE-32, TEAE-cellulose, and Sephadex G-200. The average yield by the latter method is 2.3 mg/1200 ml of serum, about 2.4% of total C1s.

(a) *Treatment of Human Plasma.* Freshly drawn human blood was collected in 400-ml lots with 2000 USP units of Lipo-Hepin (Riker Laboratories) per milliliter. To the resulting plasma, 1 M L-lysine monohydrochloride at pH 7.5 was added to a concentration of 0.06 M in order to inhibit plasmin formation. To avoid spontaneous activation to C1$\bar{s}$, C1q was precipitated early in the procedure. All steps are performed rapidly and at close to 0°. The entire procedure requires 2 to 3 days.

(b) *Isolation Procedure*

Step 1. Separation of Euglobulin and Selective Solubilization of C1s. Lots of 360 ml of fresh human plasma containing 0.06 M L-lysine are adjusted to pH 7.5 and the relative salt concentration is made equivalent to the conductance of 0.04 M NaCl by dilution with 0.005 M Tris·HCl buffer, pH 7.5. After 1 hour at 0°, the precipitate is collected and washed twice with 0.005 M Tris, 0.045 M L-lysine, conductance at 0° equivalent to 0.035 M NaCl. The precipitate is suspended to 0.1 original plasma volume in 0.02 M EDTA, 0.005 M L-lysine, pH 7.5, with conductance equivalent to 0.04 M NaCl and held for 2 hours at 0°; C1s dissolves, C1q remains insoluble. Obtain the supernatant by centrifuging at 2700 g for 20 minutes.

Step 2. Chromatography on DEAE-Cellulose. The yield from step 1 is equilibrated with 0.005 M Tris·HCl, 0.01 M EDTA at pH 8.3, at conductance at 0° equivalent to 0.140 M NaCl, and is applied to a 1.5 × 12 cm column of DE-23 in the same buffer. The initial effluent (150 ml), containing the C1s activator, is saved; the column is washed thoroughly with the same buffer. A step gradient is applied (column buffer with NaCl added to a conductance equivalent to 0.3 M NaCl). C1s is eluted in 300 ml. It is concentrated by ultrafiltration.

(c) *Purity.* C1 proesterase was homogeneous upon acrylamide gel electrophoresis with SDS and upon immunoelectrophoretic analysis with horse anti-human serum. Upon reduction and alkylation, C1s gave only 1 band in disc electrophoresis in the presence of SDS and 8 M urea.

(d) *Tests for Activity.* Hemolytic activity was measured by the C1 titration method of Borsos and Rapp.[41] 0.3–0.4 μg of C1s was required

* Section 17.D.2.a.v was compiled by the Editors.

[42] K. Sakai and R. M. Stroud, *J. Immunol.* 110, 1010 (1973).
[43] G. Valet and N. R. Cooper, *J. Immunol.* 112, 339 (1974).

to generate 1 site-forming unit, owing to trace contamination with $C1\bar{s}$ or activation during the hemolytic assay.

vi. Preparation of Human $C1\bar{s}$ $(C\bar{1}\text{-}Esterase)$ [19]*

(a) *Characteristics*. When euglobulin preparations of human or guinea pig sera are incubated in the presence of Ca^{2+} at physiological pH and ionic strength, C1 develops esterase activity. After the subunits of C1 are separated upon chelating Ca^{2+}, C1s is found to possess the catalytic site $(C1\bar{s})$. $C1\bar{s}$ is capable by itself of hydrolyzing certain amino acid esters and attacking C4 and C2 in free solution (Section 17.D.2.a.i).

$C1\bar{s}$, like its inactive precursor C1s, is an α_2-globulin with a sedimentation constant of 4 S. Neither form of this subunit will be functional in reactions requiring attachment of C1 to antigen–antibody complexes until C1q, C1r, and Ca^{2+} are added, whereupon $C1\bar{s}$ will complete formation of a macromolecular complex that will function as a unit in inducing immune hemolysis. In the case of C1s, C1 is reconstituted; with $C1\bar{s}$, $C\bar{1}$ is formed.

Purified $C1\bar{s}$ is surprisingly thermostable. It is only 50% inactivated at 64° for 30 minutes; 4% of the initial activity is still detectable after boiling for 30 minutes. $C1\bar{s}$ is stable between pH 6 and pH 9.5, losing activity above and below these values. The activity of $C1\bar{s}$ is blocked by diisopropylfluorophosphate (DFP), by serum inhibitor of $C\bar{1}$ (see Section 17.E.2) and by specific antibody to $C1\bar{s}$. C1s and $C1\bar{s}$ are antigenically indistinguishable with antisera raised in rabbits by injection of $C1\bar{s}$.

$C1\bar{s}$ hydrolyzes a limited range of amino acid esters, including N-acetyl-L-tyrosine ethyl ester (ATE), N-acetyl-L-tyrosine methyl ester, benzoyl-L-arginine ethyl ester, p-toluenesulfonyl-L-arginine methyl ester, and N-acetyl-L-phenylalanine ethyl ester. It does not act on L-lysine methyl ester. Maximal hydrolysis of ATE occurs at a final substrate concentration of 5×10^{-2} M $(K_m = 1.9 \times 10^{-2}$ $M)$, pH 6.7 to 8.0, ionic strength below 0.20, and 38.8° (apparent energy of activation = 10,400 cal/mole). Divalent cations are not required for esterolytic activity.

By all available criteria, the same catalytic site $C1\bar{s}$ which is involved in hydrolysis of amino acid esters also functions in inactivating the hemolytic activity of C4 and C2 in free solution, and in the uptake and activation of C4 and C2 on antigen–antibody complexes.[13-19, 24, 25, 28, 44]

(b) *Procedures*. Two methods are given, both starting from euglobulin in 0.1 the original volume of human serum. Thereafter, in Method A[19]

---

* Section 17.D.2.a.vi was contributed by Irwin H. Lepow.

[44] H. J. Müller-Eberhard, M. J. Polley, and M. A. Calcott, *J. Exp. Med.* **125**, 359 (1967).

the C1 is activated to $C\bar{1}$, the Ca^{2+} is chelated, and subunits are subjected to DEAE-cellulose and two successive runs on TEAE-cellulose. In Method B,[43] the euglobulin is precipitated twice in low ionic strength buffer; a third precipitation selectively *removes* C1q, and the supernatant is chromatographed on DEAE-cellulose.

Method A

A euglobulin fraction of normal human serum is prepared exactly as described in Section 17.D.2.a.ii(b) except that $Na_3H \cdot EDTA$ is *not* used at any point in the procedure. (The 10-fold concentrated euglobulin, at pH 7.4 and ionic strength 0.15, does not contain serum inhibitor ($C\bar{1}$-In) for the activated macromolecular complex.) Upon incubation in the presence of Ca^{2+} at 37° for 15 minutes, at physiological pH and ionic strength, C1 in this fraction will activate to $C\bar{1}$. Chromatographic resolution of the subunits of the activated complex on DEAE-cellulose (step 1), according to the rationale discussed earlier for C1, yields $C\bar{1}$ which is further purified on TEAE-cellulose (steps 2 and 3) by empirical methods.

Step 1. Chromatography on DEAE-Cellulose. This step follows that described [Section 17.D.2.a.ii(b)] for the separation of C1q, C1r, and C1s. Results are independent of the use of $Na_3H \cdot EDTA$ in the starting and limit buffers. In routine preparations in this laboratory, 100 ml of euglobulin solution (equivalent to 1 liter of serum) are applied to a 4.4×40 cm column of DEAE-cellulose. Linear gradient elution is accomplished with 2 liters each of starting and limit buffer. Fractions of 25 ml are collected at a flow rate of about 100 ml per hour. The resulting chromatogram is essentially indistinguishable in appearance from that found in Section 17.C.2.b.

$C1\bar{s}$, measured routinely by the esterolytic assay, is located in a single sharp peak with the small peak of protein emerging at ionic strength 0.37. Fractions from the central core of this peak are pooled, concentrated 5- to 10-fold with respect to euglobulin in an Amicon pressure ultrafiltration apparatus, and dialyzed *vs* pH 9.0, 0.02 M glycine buffer (100 ml of 0.2 M glycine and 24 ml of 0.2 M NaOH diluted to 1 liter with distilled water). Under these conditions, $C1\bar{s}$ is stable at −70° for at least 6 months.

Step 2. Chromatography on TEAE-Cellulose. $C1\bar{s}$ pooled from 4 to 6 such runs (150 to 200 mg of protein) is applied to a 1.8×30 cm column packed with TEAE-cellulose previously equilibrated with pH 9.0, 0.02 M glycine buffer at 5°. All or very nearly all of the applied protein is adsorbed and is then eluted with a linear salt gradient consisting of 1 liter each of starting buffer (pH 9.0, 0.02 M glycine) and limit buffer (0.5 M NaCl in starting buffer). Fractions of 10 ml are collected at a flow rate of 30 to 60 ml per hour.

The major peak emerges at ionic strength 0.22. It is rather broad and asymmetrical on the ascending side and is preceded by several very small, irregular protein peaks. Activity of C1s̄ is mainly confined to the central portion of the main peak. Fractions of highest specific activity are pooled, concentrated about 25-fold with respect to euglobulin by pressure ultra-filtration, and dialyzed vs pH 9.0, 0.02 M glycine buffer.

Step 3. Rechromatography on TEAE-Cellulose. Slight additional purification of C1s̄ is achieved by repetition of the second step, the yield from which (about 30 mg of protein) is applied to a 1×18 cm column of TEAE-cellulose. Conditions of chromatography are the same, except that 500-ml volumes of gradient buffers are used and fractions of 5 ml are collected.

A large, sharply defined peak of protein emerges from the column at ionic strength 0.22, with only minor asymmetry at the base on both the ascending and descending sides. Activity of C1s̄ closely parallels the protein content of all but the lowest portions of the peak. The latter fractions are discarded and the other fractions are dialyzed vs pH 7.4 phosphate buffer, ionic strength 0.15, adjusted to 100 units/ml as determined in the esterolytic assay below, and frozen in small aliquots at $-70°$. The resulting highly purified preparation is stable under these conditions for more than one year.

Method B[42]

Crude C1̄ was obtained by dialyzing serum vs a solution of 0.015 M NaCl at pH 5.5, the washed precipitate being redissolved and reprecipitated by means of dialysis vs a large excess of 0.005 M phosphate, pH 7.5, for 4 hours.[45]

Step 1. Separation of C1q. The crude C1̄ was dissolved in 0.005 M Tris·HCl, pH 7.5, with sodium chloride added to provide a conductance at 0° equivalent to 0.3 M NaCl. The solution was dialyzed vs 0.02 M EDTA, pH 7.5, conductance equivalent to 0.036 M NaCl. Precipitated C1q was removed by centrifugation, 27,000 g for 20 minutes. The supernatant, containing C1s̄, was dialyzed against 0.005 M Tris, 0.01 M EDTA, pH 8.3, conductance equivalent to 0.17 M NaCl.

Step 2. Chromatography on DEAE-Cellulose. The yield from step 1 was chromatographed on a 1.5×20 cm column of DE-23 in the same buffer, and the column was washed thoroughly. Elution of C1s̄ was made by adding NaCl to the same buffer to provide a conductance equivalent to 0.3 M NaCl.

(c) *Purity and Yield.* The yield and purification data for Method A are summarized in Table II. One liter of human serum yields 1.1 mg

[45] N. Tamura and R. A. Nelson, Jr., *J. Immunol.* **101**, 1333 (1968).

TABLE II
PURIFICATION OF C1s̄

Step	Yields[a] (% of serum)	Specific activity (units/mg N)	Purification factor (serum = 1)
Euglobulin	ca. 100[b]	32	ca. 20[b]
DEAE-cellulose chromatography	30	960	600
TEAE-cellulose chromatography	12	2800	1740
TEAE-cellulose rechromatography	5	3800	2400

[a] Based only on fractions from central core of activity peaks which are pooled for further purification or as final product.

[b] Estimated values based on hemolytic activity of C1̄.

of final product, purified 2400-fold with respect to serum with an overall yield of 5%. On this basis, the concentration in serum of C1s or C1s̄ has been calculated to be 22 μg/ml.[19]

The preparation of C1s̄ described above fulfills some, but not all, criteria for a single protein. It migrates as a single band in the α_2-globulin region in electrophoresis on paper and starch gel. In sucrose density gradient ultracentrifugation, it gives a symmetrical 4 S peak. However, in a limited number of runs in the analytical ultracentrifuge, asymmetry of the descending side of the peak has been noted or frank resolution of a smaller, slightly heavier component. Indications of heterogeneity have also been observed in immunodiffusion and immunoelectrophoresis *vs* rabbit antiserum to partially purified C1s̄. Whether these findings reflect contamination with an extraneous protein or other posssibilities such as isozymic or polymeric forms of C1s̄ is not known.

In Method B, the yield of C1s̄ is about 10%; $E_{1 \text{ cm}}^{1\%} = 16.7$ at 280 nm. Molecular size is estimated as ~110,000 daltons or as 86,200.[43] It gives a single band on acrylamide disc gel electrophoresis with SDS, and a single arc by IEA in agarose *vs* horse anti-human serum, and consistently a characteristic double arc in 1% Special Agar-Noble *vs* rabbit anti-human C1s̄. The gull-wing feature is not explained. Upon reduction and alkylation, C1s̄ showed two major chains (~36,000 and ~77,000 daltons) in disc electrophoresis in the presence of SDS or 8 M urea.

(*d*) *Tests for Activity.* (*1*) *Esterase activity.* Esterolytic activity of C1s̄ is routinely assayed with *N*-acetyl-L-tyrosine ethyl ester (ATE) as substrate. Various volumes of C1s̄ not exceeding 0.5 ml are brought to a volume of 2.375 ml with pH 7.4 phosphate buffer, ionic strength 0.15, and incubated at 37° for 5 minutes. At zero time, 0.125 ml of 1 M ATE (dissolved in ethylene glycol monomethyl ether) is added and a 1.0-ml portion is immediately withdrawn and added to 1.0 ml of 37% neutral formaldehyde. After incubation at 37° for 15 minutes, a second aliquot of 1.0 ml is similarly withdrawn. Both samples are titrated to a phenolphthalein end point with 0.05 N NaOH, employing a microburet. The net titration is a direct measure of C1s̄ activity. One unit of enzyme is arbitrarily defined as that amount which liberates 0.5 microequivalent of H^+ from ATE under these standardized conditions.

(2) *Hemolytic activity.* C1̄ activity may also be measured by assays in hemolytic systems based on reconstitution of activated macromolecular complex activity in the presence of C1q, C1r, and Ca^{2+}. The procedures are the same as those already described in Section 17.D.2.a.ii(c).

In the final preparation of Method B, the activity of C1s̄ was found to be 0.01 to 0.02 μg for generating 1 SFU (i.e., 20- to 30-fold more active than C1s tested under the same conditions). It was shown also that C1s̄, insolubilized by coupling via cyanogen bromide to Sephadex G-25, retains activity.

(3) *Inhibition of hemolysis.* C1s̄ may be assayed also by its ability to inactivate the hemolytic activity of C4 and C2 in free solution.[13, 14, 28]

b. ISOLATION OF HUMAN C2[*46]

i. *Characteristics*

C2 occurs in human serum with an average concentration of 25 to 30 μg/ml. It is a pseudoglobulin with a sedimentation coefficient of 5.2, a molecular weight of approximately 117,000, and an electrophoretic mobility in Pevikon of a β-globulin. It contains two reactive sulfhydryl groups per molecule[47] and is inactivated by treatment with p-chloromercuribenzoate (p-CMB). C2 is one of the natural substrates of C1s̄, which in the absence of C4 inactivates the molecule apparently by cleavage of a covalent bond, yielding inactivated C2 with an apparent molecular weight of 83,000. The procedure of isolation given here results in a maximal yield of about 2 mg from 800 ml of serum, i.e., 10 to 15% of the amount present in serum.

ii. *Procedure*

Outdated ACD blood has been used because it has consistently produced higher yields than freshly drawn blood. All preparative procedures have been so arranged that they can be performed at pH 5.8 to 6.0, since

* Section 17.D.2.b was contributed by Hans J. Müller-Eberhard.

[46] M. J. Polley and H. J. Müller-Eberhard, *J. Exp. Med.* **128**, 533 (1968).
[47] M. J. Polley and H. J. Müller-Eberhard, *J. Immunol.* **102**, 1339 (1969).

C2 hemolytic activity is found to be most stable at this pH. EDTA is incorporated into most buffers because C2 is readily inactivated by heavy metal ions owing to its free sulfhydryl groups. The DFP treatment of the pseudoglobulin (step 1) was needed because of the presence in these materials of a serine esterase, probably $C1\bar{s}$, which is capable of inactivating C2. The CM-cellulose chromatography (step 2) separates C2 from 97% of the pseudoglobulins. By Pevikon block electrophoresis (step 3), C2 is freed of γG-globulin, which constitutes 99% of the protein eluted from CM-cellulose together with the C2. And hydroxylapatite (step 4) eliminates C3, C4, and C5 as well as an unknown protein, which is present in trace amounts together with C2 in the electrophoretic fraction.

Step 1. Removal of Euglobulin and Treatment with DFP. Outdated human blood (21 days after drawing) is allowed to clot. The resulting 800 ml of serum is dialyzed for 48 hours against 3 portions each of 10 liters of an 8×10^{-3} M solution of EDTA (reagent 9 *at pH 5.4*, Section 17.B, Table I, diluted 1:25) and a conductance of 1.25 mS to precipitate the euglobulins, including C1. The pseudoglobulin fraction is separated from the precipitate by centrifugation at 1500 g for 30 minutes at 4°, and the pH of the supernatant is adjusted with 1 N NaOH to 7.0. This material is then incubated in a tightly stoppered Erlenmeyer flask at 37° for 1 hour with DFP at a final concentration of 1×10^{-3} M (see footnote on DFP, Section 17.D.2.a.ii). DFP is a volatile, highly toxic reagent; it is diluted with an equal volume of anhydrous isopropyl alcohol to reduce the volatility of the reagent. Add 40 μl of this dilution per 100 ml of the pseudoglobulin. Rinse the pipette with isopropyl alcohol. After the period of incubation, the flask is cooled to 0° to 4° before it is unstoppered in a chemical hood.

Step 2. Chromatography on CM-Cellulose. The DFP-treated pseudoglobulin fraction is applied to a 7.5×60 cm column containing approximately 2000 ml of packed CM-cellulose equilibrated with phosphate buffer E (Table I) pH 6, ionic strength 0.06, containing 2×10^{-3} M EDTA) having a conductance of 3.5 to 4.0 mS.* The required conductance of this starting buffer may differ slightly for different batches of CM-cellulose. It should be 0.5 mS below the value at which C2 is eluted from the CM-cellulose. After the application of the sample, 10 liters of starting buffer are passed through the column to remove proteins that are not adsorbed to CM-cellulose under these conditions. C2, together

---

* Conductivity measurements are made conveniently by a conductivity bridge, such as Model RC 16B2 of Beckman Instruments, Inc., Cedar Grove, New Jersey, together with a pair of conductivity cells with constants $K = 0.1$ and $K = 1.0$, respectively, filled by suction through a capillary. The conductivity cells, if specially ordered with a 14-cm capillary (item G 1 × 14), permit ready measurements of small volumes within fraction collector tubes—Editors.

with other basic proteins, is eluted by the application of a salt concentration gradient. The column is supplied from a 2-liter closed Erlenmeyer flask, which serves as mixing chamber containing 2000 ml of starting buffer; it is connected by siphon to a 2-liter beaker containing approximately 1900 ml of 0.7 M NaCl in starting buffer. The flow rate is adjusted to 2 ml per minute and 20-ml fractions are collected. The fractions containing C2 hemolytic activity (see below for assay method) are pooled and concentrated to 20 ml by ultrafiltration. This sample is then again treated carefully with DFP for 30 minutes at 37° as outlined above. The CM-cellulose is re-used only five or six times, then discarded.

Step 3. Preparative Block Electrophoresis. The concentrated DFP-treated chromatography fraction is divided into two 10-ml samples, each of which is separately subjected to Pevikon-block electrophoresis using phosphate buffer (A, Table I, diluted 1:2) containing 2.5×10^{-3} M EDTA (0.93 gm of $Na_2H_2 \cdot EDTA$ per liter). The polyvinyl sheeting used for the base and cover of the block must be washed with 5×10^{-3} M EDTA before use. Electrophoresis is allowed to proceed for 23 hours at 4° under a potential gradient of 4 V/cm (see Vol. II, Chap. 6.D.1 and Appendix III).

Step 4. Chromatography on Hydroxylapatite. Hydroxylapatite is prepared following the method of Tiselius et al.[48] Batches of freshly prepared hydroxylapatite usually give a very low recovery of C2 hemolytic activity. By passing 500 mg of human serum albumin through the packed hydroxylapatite column before application of the C2 preparation, this problem may be alleviated. The C2-containing fractions from the two Pevikon blocks are pooled (approximately 100 ml) and applied to a 2.5×30 cm column of hydroxylapatite equilibrated with phosphate buffer (F.a, Table I). The column is then washed with 100 ml of the same buffer, followed by 250 ml of each of two buffers having the same pH but different conductivities. The concentration of phosphate is increased to yield a conductance first of 12 mS (buffer F.b, Table I), then of 13 mS (buffer F.c, Table I). The Buffer F.b removes contaminating material, and buffer F.c elutes C2. The conductance required for optimal purification of C2 may vary slightly with each new batch of hydroxylapatite. In order to elute residual protein, the column is washed with phosphate buffer having a conductance of 68 mS (buffer F.d, Table I). The flow rate is adjusted to 1 ml/minute and 4-ml fractions are collected. At this stage, it is necessary to use siliconized tubes for collection of the effluent in order to preserve C2 activity.

The fractions containing C2 activity are pooled and, to protect C2 during subsequent concentration by ultrafiltration, monomeric carboxy-amidomethylated human serum albumin is added in an amount sufficient

[48] A. Tiselius, S. Hjertén, and Ö. Levin, Arch. Biochem. Biophys. 65, 132 (1956).

to yield 1 mg/ml in the concentrated pool. Purified C2 is divided into 0.1- or 0.2-ml aliquots contained in siliconized tubes, frozen in liquid nitrogen, and stored at $-70°$.

The albumin that is used to protect isolated C2 is prepared as follows. One gram of crystallized human serum albumin (Behringwerke A. G., Marburg/Lahn, Germany) dissolved in 10 ml of barbital buffer, pH 8.6, ionic strength 0.05 (buffer G, Table I) is subjected to Pevikon-block electrophoresis for 16 hours. The peak fractions of the major component are pooled and treated overnight at 4° with iodoacetamide at a final concentration of 10^{-2} M. After concentration and dialysis, this material is applied to a Sephadex G-100 column, and the monomeric form of the iodoacetamide-treated albumin is isolated and concentrated.

iii. Activity Assay of C2[49]

In fractions of serum separated from columns and Pevikon blocks, C2 may be *qualitatively* detected with a simple serum reagent, R2.[50]

The *quantitative assay* consists of measurement of the conversion of EAC$\overline{1}$,4 to EAC$\overline{1,4,2}$. The EAC$\overline{1}$,4 complex is required to have a minimum of 3000 bound C4 molecules/cell; i.e., it must be prepared with 100 μg of C4 per 5×10^9 EAC1 or 200 effective molecules/cell.[38] Aliquots 0.2 ml, of EAC$\overline{1}$,4 at a concentration of 1.5×10^8 cells/ml in GVB (buffer 1d, Section 17.B, Table I) are pipetted into a series of tubes, 0.4 ml of a dilution of C2 (minimal amount of C2 protein, 1 ng) is added, and the mixture is incubated at 30° for 10 minutes. Then, 2.4 ml of a 1:50 dilution of guinea pig serum in 0.04 M EDTA–VB (prepared as for GVB but omitting gelatin and including 0.04 M EDTA) is added; after incubation for 1 hour at 37°, the degree of lysis is determined spectrophotometrically at 412 nm. A sample of EAC$\overline{1}$,4 incubated with 0.04 M EDTA–VB for 60 minutes at 37° serves as control. The 100% lysis value is obtained from a water lysate of EAC$\overline{1}$,4 cells, and y, the percentage lysis in the test samples, may then be calculated. The amount of C2 present may be expressed in terms of effective C2 molecules by converting y to $-\ln(1 - y)$ and by multiplying this value by the number of cells present.

iv. Yield and Purity Criteria

The maximal yield of C2 has been 10 to 15% of the amount present in serum, i.e., approximately 2 mg from 800 ml of serum.

[49] N. R. Cooper, M. J. Polley, and H. J. Müller-Eberhard, *Immunochemistry* **7**, 341 (1970).

[50] R. A. Nelson, Jr., J. Jensen, I. Gigli, and N. Tamura, *Immunochemistry* **3**, 111 (1966).

Highly purified C2 appears as a single protein band on polyacrylamide gel electrophoresis, which, after treatment of C2 with C1s̄, is shifted *in toto* to a more anodal position. Most preparations of C2 do contain some of this inactivated C2 protein, which may be identified as such immunochemically. By immunoelectrophoretic analysis in agar (but not in agarose), native C2 has an anomalous mobility comparable to that of albumin. In contrast, the C1s̄-inactivated C2 behaves as β-globulin. In terms of hemolytic activity, 1 μg of isolated C2 contains 2 to 4 $\times$ 10^9 effective molecules.

v. Oxidation of Human C2 [44, 51]

Treatment of C2 with a critical dose of iodine was found to result in a 13-fold enhancement of its hemolytic activity. Further, the intermediate complex EACI̅,̅4̅,̅2̅ and the enzyme C4̅,̅2̅ are approximately 20 times more stable when prepared with iodine-treated C2 than they are when formed with native C2. The iodine effect was shown to be due to the oxidation of the two free sulfhydryl groups present in native C2. The molecular weight of ^{oxy}C2 is identical to that of native C2.

Highly purified C2 in a concentration of 300 μg/ml is mixed with an equal volume of a solution of 5×10^{-5} M I_2 and 2.5×10^{-3} M KI in phosphate buffer, pH 6.0, ionic strength 0.1 (buffer A, Table I). The mixture is kept for 5 minutes at room temperature, then chilled and diluted for immediate use. The iodine solution is prepared by diluting reagent Q, Table I, 1:200 in buffer A.

C2 activity in whole human serum may be enhanced approximately 6-fold by treating undiluted serum with an equal volume of 1:10 dilution of reagent Q, Table I, in buffer A (1×10^{-3} M iodine in 5×10^{-2} M potassium iodide solution). The mixture is kept at room temperature for 5 minutes and is then exhaustively dialyzed at 4° against VB (without gelatin). Since the amount of I_2 required for optimal enhancement varies slightly with each batch of serum and since an excess of I_2 will cause inactivation of the serum hemolytic activity, the optimal I_2 concentration should be determined on small aliquots of the serum to be treated, as described in Section 17.C.4.a.

c. ISOLATION OF HUMAN C4[52]*

i. Characteristics

The protein has an $s_{20,w}^\circ$ of 10 S, a molecular weight of approximately 200,000, and an electrophoretic mobility of a fast β-globulin. Its average

---

[51] M. J. Polley and H. J. Müller-Eberhard, *J. Exp. Med.* **126**, 1013 (1967).
[52] H. J. Müller-Eberhard and C. E. Biro, *J. Exp. Med.* **118**, 447 (1963).

* Section 17.D.2.c was contributed by Hans J. Müller-Eberhard.

concentration in human serum is 430 $\mu g/ml$. C4 is one of the natural substrates of C1$\bar{s}$, which activates its combining site enabling the molecule to attach to certain receptors.[28, 53, 54] Activation is transient and is effected by cleavage of the molecule. A fragment, C4a, with the molecular weight of 15,000 may be dissociated from the cleaved molecule at low pH. In the absence of receptors, C4 is inactivated by C1$\bar{s}$. In the complement reaction C4 serves as acceptor for C2,[55] and as one of the subunits of the C$\overline{4,2}$ enzyme which acts on C3 (Section 17.A, Fig. 1A).

ii. Procedure

The yield should be 10–12 mg of C4 per 100 ml of serum (7 to 8% of actual content). The rationale of the procedure is as follows. Dialysis of serum against Tris buffer at pH 7.0 separates most of the C1 complex, and thus C1$\bar{s}$, from the C4-containing supernatant (step 1). This is important because C1$\bar{s}$ can inactivate C4. By TEAE-cellulose chromatography (step 2), C4 is separated from 98% of the pseudoglobulins, and block electrophoresis at pH 8.6 (step 3) removes the contaminating γM-globulin, ceruloplasmin, and other α_2-globulins. The repeat of chromatography on TEAE-cellulose (step 4) is necessary only if step 3 has not yielded satisfactory results.

Step 1. Removal of Euglobulin. Fresh human serum, 400 ml, is dialyzed overnight against 10 liters of 0.0125 M Tris buffer, pH 7.0 (buffer H of Table I), at 4°. The euglobulin precipitate is removed by centrifugation at 1100 g for 30 minutes. The supernatant is then dialyzed for 24 hours against 2 portions of 10 liters of 0.008 M EDTA solution, pH 5.4 (reagent P, Table I, diluted 1:25). The precipitate is removed by centrifugation as above, and the pH of the supernatant is adjusted to 7.3 with 1 N NaOH.

Step 2. Chromatography on TEAE-Cellulose. The pseudoglobulin fraction is applied to a 7.5 × 59 cm column containing 2000 ml of packed TEAE-cellulose equilibrated with 0.02 M phosphate buffer, pH 7.3 (buffer I, Table I, starting buffer). When the pseudoglobulin has entered the column, the column is washed with 5 liters of the same buffer containing 0.09 M sodium chloride to yield a conductance of 10 mS, (see footnote to Section 17.D.2.b.i, step 2) and a flow rate of 200 ml per hour is established. The buffer on top of the cellulose column is then siphoned off, and 3 liters of the starting buffer, but containing 0.11 M sodium chloride to yield a conductance of 11.6 mS, is passed through the column. When the conductance of the effluent has reached 11.6 mS, elution of C4 by

[53] R. A. Patrick, S. B. Taubman, and I. H. Lepow, *Immunochemistry* **7**, 217 (1970).
[54] D. B. Budzko and H. J. Müller-Eberhard, *Immunochemistry* **7**, 227 (1970).
[55] I. Gigli and K. F. Austen, *J. Exp. Med.* **229**, 679 (1969) ; **230**, 833 (1969).

a sodium chloride gradient is started. A 2-liter closed Florence flask is used as mixing chamber, filled with 0.11 M sodium chloride dissolved in starting buffer. The flask is connected by siphon with a 2-liter Erlenmeyer flask containing 2000 ml of 0.75 M sodium chloride in starting buffer. The flow rate is adjusted to 100 ml per hour, and 14-ml fractions are collected. Every fifth fraction is analyzed for protein content and for C4 hemolytic activity as described below. C4 is usually eluted within a conductance range of 13 to 20 mS. The fractions containing C4 activity are pooled (usually 300 to 500 ml) and passed through a Millipore filter before the pool is concentrated by ultrafiltration to a volume of 10 ml.

Step 3. Preparative Block Electrophoresis. Concentrated material, 10 ml, is applied to a Pevikon block prepared with barbital buffer, pH 8.6, ionic strength 0.05 (buffer G, Table I). Application is made 7 cm away from the cathodal end of the block. Electrophoresis is carried out for 40 to 44 hours at 3.0 V/cm. The eluates from block segments are analyzed for protein and for C4 hemolytic activity. The active fractions, which correspond to a well defined protein peak in the β-globulin region, are pooled. If the yield of C4 is found to be uncontaminated, as is often the case, it is concentrated, dialyzed against phosphate buffer, pH 6.0, ionic strength 0.2 (buffer A, Table I, 2 times concentrated), and frozen in liquid nitrogen. Otherwise it is subjected to step 4.

Step 4. Chromatography on TEAE-Cellulose. The unconcentrated pool of material from the Pevikon block is applied to a 1.3 × 40 cm column containing 45 ml of packed TEAE-cellulose, which is equilibrated with starting buffer I. The chromatograph is developed by sodium chloride gradient elution. An 800-ml closed flask containing 600 ml of starting buffer is used as mixing chamber. It is connected by siphon with a 500-ml Erlenmeyer flask containing as limit buffer 450 ml of 0.7 M sodium chloride in starting buffer. The flow rate is adjusted to approximately 300 ml per hour, and 2.5-ml fractions are collected. The fractions are analyzed for protein concentration and C4 hemolytic activity. The activity distribution closely parallels the distribution of the major protein peak. The fractions containing activity are pooled and concentrated.

iii. C4 Activity Assay[56]

The formation of EAC1,4 from EAC1 is measured. Aliquots, 0.2 ml, of EAC$\overline{1}$ (see Section 17.C.2.a) at a concentration of 1.5 × 10^8 cells/ml in GVB^{2+} (buffer 1d, Section 17.B, Table I) are dispensed into a number of tubes. Then 0.2-ml portions of dilutions of C4 (ranging from 2.5 to 100 ng of C4 protein per milliliter made in the same buffer are added, and the mixtures are incubated for 15 minutes at 30°. Oxidized C2 (50

[56] N. R. Cooper and H. J. Müller-Eberhard, *Immunochemistry* 5, 155 (1968).

to 100 effective molecules/cell)[*] in a volume of 0.2 ml is then added to each tube, incubation is continued for 10 minutes at 30°, then there is added 2.4 ml of guinea pig serum diluted 1:50 in VB containing 0.04 M EDTA (buffer 7c, Section 17.B, Table I, with EDTA increased to 40 mM). After 60 minutes at 37°, the released hemoglobin is quantitated spectrophotometrically. Controls include (a) EAC1 plus C2 and 0.04 M Na$_3$H·EDTA guinea pig complement, (b) a Na$_3$H·EDTA guinea pig complement color blank, and (c) a water lysate of EAC1 cells. The optical density of (a) is subtracted from that of the experimental tubes containing the complete reaction mixture, and the difference between the optical density of (a) and of (b) is subtracted from that of (c). From this set of data the amount of C4 can be determined which yields a —$\ln(1 - y)$ value of 1.

iv. Yield and Purity Criteria

C4 protein, 10 to 12 mg, or 7 to 8% of the amount of C4 present in 400 ml of serum are usually obtained.

Isolated C4 contains approximately 1×10^{10} hemolytically effective molecules per microgram of protein. It yields a single band on disc electrophoresis. A single precipitin line is observed when isolated C4 is examined by immunoelectrophoresis or Ouchterlony test using either anti-whole human serum or anti-C4. After treatment with C1s̄ (0.5 unit of C1s̄ per 200 μg of C4, 15 minutes, 37°, two protein bands are seen, one slower, the other faster than the original band.

d. Isolation of Human C3 and C5[57][†]

i. Characteristics of Human C3

C3 is a euglobulin, having an $s^\circ_{20,w}$ of 9.5 S, a molecular weight of approximately 180,000, and an electrophoretic mobility of a β-globulin.[58] Its average concentration in serum is indeed high, 1.2 mg/ml. It is the natural substrate of the C$\overline{4,2}$ enzyme (Section 17.A, Fig. 1A) and of factor $\overline{B}$ (C3 activator, Section 17.A, Fig. 1B). When acted upon by the EAC$\overline{4,2}$ enzyme, C3 is enabled to combine with receptor sites on the erythrocyte–enzyme complex ‡ Bound C3 is split to C3a and C3b, of which a part of

---

[*] Oxidation of well purified C2 should result in 25 to 50×10^9 effective molecules per microgram, about 13-fold greater than for native C2.

[57] U. R. Nilsson and H. J. Müller-Eberhard, *J. Exp. Med.* 122, 277 (1965).

[†] Section 17.D.2.d was contributed by Hans J. Müller-Eberhard.

[58] H. J. Müller-Eberhard, U. R. Nilsson, and T. Aronson, *J. Exp. Med.* 111, 201 (1960).

‡ Owing to the large amounts of C3b which become bound to antigen–antibody complexes *in vivo*, fluorescent antisera prepared against C3 have been used to demonstrate sites of immunological reaction (Section 17.F.4.c).

the C3b is retained on the erythrocyte to form $EAC\overline{1,4,2,3b}$, opening the pathway for utilization of C5–9. When C3 encounters activated properdin factor $\overline{B}$, C3 is split likewise to C3a and C3b. C3a is one of the two anaphylatoxins generated from complement (see Section 17.A, Fig. 1A, and Section 17.E.8.b. for isolation). Bound C3 gives rise to the $\overline{C4,2,3}$ enzyme activity, the immune adherence phenomenon and to reactivity with conglutinin and immunoconglutinin.

ii. Characteristics of Human C5

C5 is a euglobulin with an $s^{\circ}_{20,w}$ of 8.7 S and an electrophoretic mobility of a fast β-globulin. Its averge concentration in human serum is 75 $\mu g/ml$. C5 is unique in being readily adsorbed to unsensitized erythrocytes.[59] The combining site of C5 which reacts with cell membrane receptors is activated by the $\overline{C4,2,3}$ enzyme. Activation is transient (half-life of 9 minutes[59]) and, failing combination with receptors, C5 is inactivated by this enzyme. Both activation and inactivation are accompanied by cleavage of the molecule and dissociation of a small fragment, C5a, which has anaphylatoxin activity as well as chemotactic activity for polymorphonuclear leukocytes. C5 displays an affinity for both C6 and C7, and thus these three proteins tend to associate in free solution.[60] This interaction appears to be functionally important because C5 cellular uptake and hemolytic efficiency are markedly enhanced in the presence of C6 and C7. Further, associated C5,6,7 after conversion by $\overline{C4,2,3}$ acquires chemotactic activity for polymorphonuclear leukocytes, apparently activating in these cells a serine esterase.[44]

iii. Procedures

In Method A, the separation of Nilsson and Müller-Eberhard[57] starts with preparation of euglobulins of human serum, which are chromatographed on TEAE-cellulose to yield a fraction containing primarily C3 and C5 and β_{1H}-globulin. This fraction also contains small amounts of C6, C7, and C8 and of γ-globulin. The major portion of γ-globulin as well as α_1- and α_2-globulins are eliminated in this step. Hydroxylapatite chromatography eliminates C6, C7, and β_{1H} and separates C5 and C3. By final block electrophoresis of the two products, γ-globulin is removed from C5, and C8 is removed from C3. The procedure should result in recovery of 80 to 120 mg of purified C3 and 5 to 10 mg of C5 per liter (up to 10% yields).

In a revised Method B, Nilsson et al.[61] precipitated euglobulin at pH

[59] N. R. Cooper and H. J. Müller-Eberhard, J. Exp. Med. 132, 775 (1970).

[60] P. A. Ward and E. L. Becker, J. Exp. Med. 125, 1001 (1967).

[61] U. R. Nilsson, R. H. Tomar, and F. B. Taylor, Jr., J. Immunol. 107, 317 (1971) (Abstract).

5.5 and low ionic strength in the presence of an inhibitor of plasmin (L-lysine). The euglobulin was chromatographed on TEAE-cellulose and then on hydroxylapatite. The final product was devoid of fibrinolytic activity, a minor problem encountered with Method A.

In Method C,[62] C3 and C5 are first separated functionally during two successive precipitations of the euglobulin, after which C3 is chromatographed alone on DEAE-cellulose and remaining impurities are removed by affinity chromatography.

Method A[57]

Step 1. Preparation of Euglobulins. Serum, 1000 ml, is dialyzed against 3×10 liters of 0.008 M EDTA solution of pH 5.4 (buffer P, Table I), having a conductance of 1.25 mS. After 40 hours of dialysis, the precipitate is harvested by centrifugation and washed three times in EDTA solution, 20 times the volume of the precipitate being used each time. After each wash the precipitate is collected by centrifugation at 1100 g for 20 minutes. It is then dissolved in 20 ml of phosphate buffer, pH 7.0, ionic strength 0.1 (buffer B, Table I), containing 0.01 M EDTA and 800 mg of sodium chloride (4%). The euglobulin fraction is cleared from lipids by ultracentrifugation in a Spinco ultracentrifuge at 30,000 rpm for 30 minutes using a No. 40 rotor. After ultracentrifugation, a hole is punctured in the bottom of each Lusteroid tube with a 20-gauge needle and the clear fluid is collected, excluding the lipid layer floating on top.

Step 2. Chromatography on TEAE-Cellulose. A 3×70 cm column containing approximately 400 ml of packed TEAE-cellulose is equilibrated with starting buffer J, Table I (0.03 M phosphate buffer, pH 8.1). The lipid-poor euglobulin is dialyzed after ultracentrifugation against 10 liters of starting buffer overnight and is then applied to the TEAE-cellulose column. The column is washed with 800 ml of starting buffer before the gradient elution procedure is begun. A Florence flask containing 1000 ml of starting buffer serves as mixing chamber, connected by siphon with 500 ml of 0.25 M NaH$_2$PO$_4$ as limit buffer in a 500-ml Erlenmeyer flask. Fractions of 10 ml are collected. Every fifth tube is analyzed for protein concentration. (Note that C9 and other euglobulins remain bound to the column.) C3 is located by an immunochemical procedure using a specific antiserum to C3. For this purpose, microscope slides are covered with a 2% agar layer (2 ml per 3×1 inch slide). Cut a longitudinal central trough and, on both sides thereof, a row of ten circular wells. The trough is filled with antiserum, the wells with aliquots of column fractions. Fractions containing C3 (and also C5) are pooled and passed through a Millipore filter before the pool is applied to a hydroxylapatite column.

[62] D. H. Vroon, D. R. Schultz, and R. M. Zarco, *Immunochemistry* **7**, 43 (1970).

Step 3. Chromatography on Hydroxylapatite. Hydroxylapatite is prepared exactly according to Tiselius *et al.*[48] The buffers to be employed for hydroxylapatite chromatography are prepared by mixing buffers K and L (Table I) in the following fashion, the number referring to mS. "8-Buffer": 5000 ml of buffer K plus 300 ml of buffer L; adjust conductance to 8 mS by addition of buffer L. "12-Buffer": 1000 ml of buffer K plus 100 ml of buffer L; adjust conductance to 12 mS by addition of small amounts of buffer L. "13-Buffer": 1000 ml of buffer K plus 120 ml of buffer L; adjust conductance to 13 mS by addition of buffer L. "14.5-Buffer": 1000 ml of buffer K plus 150 ml of buffer L; adjust conductance to 14.5 mS by addition of buffer L.

A 3 × 70 cm column, containing approximately 400 ml of loosely packed hydroxylapatite, is equilibrated with "8-buffer." The material from the TEAE column, filtered but not concentrated, is applied, and the column is washed with 600 ml of "8-buffer." C5 is then eluted with 800 ml of "12-buffer." After the elution of C5, the column is washed with 800 ml of "13-buffer," whereupon C3 is eluted with 800 ml of "14.5-buffer." The flow rate throughout the elution procedure is adjusted to 30 ml per hour and fractions of 15 ml are collected. The fractions are analyzed for protein and for C3, C5, and β_{1H} using specific antisera and the immunodiffusion technique described above. C3 and C5 may also be detected by hemolytic activity assay as outlined below.

Fractions containing C3 are pooled and the protein is precipitated by dialysis against 3 changes of 10 liters of phosphate buffer, pH 5.4, ionic strength 0.02 (buffer M, Table I), during 2 days. The precipitate is then collected by centrifugation and dissolved in 5 to 10 ml of barbital buffer, pH 8.6, ionic strength 0.05 (buffer G, Table I).

Fractions containing C5 are concentrated by ultrafiltration to a volume of 5 ml, and the material is passed through a Millipore filter.

Step 4a. Final Purification of C3 by Preparative Block Electrophoresis. C3 obtained by hydroxylapatite chromatography is applied to a Pevikon block prepared with barbital buffer G of Table I (Vol. II, Appendix III and Chap. 6.D.1). Electrophoresis is carried out for 24 hours at a potential gradient of 3.5 V/cm. The fractions are analyzed for protein content. This step removes small amounts of contaminating C8 from the highly purified C3. C8 is located cathodally from the C3 peak. The protein is concentrated and passed through a Millipore filter.

Step 4b. Purification of C5 by Preparative Electrophoresis. C5 from the hydroxylapatite column is applied to a Pevikon block, likewise prepared with barbital buffer G. Electrophoresis is carried out for 20 hours at a potential gradient of 3.5 V/cm. In this step, small amounts of contaminating IgG are separated from the otherwise highly purified C5. The fractions are analyzed for protein content, the major anodally migrating protein peak is concentrated by ultrafiltration, and the protein is filtered through a Millipore filter.

Method B

Method B of Nilsson *et al.*[61] was developed when the product from Method A was found to give fibrinolysis equivalent to low-grade contamination with plasminogen/plasmin. A C5 preparation lacking fibrinolytic activity is described, based upon addition of L-lysine to inhibit plasmin formation.

Step 1. Precipitation of Euglobin. Euglobulin is precipitated at pH 5.5 at low salt in the presence of 0.06 M L-lysine (conductance, 4.1 mS at 3°).

Step 2. Chromatography on TEAE-Cellulose. Buffer contained 0.1 M ϵ-aminocaproic acid and 0.03 M phosphate, pH 7.0. A linear NaCl gradient was established.

Step 3. Chromatography on Hydroxylapatite. Eluting gradient was formed of ascending concentrations of phosphate at pH 7.9 in the presence of ϵ-aminocaproic acid.

Method C

All purifications are relative. The published procedures for securing C3 (both functionally separated C3[62] and the preparation of C3 described in method A) were insufficiently purified for special studies. Accordingly, Molenaar *et al.*[63] produced antisera against trace impurities that can accompany C3, namely, antisera to C3c, C3d, normal euglobulin deprived of C3, and mixed C3 impurities. The globulin fractions of these antisera were coupled separately to Sepharose 4B by cyanogen bromide, and 2 columns were made up.

Normal human serum was precipitated twice according to Vroon *et al.*,[62] the supernatant then being chromatographed on DEAE-cellulose. Passage of the crude C3 preparation through the two columns yielded a product that gave only one "rocket" in Laurell's "crossed electrophoresis" in agar containing horse anti-human serum (Vol. III, Chap. 14.D.5).

iv. Assay of C3 Activity[57]

The assay cells are EAC1,4,[oxy]2 (prepared as in Section 17.C.4.a). A further reagent is guinea pig complement treated to lack both C3 and C5 activity. This guinea pig reagent is obtained by treating fresh guinea pig serum with 1 M KCNS for 5 hours at 4°,[59] followed by dialysis against VB^{2+} overnight, and by incubation with 0.02 M hydrazine for 1 hour at 37°.

For the assay, 0.2-ml portions of a suspension of EAC1,4,[oxy]2 at a concentration of 1.5 × 10^8 cells/ml in 0.01 M Na$_3$H·EDTA–GVB (buffer

---

[63] J. L. Molenaar, M. Müller, and K. W. Pondman, *J. Immunol.* **110**, 1570 (1973).

7c, Section 17.B, Table I) are dispensed in a series of tubes. Then 0.2 ml of dilutions of C3 in the same buffer, GVB, ranging from 10 to 200 ng of C3 protein per milliliter, is added, and the mixture is incubated for 20 minutes at 30°. Then, 0.2 ml of C5 at 5 μg of protein per milliliter and 2.4 ml of guinea pig serum reagent (lacking C3 and C5) diluted 1:100 in 0.04 M Na$_3$H·EDTA-GVB are added to each tube and incubation is continued for 60 minutes at 37°. Appropriate controls are included which are analogous to those described in the C4 assay (Section D.2.c.iii). The percentage of lysis is determined as before, and the amount of C3 is calculated which yields a $-\ln(1-y)$ value of unity.

v. Assay of C5 Activity[57]

The assay cells are EAC$\overline{1}$,4,^{oxy}2,3 (1.5×10^8 cells/ml) prepared as described in Section 17.C.4.b. Also required is the guinea pig reagent lacking C3 and C5 activity, described under the assay of C3 activity. EAC1,4,^{oxy}2,3 cells, 0.2 ml, are incubated with 0.2-ml dilutions of C5, ranging from 1 to 30 μg of C5 protein per milliliter, for 10 minutes at 30°. The diluent is 0.01 M EDTA–GVB (buffer 7c, Section 17.B, Table I). Then, 2.4 ml of guinea pig serum reagent diluted 1:100 in 0.04 M Na$_3$H·EDTA-GVS is added. After 60 minutes at 37°, lysis is measured, and the activity is calculated as previously described for other assays.

vi. Yield and Purity Criteria

Between 80 and 120 mg of C3 and 5 to 10 mg of C5 may be isolated from 1000 ml of serum, which is for both proteins a maximal yield of 10%.

Both C3 and C5 should yield one well defined band on disc electrophoresis and a single precipitin line when analyzed by immunoelectrophoresis or by Ouchterlony test using an antiersum to whole human serum or antisera prepared to the isolated proteins. C3 converted by C$\overline{4,2}$ is electrophoretically faster than native C3. The apparent hemolytic activities of C3 and C5 are greatly dependent on the reactivity of the assay cells used. With very large numbers of C4,2 sites per cell, fewer than 1000 C3 molecules produce one hemolytically detectable molecule. Similarly, with a very large number of C$\overline{4,2,3}$ sites per cell, fewer than 100 molecules of C5 suffice to produce one hemolytic C5 site.

e. ISOLATION OF HUMAN, RABBIT, AND GUINEA PIG C6[*64]

i. Characteristics

C6 is a β_2-globulin of 95,000 or 125,000 daltons, normally present in amounts of 55 to 65 μg/ml. Activity is lost rapidly at pH 5 to 6. C6

---

* Section 17.D.2.e was contributed by Hans J. Müller-Eberhard.
[64] C. M. Arroyave and H. J. Müller-Eberhard, *Immunochemistry* 8, 995 (1971).

complexes with C5 and C7.[65] The preparation was secured as a homogeneous protein, immunologically and physically like C6 in fresh serum but less active. A cofactor possibly may be present in fresh serum, or free sulfhydryl groups may have complexed with metal ions during the isolation. C6, although not a classical clotting factor, appears to participate in the normal coagulation mechanism of human blood.

ii. Procedure

The isolation procedure required about 20 days. All buffers contained 0.05 M chloramphenicol and 2.5 $\times$ 10^5 M kanamycin sulfate. Solutions were concentrated on an Amicon UM-50 membrane.

Step 1. Removal of Euglobulin. Fresh human blood, 400 ml, was adjusted to pH 7.0 with 1 N HCl and diluted with cold distilled water to a conductance of 3 mS. After standing at 4° for 1 hour, euglobulin was removed by centrifugation in the cold.

Step 2. Chromatography on DEAE-Cellulose. The supernatant from step 1 was equilibrated with phosphate buffer pH 7.0 of 3.0 mS conductance and applied to a 5 $\times$ 100 cm column of DEAE-cellulose in the same buffer. Elution was carried out by NaCl gradient (2 liters of starting buffer with salt to provide 30 mS, *vs* 2 liters of starting buffer) at a flow rate of 120 ml per hour. The fractions (15 ml) were analyzed for C6 activity as below. Peak activity was recovered at ca 6 to 7.5 mS.

Step 3. Rechromatography on DEAE-Cellulose. Pooled active fractions were dialyzed in starting buffer to the original conductance of 3.0 mS and applied to a 2.5 $\times$ 50 cm column in the same buffer. The NaCl gradient consisted of 1 liter of buffer with NaCl sufficient to provide 20 mS *vs* 1 liter of starting buffer. Again the fractions possessing activity (between ca 6 and 7.5 mS) were located and concentrated.

Step 4. Pevikon Block Electrophoresis. The yield from step 3 was equilibrated against pH 8.6 barbital buffer, $\Gamma/2 = 0.05$. Two 18 $\times$ 36 $\times$ 1.5 cm Pevikon blocks were used for electrophoresis (4 V/cm for 36 hours at 4°). Sections of 1.5 cm were eluted with phosphate buffer, pH 7.9, conductance being 8.0 mS. The slightly anodic eluates with C6 activity were located, pooled, and concentrated to 20 ml.

Step 5. Chromatography on Hydroxylapatite. The yield from step 4 was applied to a 1.6 $\times$ 30 cm column of hydroxylapatite,[48] and stepwise elution chromatography was performed as described previously in Section 17.D.2.d.iii, using sodium phosphate buffers at pH 7.9 with increasing conductance (8, 10, 11, 11.25 mS). Fractions were collected in siliconized tubes in view of the low protein concentration. Tubes within the 11.25 mS eluate were selected for C6 activity, pooled, concentrated, and frozen

[65] U. R. Nilsson and H. J. Müller-Eberhard, *Immunology* 13, 101 (1967).

in liquid nitrogen, either in elution buffer or in plain barbital buffer. Only about 1% of the activity applied to hydroxylapatite is recovered in the effluent.

iii. Assay of C6 Activity

Method A. Mix 10 to 15 μl of sample with 0.1 ml 1:40 dilution, in gelatin–Veronal buffer, of C6-deficient rabbit serum[66] and 0.1 ml of sensitized sheep cells (5×10^8 erythrocytes/ml). Incubate at 37° for 30 minutes, add 1.5 ml of cold saline, and centrifuge immediately. Read free hemoglobin at 412 nm or 541 nm.

Method B. From a suspension of EAC $1,4,^{oxy}2,3$ cells at 1.5×10^8 cells/ml (Section 17.C.4.b) mix 0.2 ml with 2 μg of C5, 4 μg of C7 and various amounts of test material. Incubate at 37° for 20 minutes, centrifuge, and wash cells twice with cold GVB. Suspend the cells in 0.4 ml GVB containing an excess of C8 and C9, incubate at 37° for 1 hour. Centrifuge, then read free hemoglobin as in Method A.

Method C. C6 may be quantitated by single radial diffusion in agar which contains rabbit anti-human C6.

iv. Criteria of Purity

The preparation gave rise to a monospecific antiserum when injected into a popliteal lymph node of rabbits (20 μg in CFA) with repeat injection of 100 μg subcutaneously and intramuscularly after 1 month. A single band appeared upon polyacrylamide disc gel electrophoresis. About 3000 molecules of the purified material are needed per erythrocyte to cause lysis. Hemolytically inactive samples of C6 possess a faster mobility than active samples in disc gel electrophoresis.

f. PARTIAL PURIFICATION OF HUMAN C7* [67]

i. Characteristics

C7, like C6, has an s rate of 5 to 6 S and the electrophoretic mobility of a slow β-globulin. The two also possess in common an affinity for C5. The action of C6 and C7, together with C5, on the cell surface results in formation of a very stable site, which is reactive with C8.

ii. Procedure

Step 1. Removal of Euglobulin. Euglobulin was precipitated by dialysis against EDTA (0.008 M at pH 5.4, having a conductance of 1.25 mS

---

[66] K. Rother, U. Rother, H. J. Müller-Eberhard, and U. R. Nilsson, *J. Exp. Med.* **124**, 773 (1966).

* Section 17.D.2.f was contributed by O. Götze and Hans J. Müller-Eberhard.
[67] O. Götze and H. J. Müller-Eberhard, *J. Exp. Med.* **132**, 898 (1970).

at 22°. The precipitate is removed by centrifugation. The supernatant (400 ml) was brought to pH 7.3 with 1 N NaOH, and NaCl was added to 2.2 mS.

Step 2. Chromatography on TEAE-Cellulose. The yield from step 1 was equilibrated with 0.02 M phosphate buffer pH 7.3 and applied to a 7.5 × 50 cm column of TEAE-cellulose in the same buffer. Stepwise elution was practiced, using the same buffer containing NaCl. C7 activity eluted within the range of 4.0 to 6.5 mS, as assayed below.

Step 3. Gel Filtration on Sephadex G-200. The yield from step 2 was concentrated (15 ml) and equilibrated with 0.5 M NaCl buffered with 0 5 M Tris·HCl, pH 8.0. It was applied to a 5 × 120 cm column of G-200 in the same buffer. C7 activity was detected between the second and third peaks of the profile and fractions were pooled.

Step 4. Chromatography on Cellex P (Bio-Rad, Richmond, California). The yield from step 3 was equilibrated with phosphate buffer pH 6.0, $\Gamma/2 = 0.1$, and applied to a 2 × 30 cm column of P-cellulose in the same buffer. Elution was carried out with an NaCl gradient. C7 activity was present between 17 and 23 mS.

iii. Assay of C7 Activity

C7 is assayed with EAC1–3 cells (Section 17.C.4.b) in the presence of an excess of C5, C6, C8, C9, proceeding as in Section 17.D.2.e.iii. Alternatively, C7 may be detected by the formation of heat-stable EAC1–7 from EAC1,4,^{oxy}2,3 (Section 17.C.4.b) in the presence of excess C5 and C6. After 60 minutes at 37°, the cells are washed and incubated with C8 and C9 (Section 17.D.2.g and 17.D.2.h) again for 60 minutes at 37°.

iv. Purity

The preparation as separated was functionally free of other complement components, 280 ng giving a CH_{50} value of 5 × 10^7 erythrocytes in 60 minutes at 37°.

g. ISOLATION OF HUMAN C8[*][68]

i. Characteristics

C8 has an s rate of 8.5 S, a molecular weight of 153,000, and the electrophoretic mobility of a γ_1-globulin. Its concentration in serum is estimated to be approximately 20 μg/ml. After reaction of C8 with C5,6,7 sites on the cell surface, the cell undergoes slow lysis in the absence of C9 (Section

---

[*] Section 17.D.2.g was contributed by Hans J. Müller-Eberhard.

[68] J. A. Manni and H. J. Müller-Eberhard, *J. Exp. Med.* **130**, 1145 (1969).

17.A, Fig. 1A). In the course of this reaction C8 is firmly bound to the cell surface. Thus, C8 appears to be the complement component which is directly responsible for induction of membrane injury. It is to be noted that a slow conversion of C8 to an inactive form occurs *in vitro*,[69] such inactive material, when isolated, is nonfunctional in the lytic pathway although it binds C9 and reacts with specific anti-C8 antibody. Accordingly, if present it plays the role of an inhibitor.

ii. Procedure

From 2 liters, about 1.5 to 2.0 mg of C8 can be recovered. In the method described, Rivanol precipitation (step 1) eliminates in the supernatant most of the γ-globulin from which C8 is difficult to separate. It also results in a convenient decrease in volume. Of the 100 gm of protein in the precipitate, 99% is separated on CM-cellulose (step 2), C8 being recovered together with 800 mg of contaminating protein. By means of block electrophoresis, 99% of non-C8 protein is separated from C8 (step 3). On Sephadex, C8 distributes between the theoretical positions of albumin and γG-globulin (step 4), making the technique useful in removing most of the contaminating γ-globulin, which otherwise shares identical physiochemical properties with C8. Of the 50 mg applied to the column, 5 mg are recovered together with C8 activity. Approximately 50% of this constitutes γ-globulin; the remainder is C8 protein. The amount of total protein being very small at this stage, immunoadsorption of the γ-globulin (step 5) has been selected rather than a physiochemical method.

Step 1. Precipitation with Rivanol. Pooled blood, 2000 ml, either fresh or outdated, will serve as starting material for one C8 preparation. The pH of the pool is adjusted to 7.5 with 1 N NaOH, and 500 ml are filled into each of 4 1000-ml plastic containers; an equal volume of 1% Rivanol in water is added at 0° with constant stirring. The heavy yellow-green precipitate is sedimented by centrifugation at 500 g for 30 minutes in the cold and washed with 1000 ml of 0.5% Rivanol solution in water. Approximately 100 ml of a 3% NaCl solution in water is then added to the sediment in each container, and a period of 2 hours at 4° is allowed for dissolution of the protein–Rivanol complex. Under these conditions, most of the Rivanol is insoluble and may be removed by centrifugation for 30 minutes at 500 g. The supernatant protein solution is dialyzed against two changes of 20 liters of phosphate buffer, pH 6.0, ionic strength of 0.1 (buffer A, Table I), for 24 hours.

Step 2. Chromatography on CM-Cellulose. Approximately 850 ml of packed CM-cellulose in a 4.5 × 60 cm column is equilibrated overnight

[69] R. L. Stolfi, *J. Immunol.* **104**, 1212 (1970).

with starting buffer A. Of the dialyzed Rivanol fraction, 400 ml is applied to the column, followed by a wash with 1000 to 1500 ml of starting buffer. The column is eluted with 3 liters of a linear NaCl concentration gradient in which the limiting buffer consists of 1.5 liters of buffer A brought to a conductance of 35 mS by addition of 27 gm of NaCl. The flow rate is adjusted to 60 ml per hour, and 15-ml fractions are collected. Fractions containing C8 activity are pooled and concentrated to 6 to 7 ml by ultrafiltration.

Step 3. Preparative Block Electrophoresis. Of the concentrated material, 6 to 7 ml are applied at the center of a $1 \times 18 \times 50$ cm block of Pevikon in phosphate buffer, pH 6.0, ionic strength 0.05 (buffer A, Table I, diluted 1:2 with H_2O). After electrophoresis at 3.5 V/cm for 40 hours, the block is cut into 1.25-cm segments and eluted with electrophoresis buffer. The fractions containing C8 activity are pooled and concentrated to a volume of 2 ml.

Step 4. Gel Filtration. Two milliliters of electrophoretically purified C8 are applied to a 3×10 cm column of Sephadex G-200, which is equilibrated with the limiting buffer of 35 mS used for CM chromatography. The flow rate is adjusted to 8 to 10 ml per hour, and 2-ml fractions are collected. The C8-containing fractions are pooled and concentrated by ultrafiltration to 2 to 3 ml.

Step 5. Absorption with Insolubilized Anti-γG-Globulin. Five milliliters of a rabbit antiserum to human IgG is mixed with 5 ml of 0.2 M acetate buffer, pH 5.2 (buffer 2, V ol. II, Appendix II) and the protein is insolubilized by addition of 0.8 ml of ethyl chloroformate.[70] The mixture is agitated with a magnetic stirrer for 15 minutes, the pH being maintained between 4.5 and 5.0 by addition of 1 N NaOH. After 30 minutes at room temperature, the solid protein is washed extensively, since ethyl chloroformate was found to inactivate C8 completely at a dilution of 1:40,000. It is washed 20 times with 50-ml portions of phosphate-buffered saline, pH 7.2, then with 5 portions of 50 ml of 0.1% sodium carbonate, 10 portions of 50 ml of 0.2 M glycine buffer, pH 2.2 (buffer 22, Vol. II, Appendix II) and sufficient phosphate-buffered saline to reach pH 7.2. It is finally suspended in 10 ml of saline and spun at 20,000 rpm for 1 hour in a Spinco L2 centrifuge with a No. 40 rotor. The fluid is discarded, the walls of the tube are dried with filter paper, and the wet protein (400 mg) is suspended in the C8 preparation (200 to 600 μg/ml) resulting from gel filtration step 4. The suspension is held overnight at 4° and then subjected to ultracentrifugation as described above, 2.2 ml of supernatant is recovered with a Pasteur pipette.

C8 in phosphate buffer A, Table I, containing 0.3 M NaCl is stored at −70° after quick-freezing in liquid nitrogen.

---

[70] S. Avrameas and T. Ternynck, *J. Biol. Chem.* **242**, 1961 (1967).

iii. Assay of C8 Activity

Dilutions of C8 ranging from 0.01 to 5.0 ng of C8 protein in 1 ml of total reaction mixture are incubated for 60 minutes at 37° with 5×10^7 EAC1–7 cells (Section 17.C.4.c) and an excess of C9. GVB is used as diluent. The percentage of lysis is determined, and to obtain a straight dose-response curve, the data are graphed in terms of the reciprocal of $-\ln(1 - y)$ versus the reciprocal of the dilution.

iv. Yield and Purity Criteria

The procedure allows a 5000-fold purification of C8 compared to serum. The yield is maximally 5%, i.e., 1.5 to 2.0 mg of C8 protein may be isolated from 2000 ml of serum.

Examination of 25 to 50 μg of C8 protein by disc electrophoresis yields one protein band, and C8 activity may be eluted from the position of this band. By Ouchterlony test using an anti-C8 serum, one precipitin line is seen which is slightly concave toward the antigen well. Various anti-whole human sera have failed to detect isolated C8 protein. Its behavior on immunoelectrophoresis in agar is anomalous in that it behaves like an α_2- rather than γ_1-globulin. In terms of hemolytic activity, highly purified C8 contains approximately 2×10^{11} effective molecules per microgram of protein.

h. ISOLATION OF HUMAN C9[*][71]

i. Characteristics

C9 is an α-globulin with an s rate of 4.5 S and a molecular weight of 79,000. Its concentration in serum is estimated to be 2 to 10 μg/ml. In immune hemolysis C9 enhances the lytic effect of C8 by physical attachment to the target cell surface. Its hemolytic activity is mimicked by 1,10-phenanthroline or 2,2'-bipyridine.

ii. Procedure

Although C9 activity distributes between the eu- and pseudoglobulin fractions of serum, the euglobulin (step 1) is used as starting material because it affords a considerable degree of initial purification. Furthermore, C3 and C5 may be isolated from the same material (Section 17.D.2.d). C9 is eluted from TEAE-cellulose (step 2) together with proteins that are primarily of higher molecular weight than C9 and which therefore may be separated from C9 by Sephadex filtration on G-100 (step 3). The small amount of proteins eluted along with C9 activity consists mostly of γ- and β-globulins. By block electrophoresis, these con-

---

[*] Section 17.D.2.h was contributed by Hans J. Müller-Eberhard.

[71] U. Hadding and H. J. Müller-Eberhard, *Immunology* **16**, 719 (1969).

taminants are readily removed and C9 is recovered from the α-globulin region.

Step 1. Precipitation of Euglobulin. Fresh serum, 1000 ml, is treated exactly as described in step 1 of the isolation of C3 and C5 (Section 17.D.2.d), namely, dialysis *vs* dilute, acidic EDTA.

Step 2. Chromatography on TEAE-Cellulose. The euglobulin is chromatographed as described for step 2 of the isolation of C3 and C5 (Section 17.D.2.d). After conclusion of the gradient elution procedure, C9 and remaining euglobulins are eluted in one step with 750 ml of phosphate buffer, pH 5.1, ionic strength 0.1 (buffer N, Table I), brought to a conductance of 50 mS by addition of NaCl. Fractions containing C9 activity are pooled, and the volume is reduced by ultrafiltration to 10 ml.

Step 3. Sephadex Filtration. First, 10 ml of the concentrated TEAE-cellulose fraction is applied to a 7.5 × 60 cm column containing 2500 ml of Sephadex G-100, equilibrated with VB (buffer G, Table I). The protein is eluted with VB using a flow rate of 48 ml per hour. C9-containing fractions are pooled, and the volume is reduced to 4 ml. Second, the concentrated eluate is applied to a 4.5 × 60 cm column containing 850 ml of packed Sephadex G-100 equilibrated with VB. The flow rate is adjusted to 16 ml per hour.

Step 4. Preparative Block Electrophoresis. The C9-containing effluent of the second Sephadex column is concentrated to 5 ml and applied to a Pevikon block using phosphate buffer, pH 6.0, ionic strength 0.05 (buffer A, Table I, diluted 1:2 with H_2O). Electrophoresis is carried out for 22 hours employing a potential gradient of 4 V/cm.

iii. Assay of C9 Activity

Dilutions of C9 ranging from 1 to 50 ng of C9 protein per 2 ml of total reaction volume are incubated with 5×10^7 EAC1-8 cells (Section 17.C.4.d) for 45 minutes at 37°. During this period the diluent is 0.09 M EDTA (buffer 8, Section 17.B, Table I), which inhibits lysis due to C8 and C9 without interfering with C9 action. The cells are then sedimented by centrifugation, resuspended in 2 ml of VB and incubated again for 15 minutes at 37°. Percentage of lysis is then determined.

iv. Yield and Purity Criteria

From 1000 ml of serum, 150 to 200 μg of C9 protein may be obtained.

Highly purified C9 represents one protein band on disc electrophoresis, the location of which corresponds to that of C9 activity. Anti-whole human serum does not react with isolated C9 in the Ouchterlony test. A characteristic effective molecule:protein ratio has not yet been established.

3. Complement Components from Guinea Pig Serum

a. GUINEA PIG C1

Preparations of C$\overline{1}$ are often only functionally pure; three methods are given. It is to be noted that C1q can be prepared by Method B of Section 17.D.2.a.iii.

i. Preparations

(a) Method A*

Step 1. Separation of Euglobulin. Serum, 40 ml, at 0° is adjusted to pH 5.6 by addition of 0.15 M HCl and dialyzed for 2 hours against 2 liters of distilled water at 0° to 2°: The precipitate is collected by centrifugation at 0° for 10 minutes at 900 g. The euglobulin precipitate is washed three times with 40 ml of 0.015 M NaCl at 0° and is resuspended in 40 ml of this fluid.

Step 2. Chromatography on DEAE-Cellulose.[1] A 6.5 × 60 cm column of DEAE-cellulose is equilibrated with 0.015 M NaCl at pH 7.4. The exchanger is covered with a layer of glass wool and overlaid with a layer of glass beads (diameter, 3 to 4 mm), thick enough to prevent disturbance of the surface of the column as liquids are poured into the tube. The yield from step 1 is applied to the column, which is washed thoroughly with 0.015 M NaCl, after which two 200-ml volumes of 0.06 M NaCl are passed. Next, ca 250 ml of 0.25 M NaCl is applied. After 70 ml have passed, the next 100 ml of effluent is collected since globulin dissolves and is not bound by the exchanger. Preparations of activated macromolecular complex (C$\overline{1}$) are adjusted to 0.15 M NaCl on the basis of conductivity measurements,† and may be stored at 2° to 5° [1 mM sodium azide (65 mg/liter) may be added to inhibit bacterial growth] or at −20° for up to a year without loss of activity.

Yield. The fraction eluted with 0.25 M NaCl contains most of the C$\overline{1}$

---

* Section 17.D.3a.i(a) was contributed by Louis G. Hoffmann and Manfred M. Mayer.

[1] T. Borsos and H. J. Rapp, *J. Immunol.* **91**, 851 (1963).

† Conductivity measurements are made conveniently by means of a conductivity bridge and two conductivity cells having respective constants of 0.1 (for salinity approaching 0.15 M NaCl) and of 1.0 (for measuring salt gradients). Conductivity cells in which the electrode chamber is filled through a capillary controlled with a rubber teat are recommended; they can be ordered with a 14-cm capillary, allowing measurement of small volumes within individual fraction collector tubes. Suitable bridges include Beckman Model RC 16B and (direct reading bridges) Beckman RC-19, Radiometer's Conductivity Meter Type CDM 2d, and Barnstead Model PM-70 CB.—Editors.

activity; contamination with C4 and C2 is less than $1:10^5$ in terms of site-forming units (SFU) (see assay below), but some of the components of the C3 complex may'be present. The product contains 1 to 5% of the serum proteins as estimated by absorbancy at 280 nm, and $C\bar{1}$ titers of ca 10^{13} SFU/ml commonly are obtained in our laboratory.

(b) *Method B*[*2]

Steps 1 and 2. Preparation of Euglobulin. Guinea pig serum, 100 ml, was set at pH 7.5 by adding 0.15 N HCl, and distilled water at 0° was added to reduce the conductance to 0.04 mS. Stirring at pH 7.5 was carried out 30 minutes at 4°. The precipitated euglobulin was collected, rinsed with SVB^{2+} which had been diluted to ionic strength of 0.03. The precipitate was dissolved in 40 ml of isotonic SVB^{2+} in the cold, clarified, and the procedures of step 1 repeated, the final volume being 30 ml. This product slowly precipitates; clarification by centrifugation may be necessary if storage at 0° is used.

Step 3. Filtration on Bio-Gel P-200 ("50–100 mesh"). A 2.5×85 cm column was packed in SVB^{2+} with 0.005 M sodium azide, with special attention to degassing of the gel; newly prepared columns must be conditioned by passing 1 to 2 ml of whole guinea pig serum in the same buffer. The thoroughly washed column can be used repeatedly, without undue adsorption of C1. Five milliliters of the yield from step 1 were chromatographed per column run, C1 appearing with the void volume.

To stabilize the yield, 1.5 volumes of sucrose–VB^{2+} with 2% gelatin are added (ionic strength 0.065), and aliquots are stored at −70°.

(c) *Method C. Purified Guinea Pig $C\bar{1}$*[†3]

Step 1. Collection of Euglobulin. Euglobulin from 100 ml of guinea pig serum is recovered as in 17.D.3.a.i(a) and washed twice, then dissolved in 10 ml of VB^{2+} containing about 5% sucrose. Allow the redissolved euglobulin to stand for 10 minutes at 0°, then centrifuge in the cold for 10 minutes at 27,000 g to sediment insoluble material.

Step 2. Density Gradient Centrifugations. Apply the clarified sample to a BXIV titanium preparative zonal centrifuge rotor loaded with 400 ml of an 8 to 30% sucrose gradient containing hypertonic VB^{2+}, $\Gamma/2 = 0.75$ and 2 mM sodium azide (130 mg/liter) over 115 ml of a 40% sucrose cushion. Overlay the sample with 125 ml of VB^{2+} $\Gamma/2 = 0.75$ buffer lacking sucrose. After the sample is centrifuged for 16 hours at

* Section 17.D.3.a.i(b) was contributed by the Editors.

[2] W. D. Linscott, *Immunochemistry* **5**, 311 (1968).

† Section 17.D.3.a.i(c) was contributed by Harvey R. Colten and H. E. Bond.

[3] H. R. Colten, H. E. Bond, T. Borsos, and H. J. Rapp, *J. Immunol.* **103**, 862 (1969).

36,000 rpm at 10°, collect 10-ml fractions and assay for C1 activity. Pool the fractions containing C1 but lacking 19 S protein. Dialyze overnight at 4° against 3 liters of VB^{2+} ($\Gamma/2 = 0.75$) to remove most of the sucrose, and then concentrate to 10 ml at 0° on an Amicon UM-10 membrane.

Step 3. Recycling on Density Gradient. The concentrated material is then subjected to density gradient centrifugation as in the first cycle except that the gradient, overlay, and cushion solutions are made with low ionic strength VB^{2+}, $\Gamma/2 = 0.065$. At this ionic strength the C1, which sediments as a 19 S molecule, separates from the lighter material.

ii. Purity

Between 40 and 84% of the proteins in these preparations are hemolytically active C1. Hemolytic activity is stable at 0° but is rapidly lost after two freezings and thawings. The preparation gives a single faint line in the γ-globulin region on radioimmunoelectrophoresis (developed with ^{125}I-labeled 7 S fraction of rabbit antiserum to a guinea pig euglobulin preparation).[2]

iii. Assay of Guinea Pig C1*

The assay procedure was developed by Borsos and Rapp.[1] It is based on addition of C1 to EAC4 and the formation of SAC$\overline{1}$,4, which under steady state conditions converts to SAC$\overline{1}$,4,2. The formation of SAC$\overline{1}$,4,2 is measured with guinea pig complement treated with EDTA. *The site-forming unit (SFU) of C$\overline{1}$* is defined as the amount, in milliliters, that converts one SAC4 to a SAC$\overline{1}$,4.

The reaction medium for the formation of SAC$\overline{1}$,4 and SAC$\overline{1}$,4,2 is low ionic strength MGVB^{2+} (buffer 3c, Section 17.B, Table I). A preparation of EAC4 (Section 17.C.2.c) is standardized to contain 1.5×10^8 cells/ml, and 0.5-ml portions of the suspension at 30° are mixed with equal volumes of suitably diluted samples of C1 and incubated at 30° for 10 minutes. A 0.5-ml portion of C2 (Section 17.D.3.b), diluted to 15 units/ml, is added to each tube, and tubes are held for 10 minutes at 30°. The additions of C1 and C2 may be staggered, e.g., at 1-minute intervals, to achieve the proper incubation times. SAC$\overline{1}$,4,2 is measured by addition of 6.0 ml of 1:50 fresh guinea pig serum diluted in 10 mM EDTA–buffer (buffer 7c, Section 17.B, Table I), followed by incubation at 37° for 90 minutes. The optical densities of the supernatants after centrifugation are measured at 412 nm. Controls should include: (a) a cell blank (type 1), consisting of EAC4 + 1.0 ml of MGVB buffer containing 0.01 mM EDTA; (b) a cell blank (type 2), consisting of EAC4 + 1.0 ml of MGVB

* Section 17.D.3a.iii was contributed by Louis G. Hoffmann and Manfred M. Mayer.

buffer with added 1:50 fresh guinea pig serum in 10 mM EDTA-buffer (C-EDTA); (c) a complement color blank, consisting of 1.5 ml of MGVB + 6.0 ml of C-EDTA; (d) a "CBC" or cell blank control consisting of EAC4 + 0.5 ml of MGVB to which 0.5 ml of C2 and subsequently 6.0 ml of C-EDTA are added; (e) a complete lysis control consisting of EAC4, which receives 7.0 ml of H_2O in the last step, the absorbancy of the clarified lysate being taken as 100%.

The type 2 cell blank may be slightly lower than the sum of the complement color blank (No. 3) and type 1 cell blank; in that event, it should be used to correct the optical density values of the other samples, except for the complete lysis control, which is corrected by subtracting the difference between type 2 cell blank and the complement color. The results are calculated as described in Section 17.C.3.a. The above assay produces a linear dose-response curve from 0–3 SFU of $C\bar{1}$ per cell when z' is plotted against $C\bar{1}$ concentration, subject to the important restriction that the material assayed must be $C\bar{1}$. Hoffmann[4] has found that the dose-response curve for the C1 activity of whole serum in this assay is convex with respect to the C1 axis at low concentrations of C1, i.e., at serum dilutions greater than 1/200,000, even when enough time is allowed for the activation to $C\bar{1}$ occurring after its combination with EAC4.[5]

b. GUINEA PIG C2

*i. Preparation of C2, Stage I by the Method of Borsos, Rapp, and Cook**

C2 was first isolated from guinea pig pseudoglobulin in 1961[6] by chromatography in succession on DEAE-cellulose, CM-cellulose, and DEAE-cellulose. Separation of human C2 was attained later.[7] The 1961 method usually yielded C2 products having 1000 to 2000 units/ml. Tests for contamination with C1 consist in determining residual C2 after incubation at 37° for 1 hour. The C2 is perfectly stable in the absence of $C\bar{1}$. Contamination with C4 is less than 1:10,000 in terms of SFU. Unlike human C2, guinea pig C2 does not improve with oxidation.

Methods for substantial further separation were developed in 1963,[8] starting with the stage I product; purification was attained in 1970[9] by

[4] L. G. Hoffmann, unpublished observations, 1963.
[5] T. Borsos, H. J. Rapp, and U. L. Walz, *J. Immunol.* **92**, 108 (1964).

* Section 17.D.3.b.i was contributed by Louis G. Hoffmann and Manfred M. Mayer.

[6] T. Borsos, H. J. Rapp, and C. T. Cook, *J. Immunol.* **87**, 330 (1961).
[7] M. J. Polley and H. J. Müller-Eberhard, *J. Exp. Med.* **128**, 533 (1968).
[8] M. M. Mayer, J. A. Miller, and H. S. Shin, *J. Immunol.* **101**, 813 (1963).
[9] M. M. Mayer, J. A. Miller, and H. S. Shin, *J. Immunol.* **105**, 327 (1970).

alternative techniques. The final product requires only 1.1 molecules of C2 for lysis of 1 erythrocyte.

Step 1. Separation of Euglobulin. Forty milliliters of guinea pig serum was dialyzed and centrifuged to remove euglobulin as described in Section 17.D.3.a.i. The supernatant was adjusted to ionic strength 0.08 in an ice bath and pH 7.2 with 0.1 N NaOH and 3.0 M NaCl.

Step 2. Chromatography on DEAE-Cellulose. The pseudoglobulin-containing solution from step 1 (40 ml of guinea pig serum) was applied to an 8 × 60 cm column of DEAE-cellulose (40 gm) equilibrated at pH 7.4 in 0.08 M NaCl and then washed with 200 ml of 0.08 M NaCl. The next 600 ml of effluent was collected in a 2-liter cylinder containing 1 liter of ice-cold distilled water.

Step 3. Chromatography on CM-Cellulose. From step 2, 1600 ml was applied under pressure to an 8 × 60 cm column of CM-cellulose (40 gm; 0.7 mEq/gm) equilibrated at pH 4.7 in 0.03 M NaCl. The initial 400 ml of effluent was discarded. The next 2 liters were collected.

Step 4. Chromatography on DEAE-Cellulose. DEAE-cellulose, 15 gm, was washed and equilibrated at pH 7.4 in 0.015 M NaCl in a 6.5 × 60 cm column. The charge consisted of 4 liters (2 liters from step 3 diluted with 2 liters of water to 0.015 M NaCl). The effluent plus washings with 0.015 M NaCl (200 ml) was discarded. The C2 was eluted with 0.25 M NaCl; the first 70 ml of effluent was discarded, and the next 120 ml was collected. The NaCl concentration of the preparation was adjusted to 0.15 M on the basis of conductivity measurement [see footnote to Section 17.D.3.a.i(a), Step 2], and divalent cations were added to provide 0.15 mM Ca^{2+} and 1.0 mM Mg^{2+}. The product is stored at −20°.

ii. Preparation of C2, Stages II to IV*[9]

The following procedure for purifying C2 from pseudoglobulin yields an essentially homogeneous protein, with a yield of ca 300 μg from 160 ml of guinea pig serum. The starting material utilizes EAC4 cells (Section 17.C.2.c) and the stage I preparation of C2 described above (Section 17.D.3.b.i).

Step 1. Absorption and Elution on Treated Erythrocytes. Introduce 235 ml of 1 × 10^9 EAC4 cells/ml (high multiplicity), prepared with sheep erythrocytes, rabbit anti-Forssman antibody, and guinea pig C4 (see Section 17.C.2.c), into each of six 250-ml centrifuge bottles. Centrifuge, strip, and warm the cells (ca 12 ml) to 30°. Dilute 250 ml of stage I C2 (approximately 1000 to 1500 units/ml) to 1250 ml with buffer A, Table III. After equilibration at 30°, 208 ml of the diluted C2 is added to each of the centrifuge bottles and mixed with the cells; the reaction is allowed

* Section 17.D.3.b.ii was contributed by Manfred M. Mayer.

TABLE III
SPECIAL BUFFERS FOR PREPARING GUINEA PIG C2

A. Gelatin–Veronal–Sucrose, pH 8.5, with increased Ca^{2+} and Mg^{2+}, $\Gamma/2 = 0.0544$: Dissolve 68.1 gm of sucrose (reagent grade), 1.019 gm of barbital sodium, 2.49 gm of NaCl in ca 700 ml of distilled water. Adjust the pH to 8.5 with 1 N HCl, add 5 ml of additive mixture and 1 gm of USP gelatin. Bring volume to 1 liter (2.0 mM $MgCl_2$ and 0.3 mM $CaCl_2$). *Additive Mixture:* Dissolve 40.65 gm of $MgCl_2 \cdot 6H_2O$ (0.4 M) and 4.41 gm of $CaCl_2 \cdot 2H_2O$ (0.06 M) in 500 ml of distilled water.

B. Gelatin–Veronal–Sucrose, pH 8.5 with increased Ca^{2+} and Mg^{2+}, $\Gamma/2 = 0.0686$: Prepare exactly like buffer A, but use instead 58.2 gm of sucrose and 3.32 gm of NaCl per liter.

C. Gelatin–Veronal–Saline, pH 6.5, $\Gamma/2 = 0.147$, 0.006 M barbital. Dissolve 1.019 gm of barbital sodium and 8.3 gm of NaCl in ca 700 ml of distilled water. Adjust the pH to 6.5 (ca 4.5 ml of 1 N HCl) and bring the volume to 1 liter including 0.5 gm of gelatin (0.05%). (This formulation represents the toe of the buffer curve.)

D. Special Gelatin–Veronal–Saline, pH 7.3, $\Gamma/2 = 0.147$: Dilute 5× concentrate of stock VBS (buffer 1a, Section 17.B, Table I) to 1 liter, adding only 0.01% of gelatin (2 ml of 5% gelatin) and NaF to a final concentration of 0.075 M. If photometric scanning is intended, replace the gelatin with 2% L-lysine, of somewhat lesser protective activity. The lysine is removed by dialysis prior to scanning.

E. Tris–H_3PO_4, pH 7.0: Dissolve 7.11 gm of "Trizma Base" (Sigma Chemical Company) in 750 ml of water and titrate to pH 7.0 using a solution of 5 gm of 85% phosphoric acid in 50 ml of water. Bring volume to 1 liter (0.0587 M Tris).

---

to proceed at 30° for 10 minutes. The resulting EAC4,2 cells are then sedimented by centrifugation at room temperature and washed twice with 1250 ml of buffer B, Table 3 at 25–30°.

After removal of the second wash fluid, the C2 is eluted from the C4,2 cells with 450 ml of buffer C at 0°. After 10 minutes, the EAC4 are removed by centrifugation at 0°.

Another batch of 250 ml of stage I C2 is subjected to the same adsorption and elution procedure, using the same EAC4 cells. Combine the two 450-ml eluates, centrifuge to remove any remaining cells, and add 0.1 volume of 0.75 M NaF to retard microbial growth. Concentrate at 5° by ultrafiltration to approximately 10 ml, dialyzing simultaneously against buffer E (Table III). Owing to the high gelatin concentration, the contents of the collection bag will solidify. The gelatin is melted by immersing the collodion bags in Tris-phosphate buffer E (Table III), warmed to 37°, and the bag contents with buffer rinsings are transferred to a suitable container for storage at about −20 to −30° (volume ca 15 ml). This product (designated stage II of C2) is essentially free of guinea pig serum proteins other than C2, but it does contain erythrocyte proteins. For most purposes erythrocyte proteins do not interfere. However, for experiments requiring highly purified C2, these proteins are removed in steps 2 and 3.

Step 2. Disc Electrophoresis on a Slab of Polyacrylamide Gel and Elu-tion (Stage III). The vertical electrophoresis chamber of the EC Corporation (Philadelphia, Pennsylvania) (Vol. II, Chap. 6.C.5) is modified for preparative polyacrylamide electrophoresis by making a gel chamber ca 6 mm deep. The gasket of sponge rubber is removed, and a Plexiglas spacer, 3 mm $\times$ 8 mm $\times$ 200 mm, is cemented in place of the gasket. A compressible gasket of pure gum rubber (3 $\times$ 8 $\times$ 200 mm) is placed on the spacer. The entire cross section of the resulting chamber is 120 mm $\times$ ~6 mm. The polyacrylamide gel and buffers are used as described in Vol. II, Chap. 6.C.4.b, excepting that, in the stacking gel, the TEMED is reduced to 0.1 ml and the sucrose to 40 gm/400 ml of solution.

Stage II material, 15 ml warmed to 37°C, is placed on the stacking gel in the modified vertical electrophoresis chamber, followed by a carefully applied overlay of Tris buffer to fill the remaining space at the top of the chamber. Coolant at 5° to 8° is circulated around the chamber. A current of 30 to 40 mA (200 to 250 V) is applied until the sample has become stacked at the top of the separating gel. At this time, the current is increased to 70 to 80 mA (400 to 450 V) and kept at this value until the separation is complete (6 to 7 hours). At the end of the run, the separating gel (12 cm wide $\times$ 10 cm high $\times$ 0.6 cm thick) is removed from the chamber and placed on a glass plate. A 2.5-mm strip is trimmed away from each edge. The gel is cut into 0.5-cm strips across the electrophoretic pathway. Each lateral segment is chopped finely into as many small pieces as possible and placed in a 40-ml tube. Four successive elutions are made in the cold, each with 5 ml of buffer D (Table III)[*] for 2 days, and combined. The eluates are checked for C2 activity, and active fractions are pooled. This material is designated stage III. It still contains some contaminating erythrocyte proteins. It is concentrated to approximately 0.5 to 0.1 ml and dialyzed against Tris-phosphate buffer E.

Step 3. Disc Electrophoresis and Elution (Stage IV). The concentrated stage III material (25 to 100 μl) is placed on the stacking gels of 4 or 5 cylindrical, analytical gels (Vol. II, Chap. 6.C.4), 25 μl of buffer E containing 50% sucrose, and 2 μl of 0.1% aqueous bromophenol blue are added, and finally an overlay of the Tris buffer as used in the cathode chamber. Electrophoresis stacking is carried out with a field of 100 V and a current of 1 mA per tube. When the sample enters the small-pore

---

[*] An alternative and speedier extraction system is described by U. J. Lewis and M. O. Clark, *Anal. Biochem.* 6, 303 (1963). These workers obtained proteins from segments of polyacrylamide gel by dispersal within large-pore gel (Vol. II, Chap. 6.C.4.e, Table II) and discharged the protein into Cellophane sacs by secondary electrophoresis—Editors.

gel, the field is increased to 400 V and current of 3 mA per tube is maintained until the bromophenol blue tracking dye migrates to the bottom of the separating gel. At the end of the run, each of the 4 or 5 separating gels (5 × 40 mm) is cut into 1.25-mm segments and eluted in 4 ml of buffer D (Table III) for 24 hours at 3° to 5°. Corresponding segments from each of the four gels are eluted together and considered as one fraction. The gel segments are eluted a second time with 1.5 ml of buffer for 18 hours, and the first and second eluates of each fraction are pooled and checked for C2 activity.* The active fractions are combined (volume approximately 50 ml), concentrated by ultrafiltration to about 0.5 to 1 ml, and stored at −20 to −30°C.

iii. Purity

On disc electrophoresis, the product yields a single stained band at the locus of elutable C2 activity and gives rise to a monospecific rabbit anti-GP C2.[9] On immunoelectrophoresis, it yields a single arc. All the protein in purified C2 is absorbable on EAC4. Contamination with the other eight C components is less than 1 part in 20,000. The molecular weight of the product is about 130,000. Approximately 1.1 molecules are required for lysis of one erythrocyte.

A yield of about 300 μg of protein (16–22% of C2 of stage I material) is usually obtained from 160 ml of serum.

iv. Assay of Guinea Pig C2†

The assay for C2 is based upon formation of SAC142 from EAC1,4 by adding C2.

Because EAC1,4,2 decays, this reaction exhibits a maximum with respect to time in the presence of a limited amount of C2. The time at which this maximum occurs, t_{max}, is determined by temperature and effective SAC1,4 concentration, but is independent of C2 concentration. It will therefore vary from one EAC1,4 preparation to the next and must be measured for each preparation. In other words, the number of site-forming units (SFU) of C2[10] originally added for the titration is greater than the number of SAC1,4,2 formed during the reaction.

The first assay developed (Borsos et al., 1961[10]) predicted a linear relationship between the number of SAC1,4,2 formed and concentration of

---

* One SFU of C2 is defined as the volume of a particular preparation, in milliliters, that will convert one SAC1,4,2 in the absence of decay of the latter.

† Section 17.D.3.b.iv was contributed by Louis G. Hoffmann and Manfred M. Mayer.

[10] T. Borsos, H. J. Rapp, and M. M. Mayer, J. Immunol. 87, 310 (1961).

C2. In fact, the dose response curve is slightly concave with respect to the C2 axis and the extent of deviation from linearity varies somewhat. Accordingly, it is convenient to reserve a reference lot of C2 and include it as a standard in all titrations of C2 samples.

A unit of C2 activity has been defined as 1:1000 of the activity of a particular reference lot of C2; the corresponding value has been found to be equivalent to about 4 to 6 $\times$ 10^8 SFU of C2.[11]

(a) *Determination of t_{max}.* A 125-ml Erlenmeyer flask, containing 1.5 $\times$ 10^9 EAC1,4 cells (Section 17.C.2.b) in 19.0 ml of GVB^{2+} (buffer 2, Section 17.B, Table I), is suspended from a wrist-action shaker in a water bath maintained at 30.0°. The contents of the flask and a sample of C2 diluted to 3 to 6 units/ml are brought to this temperature separately and then 1.0 ml of the C2 dilution is added to the cell preparation. Samples of 1.0 ml are removed periodically into 15 $\times$ 125 mm tubes containing 1.5 ml of C-EDTA diluted 1:37.5 in EDTA-buffer 10 mM in EDTA (buffer 7c, Section 17.B, Table I). The contents of these tubes are mixed immediately and incubated at 37° for measurement of the number of SAC1,4,2 per cell, as described in Section 17.C.3.a. For the purpose of determining t_{max}, it is not necessary to calculate z'; it is sufficient to plot optical density values against time. The value of t_{max} is determined by inspection of the graph.

(b) *Titration of C2.* The problem of decay of the end product of SAC1,4,2 during the titration of C2 has been noted above. One approach has been to take account of the extent of decay in terms of t_{max}. The mathematical model formulated by Borsos et al.[10] leads to a good first approximation and provides a correction factor if t_{max} is known (Table IV).

Another procedure was developed by Mayer and Miller.[11] Portions of 1.0 ml of EAC1,4 containing 1.5 $\times$ 10^8 cells are pipetted into 40-ml centrifuge tubes. After warming to 30.0°, 1.0 ml of a suitable dilution of C2, also at 30.0°, is added to each tube, and the mixture is incubated for a period equal to the t_{max} of the EAC1,4 preparation as ascertained in (a). The diluent is buffer containing 0.15 mM Ca^{2+} and 1.0 mM Mg^{2+}. If a number of samples are to be assayed, addition of C2 to the tubes should be staggered, e.g., at equal intervals of 1 minute, so that all tubes are incubated exactly the same period. The reaction is terminated by addition to each tube of 1.0 ml of ice-cold 10 mM EDTA-buffer followed immediately by 2.0 ml of complement diluted 1:25 in 10 mM EDTA-buffer (C-EDTA). The tubes are transferred at once to a water bath at 37.0° for determination of the number of SAC1,4,2 sites per cell, as

[11] M. M. Mayer and J. A. Miller, *Inter. J. Immunochem.* **2,** 71 (1965).

described in Section 17.C.3.a, which also lists the procedure and the necessary controls.

Further reaction between EAC1,4 and C2 must be terminated by adding EDTA-buffer *before* addition of C-EDTA, otherwise the divalent cations in the reaction mixture would bind all the EDTA in the first fraction of a milliliter of C-EDTA added, allowing the cells to be exposed for a very brief interval to a high concentration of C2 (from the C-EDTA) under conditions where reaction will occur. Willoughby[12] has observed that omission of the EDTA-buffer as stop-diluent leads to a small increase in the value of the "CBC" blank.

Since the dose-response curve is not linear but is slightly concave with respect to the C2 axis, the number of SFU of C2 in a given sample must therefore be based not on the volume of the sample giving a $z' = 1.00$, but on the slope of the plot of z' *vs* C2 concentration near the origin.

To obtain the C2 content of the sample assayed in terms of SFU/ml, a number of dilutions must be examined, particularly at low levels of lysis (z' below 0.5). The number of SAC1,4,2 per cell (z') is plotted against the reciprocal of the dilution, and a tangent is drawn to the resulting line at the origin. The tangent is extrapolated to a value of z' equal to the appropriate correction factor for the EAC1,4 preparation used, obtained by interpolation of values shown in Table IV. The dilu-

TABLE IV
CORRECTION FACTOR DECAY OF
SAC1,4,2

t_{max} (min)	Correction factor[a]
2	0.94
4	0.89
6	0.83
8	0.78
10	0.74
15	0.64
20	0.55

[a] The factor represents the ratio between the maximal number of SAC1,4,2 formed and the (higher) original number of site-forming units in the C2.

[12] W. F. Willoughby, unpublished observations, 1961.

tion of the sample corresponding to this value of z' contains 1.5×10^8 SFU/ml.

If the result is to be expressed in terms of units of C2, a calibration curve is prepared by including in the assay at least four evenly spaced dilutions of a standard lot of C2; the values of z' obtained for the unknown samples can then be converted directly to units of C2 by reference to this curve.

The method described here has been used in our laboratory to measure C2 in purified fractions as well as in whole serum of the guinea pig; in the latter case the high dilutions employed (1:10,000 to 1:40,000) reduce to a negligible level the amounts of C1 and C4 contributed by the sample, compared to the amounts of these components present in good EAC1,4 preparations. An application of the method to the assay of human C2* requires C4 contributed by the human serum. Thus, the method is suitable for the determination of C2 in human serum only if the C4 content is normal, or with EAC1,4 made with human C4.

c. ISOLATION OF GUINEA PIG C3†[13]

Guinea pig serum (150–200 ml) was adjusted to pH 7.5 with 1 M acetic acid and diluted with ice-cold distilled water until the conductivity corresponded to that of 0.04 M NaCl (see text footnote to Section 17.D.3.a.i(a) step 2). The resulting precipitate was allowed to aggregate for 30 minutes and then removed by centrifugation at 1500 g, 0°, for 45 minutes.

i. Procedure

Step 1. DEAE-Cellulose Chromatography. The clear supernatant was applied at a flow rate of 250 ml per hour to a DEAE-cellulose column 5.0×70 cm, equilibrated with pH 7.5 starting buffer containing 0.005 M phosphate, 0.033 M NaCl, and 0.001 M EDTA. The column was washed with 1500 ml of starting buffer. A linear NaCl gradient was then developed (limit buffer, 1500 ml of a pH 7.5 buffer containing 0.005 M phosphate, 0.243 M NaCl, and 0.001 M EDTA). Eluates containing C3 (ca 400 ml) were pooled, concentrated to 10 ml by ultrafiltration, and diluted to 20 ml with NaCl solution to adjust the conductivity to that

---

* The technique of A. S. Townes and C. R. Stewart, Jr. [*Bull. Johns Hopkins Hosp.* **117**, 331 (1965)], using as it does human EAC1 and human C4, does not suffer from this difficulty. But because it requires the daily preparation of human EAC1,4, it is impractical to use it for the routine analysis of C2 in whole human serum.

† Section 17.D.3.c was contributed by Manfred M. Mayer.

[13] H. S. Shin and M. M. Mayer, *Biochemistry* **7**, 2991 (1968).

of 0.08 M NaCl. The pH was brought to 5.0 with 1 M acetic acid. No precipitate appeared.

Step 2. Chromatography on CM-Cellulose. The material was applied at a rate of 20 ml/hr to a CM-cellulose column, equilibrated with pH 5 starting buffer containing 0.02 M acetate and 0.07 M NaCl. The column was washed with 150 ml of starting buffer. A linear gradient was then developed by gradual addition (75 ml/hr) of 450 ml of pH 5 buffer containing 0.02 M acetate and 0.19 M NaCl to a mixing chamber containing 450 ml of starting buffer. Fractions from CM-cellulose columns were collected in tubes containing an appropriate amount of 0.5 M Tris to bring the pH to 7.5. A volumetric collecting device was used since its rapid discharge of each fraction promotes mixing with the Tris buffer.

Step 3. Preparative Block Electrophoresis. Approximately 400 to 500 ml of eluate containing C3 was concentrated to 1 ml by ultrafiltration and dialyzed for 4 hours against 500 ml of Tris buffer (pH 8.6) and ionic strength 0.05. The material was applied, 12 cm from the cathode, to a Pevikon block $(1 \times 10 \times 50$ cm$)$ equilibrated with the pH 8.6 Tris buffer. The electrophoresis was run for 48 hours at 400 V, with a current of 20 mA and a gradient of 2.5 V/cm of Pevikon block. After the electrophoresis, the block was sliced into $1 \times 1 \times 10$ cm segments, and each segment was eluted four times in 10 ml of pH 7.5 buffer containing 0.005 M phosphate, 0.15 M NaCl, and 0.001 M EDTA. Only the first eluate of each fraction was analyzed for C3 activity, but all four eluates were pooled if the first eluate contained C3.

For further purification, the three fractionation procedures just described were repeated, but in a different order.

Step 4. DEAE-Cellulose Chromatography. A pool of about 300 to 500 ml of the electrophoretically fractionated C3 was concentrated to 30 ml and diluted with 0.005 M phosphate buffer pH 7.5 until the conductivity corresponded to that of 0.035 M NaCl. The pH was adjusted to 7.5 if necessary. The material was applied at a rate of 15 ml per hour to a DEAE column $(2 \times 30$ cm$)$ equilibrated with pH 7.5 starting buffer, containing 0.005 M phosphate, 0.028 M NaCl, and 0.001 M EDTA. The column was washed with 100 ml of this starting buffer, and then a linear gradient was developed by the addition (30 ml per hour) of 250 ml of pH 7.5 buffer, containing 0.005 M phosphate, 0.193 M NaCl, and 0.001 M EDTA to a mixing chamber containing 250 ml of starting buffer.

Step 5. Preparative Block Electrophoresis. Eluate (40 to 50 ml) containing C3 was concentrated to 0.2 ml, followed by dialysis and electrophoresis on a $1 \times 5 \times 50$ cm Pevikon block, as before, except that the current was 10 mA and segments of $1 \times 1 \times 5$ cm were eluted in 5-ml portions of pH 7.5 buffer.

Step 6. Chromatography on CM-Cellulose. About 100 ml of eluate containing C3 was concentrated to about 0.5 ml and dialyzed for 12 hours against 500 ml of pH 7.5 buffer, containing 0.005 M phosphate and 0.035 M NaCl. After dialysis, the contents of the dialysis bag were diluted with 6 ml of pH 5.0 starting buffer containing 0.02 M acetate and 0.07 M NaCl. The material was applied to a CM-cellulose column (1×20 cm) equilibrated with the pH 5.0 starting buffer. The column was washed with 50 ml of the starting buffer, and a linear gradient was applied by gradual addition (12 ml per hour) of 120 ml of pH 5.0 buffer containing 0.02 M acetate and 0.24 M NaCl to a mixing chamber containing 120 ml of starting buffer. The fractions containing C3 were pooled, concentrated to at least 5 mg of protein per milliliter, and stored at $-70°$.

ii. Characteristics of Isolated C3

Immunoelectrophoretic analyses of C3 preparations using anti-C3 and anti-whole guinea pig serum showed single precipitation lines in every case. Furthermore, immunoelectrophoresis of whole guinea pig serum with anti-C3 gave a single precipitation line. Disc electrophoresis also showed a single fuzzy band, and C3 activity could be eluted from the segment corresponding to this band. Purified C3 was eluted from a hydroxylapatite column as a single symmetric peak at a phosphate concentration of 0.17 M. All fractions across the peak had the same specific activity.

Analysis by ultracentrifugation showed a single symmetric peak. The sedimentation coefficient of C3 at 20° was 7.4×10^{-13} second at four different concentrations, namely, 0.1, 0.125, 0.2, and 0.4%. Molecular weight values of 179,000 and 179,600 were obtained from sedimentation equilibrium analyses at concentrations of 0.05 and 0.015%, respectively. Partial specific volume of 0.725 was assumed.

No other complement components were detected by hemolytic tests. C3-inactivator was also absent.

A yield of 5 to 7 mg of protein is usually obtained from 150 to 200 ml of serum.

iii. Assay of C3[14]

A converting agent was prepared to contain, per milliliter, C2 (80 units), C5 (100 units), C6 (100 units), C7 (300 units), C8 (200 units), and C9 (300 units) in DGVB^{2+}. Partially purified C2 was made by the method of Borsos *et al.,*[6] C9 was purified (Section 17.D.3.h), while C5 through C8 were functionally separated according to Nelson *et al.*[15]

[14] H. S. Shin and M. M. Mayer, *Biochemistry* **7**, 2997 (1968).
[15] R. A. Nelson, Jr., J. Jensen, I. Gigli, and N. Tamura, *Immunochemistry* **3**, 111 (1966).

Two parts of C3 for titration were mixed with two parts of the converting reagent at 0° and one part of (0°) EAC1,4 (1.54 × 10^8/ml) was added. The mixture was incubated at 37° for 90 minutes with frequent shaking; 10 parts of 0.15 M NaCl were then added, tubes were centrifuged, and oxyhemoglobin was read at 412 nm and converted into SAC4,2,3 per cell.

d. GUINEA PIG C4[*]

Presently guinea pig C4 is obtained only as a functionally separated fraction from other complement components of guinea pig serum.[15, 16]

e. ISOLATION OF GUINEA PIG C5[†][17]

All steps were performed at 3° unless mentioned otherwise. The conductivity of solutions was measured at 0°.

i. Procedure

Step 1. Removal of Euglobulin. Pooled guinea pig serum, 250 ml, was adjusted to pH 7.5 with 1 M acetic acid, and diluted with water at 0° until the conductivity was 2.4 mS at 0°. After 30 minutes, the precipitate (containing C1) was centrifuged at 1300 g for 1 hour.

Step 2. Chromatography on DEAE-Cellulose. The supernatant was applied to a 5 × 65 cm column of DEAE-cellulose, 0.82 mEq/gm, equilibrated with 0.005 M pH 7.5 phosphate buffer containing 0.035 M NaCl. After the column was washed with 800 ml of starting buffer, a linear salt gradient was developed (limit buffer, 1500 ml of 0.005 M pH 7.5 phosphate buffer containing 0.245 M NaCl). A flow rate of 150 ml per hour was maintained. Fractions containing C5 were pooled and concentrated to about 10 ml under negative pressure in collodion bags (Schleicher and Schuell, Keene, New Hampshire).

Step 3. Precipitation at Low Ionic Strength. The conductivity was adjusted to 2.4 mS with distilled water and pH to 5.0 with 1 M acetic acid. After 30 minutes the precipitate was sedimented by centrifugation at 11,000 g for 20 minutes. The precipitate was washed once with 40 ml of

---

[*] Section 17.D.3.d was contributed by the Editors.

[16] R. M. Zarco, R. A. Cort, and D. R. Schultz, Cordis Corporation, under contract with NIAID and NCI, scheme reproduced by H. J. Rapp and T. Borsos *in* "Molecular Basis of Complement Action," p. 98. Appleton-Century-Crofts, New York, 1970.

[†] Section 17.D.3.e was contributed by Manfred M. Mayer.

[17] C. T. Cook, H. S. Shin, M. M. Mayer, and K. A. Laudenslayer, *J. Immunol.* **106**, 467 (1971).

0.02 M pH 5.0 acetate buffer containing 0.03 M NaCl and then dissolved over a 12-hour period in 20 ml of 0.005 M pH 7.5 phosphate buffer containing 0.2 M NaCl. Insoluble residue was removed by centrifugation. The pH of the supernatant was adjusted to 5.0 with 1 M acetic acid, and the conductivity to 7.3 mS with distilled water.

Step 4. Chromatography on CM-Cellulose. The adjusted C5 pool was applied to a 2 × 35 cm column of CM-cellulose (0.7 mEq/gm) equilibrated with 0.02 M pH 5.0 acetate buffer containing 0.12 M NaCl. After the column was washed with 100 ml of starting buffer, a linear gradient was developed (limit buffer, 200 ml of 0.02 M pH 5.0 acetate buffer containing 0.30 M NaCl). The flow rate throughout the procedure was 70 ml per hour. Fractions were discharged from a volumetric head into tubes containing enough 0.5 M Tris base to bring the pH from 5.0 to 7.5.

Step 5. Preparative Block Electrophoresis. The fractions with C5 activity were pooled, concentrated to about 1 ml, dialyzed against pH 8.6 Tris·HCl buffer, ionic strength 0.05, and applied to a 1 × 5 × 50 cm Pevikon block equilibrated with the same Tris buffer, for electrophoresis lasting 65 hours at 3.2 V/cm. Segments of 1 × 1 × 5 cm were cut, and each was eluted repeatedly with 5 ml of 0.005 M pH 7.5 phosphate buffer containing 0.15 M NaCl. The first set of eluates was analyzed for absorbancy at 280 nm and hemolytic activity. The final pool consisted of 4 successive eluates of each segment containing C5.

Step 6. Chromatography on Hydroxylapatite. The pool was concentrated to about 3 to 4 ml, dialyzed against 0.08 M pH 6.8 potassium phosphate buffer and applied to a 1 × 16 cm column of hydroxylapatite (Hypatite C, Clarkson Chemical Co., Inc., Williamsport, Pennsylvania), equilibrated with the same phosphate buffer. After washing with 80 ml of starting buffer, a linear phosphate gradient was made by mixing 120 ml of starting buffer with 120 ml of 0.25 M pH 6.8 potassium phosphate buffer. The flow rate was 15 ml per hour.

Step 7. Chromatography on DEAE-Cellulose. The fractions with C5 activity were concentrated to 1 ml, dialyzed against 0.005 M pH 7.5 phosphate buffer containing 0.045 M NaCl and applied to a 1 × 30 cm column of DEAE-cellulose, equilibrated with the same buffer, and then washed with 100 ml of starting buffer. A linear gradient was developed by mixing 100 ml of starting buffer with an equal volume of 0.005 M phosphate buffer, pH 7.5, containing 0.245 M NaCl at a flow rate of 70 ml per hour. The active fractions were pooled, concentrated to at least 2 mg/ml and stored at −70°. Alternatively, lower concentrations may be stored safely at −40° to −70° in the presence of 1% gelatin. This product is checked for purity by immunoelectrophoretic analysis against a rabbit anti-guinea pig serum and a rabbit anti-GP C5 serum. The product is essentially homogeneous, with 2 minor noncomplement contaminants.

Step 8. Electrophoresis on Agarose. The final product sometimes contained a minor noncomplement contaminant which could be eliminated by electrophoresis on 1% agarose gel in 0.05 M pH 8.6 barbital buffer. The agarose gel was made in a glass tube (0.7 cm i.d.) plugged at the anodal end with 1 cm of 7.5% acrylamide gel. A 4-cm layer of melted agarose was poured, and barbital buffer was layered to obtain a flat meniscus.

After solidification of the agarose, the overlying buffer was removed and 10 μl of C5 (120 μg) and 10 μl of 25% sucrose were introduced. The barbital buffer head was restored. Electrophoresis was performed at 150 V for 1.5 hours at 3°. The agarose gel was sectioned into 1.3-mm segments, and each segment was eluted for 24 hours in 1 ml of 0.005 M phosphate buffer, pH 7.5, containing 0.15 M NaCl.

ii. Characteristics of Isolated Guinea Pig C5

The product has a sedimentation coefficient of 7.8 S and a molecular weight of about 180,000. It is free of the other eight complement components and no substantial noncomplement contamination is present, as indicated by immunoelectrophoretic tests.

A yield of 1 to 2 mg is usually obtained in step 7 from 250 ml of serum. On disc electrophoresis in polyacrylamide gel, C5 produced a single diffuse smear.

iii. Assay

Titration for C5 activity was made by mixing 2 parts of C5 sample with 2 parts of a mixture of C2, C3, C6, C7, C8, and C9 in DGVB^{2+} and 1 part of EAC$\overline{1,4}$ at 0°. After incubation at 37° for 70 minutes, 10 parts of 0.15 M NaCl were added, and the supernatant was read for absorbancy at 412 nm.[18]

A rabbit anti-C5 was prepared against the partially purified step 6 product, useful particularly because it served to detect contaminants in the final product.

EAC$\overline{1,4,2,3}$ cleaves C5 into 2 fragments, C5a (1.5 S) causing direct contraction of guinea pig ileum (Section 17.E.9) and C5b (7.4 S).

f. PURIFICATION OF GUINEA PIG C6

The method given for human C6 is stated to be applicable also to guinea pig C6 (Section 17.D.2.e)

[18] H. S. Shin, R. J. Pickering, and M. M. Mayer, *J. Immunol.* **106**, 473 (1971).

g. GUINEA PIG C7 AND C8

Guinea pig C7 and C8 are presently obtained only as functionally separated fractions from other complement components.[15, 16]

h. ISOLATION OF GUINEA PIG C9*[19]

i. Preparation

Step 1. Removal of C1 and Preparation of Ammonium Sulfate Fraction (2.0 to 2.6 M). Guinea pig serum (250 ml) was brought to pH 7.5 and diluted with 3 volumes of 0.005 M phosphate, pH 7.5. The precipitate containing C1 was removed. The clear supernatant fluid was brought to 2.0 M $(NH_4)_2SO_4$ by adding solid salt (303 gm/liter), after which the precipitate was removed by centrifugation. The 2.0 M supernatant was brought to 2.6 M by adding further solid ammonium sulfate (96.3 gm/liter). This precipitate was collected, dissolved in water, and dialyzed vs 0.005 M phosphate, pH 7.5, containing 0.001 M EDTA and NaCl to provide 0.06 M.

Step 2. Chromatography on DEAE-Cellulose. The yield from step 1 was applied to a 5 × 48 cm column of DEAE-cellulose in the same buffer. The first effluent contained C2; the column was washed thoroughly. Elution was carried out by a linear NaCl gradient to 0.3 M, C9 appearing between 0.1 and 0.15 M. Fractions were pooled (800 ml) and adjusted to pH 6.0.

Step 3. Chromatography on CM-Cellulose. The yield from step 2 was diluted with 0.005 M phosphate buffer, pH 6.0, containing 0.001 M EDTA, and conductance was adjusted to be equivalent to 0.08 N NaCl. The adjusted yield was applied to a 2.5 × 40 cm column of CM-cellulose equilibrated with the same solution; the column was washed thoroughly. Elution was carried out with a linear NaCl gradient, C9 eluting between 0.17 and 0.24 M NaCl. Fractions were pooled (480 ml) and dialyzed against 0.005 M phosphate, 0.001 M EDTA at pH 7.5, with NaCl added to conductance equal to 0.06 M NaCl.

Step 4. Rechromatography on DEAE-Cellulose. The yield from step 3 was applied to a 2.5 × 26 cm column of DEAE-cellulose in the same buffer, and step 2 was repeated. Recovery of C9 was not improved.

Step 5. Separation by Pevikon Block Electrophoresis. The concentrated yield from step 4 (2.5 ml), equilibrated with barbital buffer, $\Gamma/2 = 0.05$, pH 8.6, was electrophoresed on a Pevikon block (1 × 10 × 40 cm) for 40 hours at 3.5 V/cm, 20 mA. One centimenter segments were eluted by VB, pH 7.5, 0.15 M. This step entailed a 67% loss in recovery.

* Section 17.D.3.h was compiled by the Editors in consultation with Manfred M. Mayer.

[19] N. Tamura and A. Shimada, *Immunology* **20**, 415 (1971).

ii. Purity

No arc could be detected in direct IEA tests vs rabbit anti-guinea pig serum. However, antiserum developed to C9 showed one arc in the α_2-globulin position by radioimmunoelectrophoresis using ^{125}I-labeled C9 (37,000 cpm/ml) diluted in guinea pig serum. C9 was subjected to electrophoresis and tested with IgG globulin fractions of antisera; then an overlay of agar containing EAC1-8 was applied. Hemolysis occurred in the α_2 position ("immunolysoelectrophoresis"). It will be recalled that human C9 is also an α-globulin (Section 17.D.2.h).

E. Complement-Related Proteins

1. INTRODUCTION*

Certain factors other than complement components react to control the "complement-cascade" and the utilization of later complement components by the alternative pathway (Section 17.A). Methods are described for preparation of the $\overline{C1}$-inhibitor (Section 17.E.2), the C3b-inactivator, or KAF (Section 17.E.3), properdin (Section 17.E.4), properdin factor D (the proenzyme of C3-proactivator-convertase) from human and guinea pig serum, and factor $\overline{D}$ (the activated form of D, known as C3-proactivator convertase, C3PA*ase* or GBG*ase*) (Section 17.E.5), and properdin factor B (C3-proactivator or C3PA) from human and guinea pig serum (Section 17.E.6). In addition, methods are given for preparing the cobra venom factor, CoF (Section 17.E.7), C3a anaphylatoxin, and C5a exhibiting anaphylactic and chemotactic factors (Sections 17.E.8 and 9). One among the many known inherited defects in the complement system (lack of functional $\overline{C1}$-inhibitor), which causes the disease hereditary angioneurotic edema, is described (Section 17.E.2.a.ii).

2. ISOLATION OF HUMAN SERUM $\overline{C1}$-INHIBITOR ($\overline{C1}$-INH)†‡

The existence of an inhibitor of the complement enzyme $\overline{C1}$ in serum (Section 17.A, Fig. 1) was first demonstrated by Ratnoff and Lepow in 1957.[1] It was identified as α_2-neuraminoglycoprotein in 1969.[2]

* Section 17.E.1 was contributed by the Editors.
† Section 17.E.2 was contributed by Jack Pensky and Irwin H. Lepow.
‡ This work was supported by U.S. Public Health Service Grants AI-106345 and AI-01255 and was performed in part during tenure of a Research Career Development award (J. P.) (1-K3-AI-21,722) and a Research Career Award (I. H. L.) (Gm-K6-15,307) of the National Institutes of Health.
[1] O. D. Ratnoff and I. H. Lepow, *J. Exp. Med.* **106**, 327 (1957).
[2] J. Pensky and H. G. Schwick, *Science* **163**, 698 (1969).

The inhibitor blocks the action of $\overline{\text{C1}}$ both in C1$\bar{\text{s}}$-catalyzed esterolysis of synthetic amino acid esters and in inactivation of C4 and C2 by $\overline{\text{C1}}$ in free solution (Section 17.A, Fig. 1). The reaction between $\overline{\text{C1}}$-inhibitor and $\overline{\text{C1}}$ is stoichiometric and very rapid.[3] Similarly, "$\overline{\text{C1}}$-inhibitor," formerly termed "C'1a-esterase inhibitor" or "C'1a esterase inactivator," blocks $\overline{\text{C1}}$ contained in the intermediate complexes $\text{EAC}\overline{\text{1}}$ and $\text{EAC}\overline{\text{1,4}}$ but has no effect on the lysis of $\text{EAC}\overline{\text{1,4b,2a}}$ by later-acting components of complement.[4, 5]

Partial purification of the inhibitor of $\overline{\text{C1}}$ was described by Pensky et al.[6]; it has since been obtained as a homogeneous protein.[2]

a. CHARACTERISTICS

$\overline{\text{C1}}$-inhibitor is a glycoprotein containing about 12% hexose, with a sedimentation constant of about 4.2 S and a molecular weight of 139,000 ± 13,000.[6] Its concentration in serum is 24 ± 4 μg/ml.[7] Electrophoretically, $\overline{\text{C1}}$-inhibitor migrates on paper as an α_2-globulin, and in the β region in agar and in polyacrylamide gel. Its mobility is greatly decreased by treatment with purified bacterial neuraminidase, indicating loss of neuraminic acid groups, yet the inhibitory activity remains unaffected.[6]

Several parameters of $\overline{\text{C1}}$-inhibitor—$E_{1cm}^{1\%}$ of 4.05 at 280 nm, sedimentation constant, electrophoretic mobility, and hexose content—closely resemble those of the α_2-neuraminoglycoprotein obtained from plasma in perchloric acid filtrates in 1962.[8] The latter protein is biologically inactive because of exposure to acid conditions, yet it is indistinguishable from $\overline{\text{C1}}$-inhibitor both antigenically[9] and upon immunoelectrophoresis.[6]

Approximately 90% of $\overline{\text{C1}}$-inhibitor is destroyed by heating at 56° for 30 minutes and 100% is destroyed by 60° for 30 minutes.[2] $\overline{\text{C1}}$-inhibitor is not identical with α_1-antitrypsin. It is rapidly inactivated below pH 5.5[2] or by treatment of serum at 0° with low concentrations of methanol[10] or ether.[11]

Complement-fixed serum, derived from mixtures of immune aggregates incubated in fresh serum, contains about 12% of its original active $\overline{\text{C1}}$-inhibitor. Serum after activation of plasmin by streptokinase treatment shows a reduction of $\overline{\text{C1}}$-inhibitor activity to about 40% of the

[3] J. Pensky, L. R. Levy, and I. H. Lepow, *J. Biol. Chem.* **236**, 1674 (1961).
[4] I. H. Lepow and M. A. Leon, *Immunology* **5**, 222 (1962).
[5] M. A. Leon and I. H. Lepow, *Immunology* **5**, 235 (1962).
[6] J. Pensky, L. R. Levy, and I. H. Lepow, *J. Biol. Chem.* **236**, 1674 (1961).
[7] F. S. Rosen, P. Charache, J. Pensky, and V. Donaldson, *Science* **148**, 957 (1965).
[8] H. E. Schultze, K. Heide, and H. Haupt, *Naturwissenschaften* **49**, 133 (1962).
[9] H. G. Schwick, personal communication.
[10] L. R. Levy and I. H. Lepow, *Proc. Soc. Exp. Biol. Med.* **101**, 608 (1959).
[11] V. H. Donaldson, *J. Clin. Invest.* **40**, 673 (1961).

original value.[1] In the classical complement reagents R1, R3, and R4, concentration of C$\bar{1}$-inhibitor is essentially unchanged from serum levels; the euglobulin reagent R2, however, lacks C$\bar{1}$-inhibitor.

C$\bar{1}$-inhibitor blocks the action of C$\bar{1}$ in paroxysmal cold hemoglobinuria (Donath–Landsteiner reaction),[12] and in the immune cytotoxic action of complement and antibody on human amnion cells.[13] The C$\bar{1}$-inhibitor retards but does not completely stop the spontaneous activation of the proenzyme C1 to the enzyme C1$\bar{s}$.[14] In studies on the rate of C$\bar{1}$ activation in a euglobulin preparation, it was found that (a) increasing the amounts of C$\bar{1}$-inhibitor in the reaction mixture increased progressively the lag period before formation of C$\bar{1}$ was detected and (b) C$\bar{1}$-inhibitor was shown to be consumed in the reaction.

Preincubation of C$\bar{1}$-inhibitor with rabbit anti-inhibitor serum will overcome the normal effect of C$\bar{1}$-inhibitor in blocking esterolysis of synthetic substrates by C1$\bar{s}$,[6] indicating closeness or identity of the inhibitory group(s) and antigenic groups(s) on the C$\bar{1}$-inhibitor molecule.

i. The Effect of C$\bar{1}$-Inhibitor in Other Enzyme Systems

Highly purified C$\bar{1}$-inhibitor can inhibit several other enzymes, such as chymotrypsin,[6] kallikrein,[15,16] and permeability globulins.[15–17] In agreement with earlier results[16,18] obtained by Kagan and Becker with partially purified preparations of C$\bar{1}$-inhibitor, a homogeneous preparation of C$\bar{1}$-inhibitor is able to block the generation of the permeability factor, PF/dil, from plasma and, to a lesser extent, the effects of pregenerated PF/dil on vascular permeability. Higher concentrations of C$\bar{1}$-inhibitor block the kallikreinlike activity generated in plasma by ellagic acid in the presence of EDTA.[15]

C$\bar{1}$-inhibitor blocks the fibrinolytic and caseinolytic activities of human plasmin, both streptokinase-activated or—when highly purified—spontaneously activated.[15] Partially purified preparations of plasmin, however, destroy C$\bar{1}$-inhibitor activity,[19] this loss of activity being accompanied by fragmentation of the inhibitor molecule.

The effect of C$\bar{1}$-inhibitor on trypsin is difficult to measure because the

[12] C. F. Hinz, Jr., M. E. Picken, and I. H. Lepow, J. Exp. Med. 113, 177 (1961).

[13] I. H. Lepow and A. Ross, J. Exp. Med. 112, 1107 (1961).

[14] I. H. Lepow, G. B. Naff, and J. Pensky, Complement. Ciba Found. Symp. 1964, p. 74 (1965).

[15] O. D. Ratnoff, J. Pensky, D. Ogston, and G. B. Naff, J. Exp. Med. 129, 315 (1969).

[16] L. J. Kagen and E. L. Becker, Fed. Proc. Amer. Fed. Exp. Biol. 22, 613 (1963).

[17] N. S. Landerman, M. E. Webster, E. L. Becker, and H. E. Ratcliffe, J. Allergy 33, 330 (1962).

[18] L. J. Kagen, Brit. J. Exp. Pathol. 45, 604 (1964).

[19] P. Harpel, J. Clin. Invest. 49, 568 (1970).

inhibitor is subject to tryptic digestion; nevertheless, it could be shown by immunodiffusion that highly purified $C\bar{1}$-inhibitor is free of α_1-antitrypsin.[6]

Highly purified $C\bar{1}$ inhibitor is without effect on the clotting time of whole blood in glass tubes, on the clotting time of recalcified citrated plasma in plastic tubes, on the formation of fibrin by the action of purified bovine thrombin upon purified fibrinogen, on esterolysis of acetyl lysine methyl ester by urokinase,[15] or on the activation of plasmin in a euglobulin fraction of human serum by kaolin.

ii. Hereditary Angioneurotic Edema (HAE)

HAE is a disease characterized by episodes of localized, noninflammatory edema and is inherited as an autosomal dominant trait. $C\bar{1}$-inhibitor is missing or is present only in small amounts in the sera of these patients.[20] Their sera fail to inhibit esterolysis of N-acetyl-L-tyrosine ethyl ester by $C\bar{1}$. The concentration of $C\bar{1}$-inhibitor in normal serum was found to be 2.4 ± 0.4 mg per 100 ml by agar-gel diffusion titration; in HAE sera, the value varied from 0.16 to 0.64 mg per 100 ml. Affected members of families with HAE always had little or no detectable $C\bar{1}$-inhibitor by esterolytic assay, but in some families a nonfunctional protein, antigenically identical with $C\bar{1}$-inhibitor, was detected by immunodiffusion.[7] Serum titers of $C\bar{1}$-inhibitor in heterozygotes exhibiting HAE are always near zero; unaffected members of these families have normal amounts of $C\bar{1}$-inhibitor. The presence of $C\bar{1}$-esterase in plasma and serum of affected individuals between attacks of edema, and its marked increase during attacks have been noted; between attacks the activity of C2 and C4 in serum is diminished, and it is absent during attacks.[21-25]

The genetic defect resulting in HAE does not appear to involve any factor in HAE serum which destroys $C\bar{1}$-inhibitor, since mixtures of normal and HAE sera have the expected amount of $C\bar{1}$-inhibitor as determined by the esterolytic assay.[20] Nor does the rate of catabolism of ^{131}I-labeled inhibitor in HAE patients differ significantly from that in normal subjects,[26] suggesting that in HAE there is a defect in protein synthesis which in some subjects may result in deficiency of synthesis

[20] V. H. Donaldson and R. R. Evans, Amer. J. Med. **35**, 37 (1963).
[21] V. H. Donaldson and F. S. Rosen, J. Clin. Invest. **43**, 2204 (1964).
[22] K. F. Austen and A. L. Sheffer, N. Engl. J. Med. **272**, 649 (1965).
[23] R. Siboo and A. B. Laurell, Acta Pathol. Microbiol. Scand. **65**, 413 (1965).
[24] A. B. Laurell, B. Lundh, J. Malmquist, and R. Siboo, Clin. Exp. Immunol. **1**, 13 (1966).
[25] H. G. Boman and L. E. Westlund, Arch. Biochem. Biophys. **64**, 217 (1956).
[26] F. S. Rosen and P. Fireman, unpublished experiments, 1968.

of the inhibitor, while in others an aberrant, nonfunctional protein is synthesized.

b. PROCEDURE

Recovery from 1000 ml of serum should be 3 to 4 mg. Ammonium sulfate precipitation (step 1) effectively removes about half of the inactive serum protein without loss of $C\overline{1}$-inhibitor activity. Although serum euglobulin contains no $C\overline{1}$-inhibitor, its preparation risks coprecipitation[14] of inhibitor at low pH, at which acidity the inhibitor is unstable, and all $C\overline{1}$-activity is removed in the ammonium sulfate precipitate. Since $C\overline{1}$-inhibitor binds to Dowex 2-X10, while more than 99% of applied protein cannot bind to Dowex 2-X10 (possibly because of the anionic structure conferred upon $C\overline{1}$-inhibitor by its high neuraminic acid content), chromatography on Dowex 2-X10 constitutes step 2. (Proteins still more anionic, such α_1-acid glycoprotein and prealbumin, are more avidly bound and these are removed by 1 N HCl only in the regeneration step.) By chromatography on DEAE-cellulose with gradient elution (step 3), $C\overline{1}$-inhibitor emerges on the trailing side of the main peak and is substantially purified over the starting material, the main contaminant apparently being ceruloplasmin. Finally, on hydroxylapatite (step 4), all contaminating proteins appear fortuitously to be bound to hydroxylapatite; only $C\overline{1}$-inhibitor appears not to be bound.

Step 1. Ammonium Sulfate Fractionation. Pooled human serum is cooled to 1°. Powdered ammonium sulfate (242 gm per liter of serum to about 40% saturation) is added in portions and stirred until all ammonium sulfate is dissolved, and then occasionally. After the preparation has stood overnight at 1°, it is centrifuged at 33,000 g (Spinco type 19 rotor, 15,000 rpm) for 60 minutes at 1°. The supernatant protein, containing $C\overline{1}$-inhibitor, is filtered through glass wool and dialyzed against 15 volumes of cold distilled water with three changes over a period of 48 hours, frozen, and stored at $-60°$. This material is referred to as "40% supernatant."

Step 2. Chromatography on Dowex 2-X10.[25] A glass chromatography column 4.7 × 48 cm of 1-liter capacity is packed with Dowex 2-X10 (AG2-X10 available from Bio-Rad, Richmond, California) equilibrated with 0.06 M Tris·HCl buffer, pH 7.3 ± 0.1 at 25° (dilution of buffer A, Table I).

The column is charged with the 40% supernatant (50 to 75 ml); after it has entered the column, the column walls are washed with 2 × 5 ml of the same buffer, and buffer is allowed to flow through the column at the rate of 1 to 2 ml/minute. At the void volume of the column (about 0.5 column volume), ca 99% of unbound serum protein emerges from the

TABLE I
STOCK BUFFERS FOR COLUMN CHROMATOGRAPHY[a]

A. Tris·HCl pH 7.3, 1 M: Dissolve 242 gm of "Trizma Base" (Sigma Chemical Company) in 1500 ml of distilled water and titrate at 20° to pH 7.3 with 6 N HCl (ca 300 ml); bring volume to 2 liters.

B. Tris·HCl pH 8.6,1 M: Dissolve 242 gm of "Trizma Base" in 1500 ml and titrate to pH 8.6 with 6 N HCl (ca 81 ml); bring volume to 2 liters.

C. NaH_2PO_4–Na_2HPO_4 pH 6.7, 0.2 M: Mix 1 volume of 0.2 M Na_2HPO_4 and 1.08 volumes of 0.2 M NaH_2PO_4.

D. NaH_2PO_4–Na_2HPO_4 pH 7.4, $\Gamma/2 = 0.15$: Mix 50 ml of 0.2 M NaH_2PO_4 and 235 ml of 0.2 M Na_2HPO_4 and dilute to 1 liter (1.38 gm of $NaH_2PO_4·H_2O$ and 12.6 gm of $Na_2HPO_4·7\ H_2O$).

[a] Readings of pH are made at 20°.

column. The composition of the eluting buffer is then changed to 0.09 M NaCl in the same 0.06 M Tris buffer. More inactive protein emerges from the column in the next two void volumes. The eluting buffer is then changed to 0.19 M NaCl in the same 0.06 M Tris buffer. The protein eluted in about 1.5 column volumes contains about 80% of the $C\overline{1}$-inhibitor. If column effluent is monitored in an ultraviolet flow analyzer, regions of protein emerging from the column can be collected in 10 to 20-ml aliquots for assay. With practice, the timing of each buffer shift can be brought closer so that the entire chromatographic run will require only about 1 column volume of liquid flow.

The same results are obtained in large-scale chromatography, when a column of 15 × 110 cm packed with 16 liters of Dowex 2-X10 is used, having a void volume of 7 liters and capable of processing 1 liter of starting material.

The resin is regenerated by passing through the column in succession 1 column volume of 1 N HCl, 3 column volumes of distilled water and 2 column volumes or more of 0.06 M Tris·HCl buffer, until the pH of the effluent is 7.3.

Different lots of resin have different retention characteristics for $C\overline{1}$-inhibitor[2]; some lots may release inhibitor protein when 0.09 M salt is passed through the column, and others may retain it until 0.19 M NaCl is passed through. Furthermore, the ability of the column to retain inhibitor can change markedly when a column is subjected to repeated regenerations. This change is evident as an appearance of inhibitor in the 0.09 M NaCl eluate when formerly it would be present only in the 0.19 M NaCl eluate. (Such a change will be partly reversed by batch-washing of the resin with 1 column volume of 0.1% (v/v) nonionic detergent (Triton X-100, Rohm and Haas, Philadelphia, Pennsylvania). After about 12 column volumes of starting material have been processed on the same column, the purity and yield of C$\overline{1}$-inhibitor begins to deteriorate and the resin requires regeneration by cycling through its hydroxyl form, with warming to 50° for regeneration.

The C$\overline{1}$-inhibitor from step 1 may be lyophilized or stored frozen at $-20°$ for about a month with little loss of activity, but dialysis against distilled water at this stage will result in some instability of inhibitor activity.

Step 3. Chromatography on DEAE-Cellulose. The pool of fractions containing C$\overline{1}$-inhibitor from Dowex 2-X10 chromatography is concentrated 20-fold in a pressure ultrafiltration apparatus (Amicon Corporation, Cambridge, Massachusetts), dialyzed overnight against 20 volumes of 0.06 M Tris·HCl buffer, pH 8.6 (dilution of buffer B, Table I), and applied to a 1.5 × 20-cm column packed with DEAE-cellulose (Whatman DE-52) equilibrated in the same buffer. Characteristically, the protein bound at the top of the column appears as a blue band lying atop a yellow band. Inert protein is washed from the packing by several column volumes of equilibration buffer.

A linear gradient of NaCl is then passed through the column under gravity flow. Gradient vessels are 1-liter cylinders of equal cross section connected at the bottom by narrow tubing. The limit vessel contains 0.15 M NaCl dissolved in 1 liter of the equilibration buffer. The mixing vessel contains 1 liter of equilibration buffer in hydrostatic equilibrium with the liquid in the limit reservoir, its contents being mixed by a magnetic stirrer. The bottom exit tube is connected to the top of the column. The flow rate is adjusted to 1–2 ml/minute and fractions of 10–15 ml of effluent are collected. Usually one major protein peak is eluted from the column under these conditions. The C$\overline{1}$-inhibitor emerges at about 0.10 M NaCl, on the trailing side of the major peak. C$\overline{1}$-inhibitor protein at this stage of purification is stable for several days at 0° and for several weeks when frozen at $-20°$C.

Step 4. Chromatography on Hydroxylapatite. The pool of active fractions containing C$\overline{1}$-inhibitor from step 3 (40–80 ml) is concentrated 20-fold by pressure ultrafiltration and dialyzed overnight against 100 volumes of 0.005 M sodium phosphate buffer at pH 6.7 (1:50 dilution of buffer C, Table I).

The dialyzed, concentrated C$\overline{1}$-inhibitor solution is applied to a 1 × 15-cm column packed with hydroxylapatite (Hapatite-C, Clarkson Chemical Co., Williamsport, Pennsylvania) previously washed and equilibrated with the pH 6.7, 0.005 M phosphate buffer. After the sample has entered the column, flow of this buffer through the column is adjusted to 6–12 ml per hour and 3-ml aliquots of effluent are collected. Almost all contaminating proteins are retained on the column and highly purified C$\overline{1}$-inhibitor emerges at the void volume of the column. The inhibiting material of highest purity, within limits of experimental error, coincides with the fraction of highest optical density emerging at the void volume. (Fractions of lower purity from the sides of the main peak may be concentrated and recycled through a fresh hydroxylapatite column with further purification.) The C$\overline{1}$-inhibitor of highest purity in this step can be stored for about 4 days at 0° or about 1 month at $-20°C$ without significant loss of activity; thereafter, a slow decline of activity is observed, amounting to about 50% after 6 months of storage at $-20°C$.

c. YIELD AND ASSAY OF ACTIVITY

The above steps under average conditions of yield will provide 3 to 4 mg of pure C$\overline{1}$-inhibitor per liter of serum. The purification attained in these steps is shown in Table II.

The assay of C$\overline{1}$-inhibitor is based on its ability to inhibit the esterolysis of N-acetyl-L-tyrosine ethyl ester (ATE) by C1$\overline{s}$.[10] The source of C1$\overline{s}$ is the fraction obtained from DEAE-cellulose chromatography of serum euglobulin as described by Haines and Lepow.[27] The assay employs a standardized preparation of C1$\overline{s}$, diluted to contain 40 ± 4 units of esterase activity per milliliter. One unit of esterase activity is defined as that amount which will cause the liberation of 0.5 mEq of H^+ from ATE under standard conditions (15 minutes, 37°, pH 7.4). A series of 12×75 mm tubes is set up and charged with 1.375 ml of sodium phosphate buffer, pH 7.4 and ionic strength 0.15 (buffer D, Table I). To each tube is added the desired volume of C$\overline{1}$-inhibitor, 0.5 ml of standardized C1$\overline{s}$ and 0.15 M NaCl to a volume of 2.375 ml. After 5 minutes of incubation at 37°, 0.125 ml of 1 M ATE (dissolved in ethylene glycol monomethyl ether) is added to each tube at 1-minute intervals. The tube is mixed after addition of ATE, and 1.0 ml is immediately withdrawn (zero time) and mixed with 1.0 ml of 37% neutral formaldehyde. After 15 minutes a second

TABLE II
PURIFICATION OF SERUM INHIBITOR OF C1$\overline{s}$

Step	Yield (%)	Specific activity (units/OD unit at 280 nm)	Purification factor (serum = 1)
1. Ammonium sulfate	Ca. 100	0.4	3
2. Dowex 2-X10 chromatography	80	15	115
3. DEAE-cellulose chromatography	60	70	540
4. Hydroxylapatite chromatography	30	220	1770

[27] A. L. Haines and I. H. Lepow, J. Immunol. **92**, 456 (1964).

1.0 ml of reaction mixture is withdrawn and mixed with 1.0 ml of neutral formaldehyde. The acid liberated from ATE in each mixture is titrated with 0.05 N NaOH to a phenolphthalein end point or to pH 7.50 using an expanded-scale pĤ meter. The difference in titration between zero-time and 15-minute samples is a measure of C1s̄ activity remaining in each reaction mixture. A duplicate set of tubes containing all reactants but no C1̄-inhibitor indicates the amount of C1s̄ activity present. One unit of inhibitor is defined as that amount which will inhibit the action of 10 units of C1s̄. Under conditions of this assay, 1 ml of serum contains 7–10 units of C1̄-inhibitor.

Alternatively, the inhibitor may be assayed by inhibition of C1s̄ on intermediate complexes. Extending the observations of Lepow and Leon,[4, 5] Gigli et al.[28] have used the consumption of C1̄-inhibitor by EAC1̄,4 complexes as a sensitive, stoichiometric assay.

The concentration of C1̄-inhibitor in serum has been measured by immunodiffusion by Rosen et al.,[7] using antiserum specific for the inhibitor.

d. PURITY CRITERIA

In the analytical ultracentrifuge C1̄-inhibitor exhibits a single, hyper-sharp boundary characteristic of glycoproteins. It migrates as a single, broad band in analytical disc-gel electrophoresis in 10% polyacrylamide gels at pH 8.4. Inhibitor protein inactivated at low pH yields several bands in such gels, indicating an acid-induced fragmentation.[6] Upon immunoelectrophoresis at pH 8.6, highly purified C1̄-inhibitor gives a single skewed precipitate arc in the β region against rabbit serum specific for C1̄-inhibitor. A similar precipitate is seen upon immunoelectrophoresis of C1̄-inhibitor against rabbit or horse anti-whole human serum.

Neuraminidase treatment of the inhibitor produces a less anodic, symmetrical arc against rabbit anti-C1̄-inhibitor serum. Immunoelectrophoresis of whole human serum against currently available rabbit anti-C1-inhibitor serum does not, however, result in a demonstrable inhibitor precipitate arc.

3. PURIFICATION OF HUMAN C3b-INACTIVATOR (C3b-In, OR CONGLUTINOGEN-ACTIVATING FACTOR, KAF)*

A C3-inactivator was described in 1967,[29] and a conglutinogen-activating factor in the same year (see Lachmann and Müller-Eberhard[30]).

[28] I. Gigli, S. Ruddy, and K. F. Austen, *J. Exp. Med.* **130**, 833 (1969).

* Portions of Section 17.E.3 were contributed by Hans J. Müller-Eberhard, the remainder by the Editors.

[29] N. Tamura and R. A. Nelson, Jr., *J. Immunol.* **99**, 582 (1967).
[30] P. J. Lachmann and H. J. Müller-Eberhard, *J. Immunol.* **100**, 691 (1968).

(The conglutinin of bovine serum will not react with the complement intermediate EAC$\overline{1,4}$,^{oxy}2,3 unless C3-In is present, and if present there is gradual dissociation of C3 from the intermediate.) In 1969, the two "factors" were shown to be identical.[31]

C3-In is a heat-stable β-globulin, with MW $\sim$100,000 and sedimentation rate of 5.5 S. It was first purified in 1968,[30] a chief difficulty being complete separation from transferrin. A new method has been devised,[32] based on the different distribution of proteins in euglobulin precipitated by 20% Na$_2$SO$_4$ as compared to the euglobulin secured at pH 5.4 and low ionic strength. Another method for purification is given by Ruddy et al.[33]

a. PROCEDURE

Step 1. Preparation of Euglobulin by 20% Na$_2$SO$_4$. Human serum at pH 6.0 is precipitated with sodium sulfate and washed. It is dissolved and then dialyzed *vs* 0.002 *M* phosphate, pH 5.4. The second precipitate is washed, dissolved and equilibrated with 0.01 *M* phosphate, pH 7.0, with 0.05 *M* NaCl.

Step 2. Exclusion Chromatography on DEAE-Cellulose. The yield from step 1 is passed through a column of the exchanger in the same buffer. C3-In is excluded at this ionicity; it is concentrated and equilibrated with 0.01 *M* phosphate, pH 7.0, containing 25% glycerol.

Step 3. Chromatography on DEAE-Cellulose. The concentrate from step 2 is applied to DEAE-cellulose in the same buffer, and the column is washed. A linear salt gradient is established (limit buffer, 0.3 *M* NaCl). C3-In elutes in the salt gradient rising to 0.1 *M* NaCl. Active fractions are pooled, dialyzed free of glycerol and concentrated on an Amicon membrane and equilibrated *vs* 0.5 *M* NaCl, pH 7.2.

Step 4. Gel Filtration on Sephadex G-200. The yield from step 3 is passed through a 5 $\times$ 100 cm column of G-200. Active fractions are pooled and concentrated and equilibrated with phosphate-saline, pH 7.9, conductance of 3.0 mS.

Step 5. Chromatography on Hydroxylapatite. The material from step 4 is run through hydroxylapatite in buffer of 3.0 mS in which C3b-In binds to the exchanger. Elution is done by a phosphate gradient to 17.0 mS. Active fractions are dialyzed and concentrated.

Step 6. Absorption by Insolubilized Anti-IgG. The antibody is insolubilized with ethyl chloroformate (Section 17.D.2.g.ii),[34] and the yield from step 5 is absorbed to remove a small amount of γ-globulin.

[31] S. Ruddy and K. F. Austen, *J. Immunol.* **102**, 533 (1969).

[32] P. J. Lachmann, P. Nicol, and W. P. Aston, *Immunochemistry* **10**, 695 (1973).

[33] S. Ruddy, L. G. Hunsicker, and K. F. Austen, *J. Immunol.* **108**, 657 (1972).

[34] S. Avrameas and T. Ternynck, *J. Biol. Chem.* **242**, 1651 (1967).

b. Purity

Titers of 50 units/μg were obtained. The product is a unique protein, moderately heat labile. It produced a rabbit anti-C3b-In which gave a single arc with anti-human serum.

c. Assay of Activity

Five different methods may be used.

Method 1. Conglutination. Titrations of C3b-In (KAF) are performed in 0.025-ml volumes using titration loops and plastic titration trays.* One drop (0.025 ml) of a 1.25% suspension (6×10^6 cells) of EAC$\overline{1,4,}^{\text{oxy}}\overline{2,3}$ cells (Section 17.C.4.b) is added to each dilution, and the mixture is kept for 5 minutes at room temperature, whereupon 10 minimal conglutinating doses of bovine conglutinin[35] are added and the trays are then transferred to 4°. The reaction is evaluated after 2 hours by reading the sedimentation pattern.

Method 2. Immune Adherence. EAC$\overline{1,4,}^{\text{oxy}}\overline{2,3}$ cells are first treated with various dilutions of C3b-In for 5 minutes at room temperature, then the treated cells are titrated in 0.025-ml volumes (see above) and 0.05 ml of 0.5% human group O erythrocytes is added as an indicator. After 30 minutes at 37°, the results are read by sedimentation pattern.

Method 3. Reaction with Immunoconglutinins. The injection of precipitates formed of antigen–antibody rabbit complement into rabbits gives rise to autoantibodies against fixed complement components. These antibodies, predominantly IgM, increase agglutination of complement-coated red cells or yeast. Rabbit immunoconglutinin sera can be found that will distinguish between EAC43 and EAC43(C3b-In), only the former cells reacting. This reagent may be used as in Method 1.

Method 4. Inhibition of the Hemolytic Activity of C3. Treatment of EAC4,3 with C3b-In markedly enhances the titer when *rabbit serum* is used as complement. Dilutions of C3b-In are incubated with EAC4,3 for 15 minutes at 37°, then the reaction is stopped by adding antrypol (Suramin, Imperial Chemical Industries) to 1 mg/ml. The cells are washed free of antrypol and a suitable dilution of fresh rabbit serum (usually 1:100) which is found to be without effect on EA or EAC4,3(C3b-In) is added. Lysis is conducted by incubation at 37° for 30 minutes.

Method 5. Inhibition of Immune Adherence. For this special test, the reader is referred to Lachmann et al.[32]

---

* The Takatsy system (spiral windings), or the Cooke "Microtiter System" (slotted metal wands) available from Microbiological Associates, Bethesda, Maryland; these transfer either 0.05 ml or 0.025 ml.

[35] P. J. Lachmann, *Immunology* **5**, 687 (1962).

4. ISOLATION OF HUMAN PROPERDIN ($\overline{P}$)*

The original isolation by Pensky et al.[36] given here is based on adsorption to zymosan. This product has been studied structurally in detail.[37] A pure preparation made without use of zymosan, but requiring volumes of 5 to 7 liters of serum, is given by Götze and Müller-Eberhard.[38] A further method employing affinity chromatography is currently being studied.[39]

Properdin is a highly basic euglobulin. Purified, it is not active on C3, but requires the presence of both C3 and factor B. Recent studies show a molecular size of 184,000 daltons,[37] with 4 subunits of 45,000 daltons. Carbohydrate is 9.8%, with 3.8% hexose, 3.8% sialic acid, and smaller amounts of hexosamine and fucose.

a. PROCEDURE

Step 1. Adsorption on Zymosan. Serum was mixed with zymosan in pH 7.4 barbital buffer to provide 2 mg/ml and held at 15° for 60 minutes (resulting pH ∼ 7.6). The properdin–zymosan complex was collected by centrifugation at 1°. The sediment was washed 3× with 0.5 serum volume of ice-cold 0.15 M NaCl. At 0° the complexes could be kept for 3 days.

Step 2. Dissociation of the Complex. The yield from step 1 was eluted in one-eighth serum volume with barbital buffer, at pH 7.4, adjusted with 2 M NaCl to $\Gamma/2 = 0.6$, by holding at 37° for 30 minutes, then centrifuging at 1° to remove the zymosan.

Step 3. Dialysis, Precipitation, and Extraction. The eluate was dialyzed *vs* distilled water at 1° for 2–3 days, then the sac contents were pooled and brought to pH 5.6 ± 0.1 with 1 N HCl. After standing for 1 hour at 1°, the precipitate was sedimented at 53,000 g for 1 hour and redissolved to 0.01 serum volume with phosphate, pH 8.0, $\Gamma/2 = 0.15$ and clarified at 105,000 g for 1 hour at 2°, then filtered through glass wool.

Step 4. Chromatography on DEAE-Cellulose. In the same phosphate buffer, 145 ml representing 21.7 liters of serum was passed through a 4.4 × 45 cm column of DEAE-cellulose at 30 ml per hour. Properdin is not bound by the exchanger, but 73% of contaminating protein is retained. The properdin peak (195 ml) was concentrated at 5° and equilibrated with phosphate buffer, pH 5.9, $\Gamma/2 = 0.025$.

* Section 17.E.4 was contributed by the Editors.

[36] J. Pensky, C. F. Hinz, Jr., E. W. Todd, R. J. Wedgwood, J. T. Boyer, and I. H. Lepow, *J. Immunol.* **100**, 142 (1968).
[37] J. O. Minta and I. H. Lepow, *Immunochemistry* **11**, 361 (1974).
[38] O. Götze and H. J. Müller-Eberhard, *J. Exp. Med.* **139**, 44 (1974).
[39] J. O. Minta and I. H. Lepow, *J. Immunol.* **111**, 286 (1973) (Abstract).

Step 5. Chromatography on CM-Sephadex. The yield from step 4 was loaded on a 1.4 × 38 cm column of CM-Sephadex (C50, medium) in the same buffer; 5-ml portions were collected at 20 ml per hour. After 90 ml had passed, a linear salt gradient was applied (250 ml of limit buffer with 0.4 M NaCl). Properdin emerged at conductance equal to 0.2 to 0.22 M NaCl. The contents of two tubes were pooled for analysis.

b. YIELD AND PURITY

The yield was 18%, 7000-fold concentrated over the level in serum. Sedimentation rate was 5.1 to 5.3 S, weight now calculated as 184,000 daltons. One cathodally migrating band was seen on disc gel electrophoresis, and a single arc with rabbit anti-properdin serum in IEA. Note: Götze and Müller-Eberhard[38] found 1% agarose to be necessary for IEA, and they described a special technique for disc electrophoresis at pH 9.5.

c. ASSAY

The assay given here follows Götze and Müller-Eberhard.[38] Heated serum (factor B-depleted) was incubated with $\overline{P}$ (10 μg/ml serum) and isolated factor B (100 μg/ml serum), at 37° for 30 minutes. Mixtures were then assayed for conversion of C3 by IEA in 1% ionagar *vs* monospecific anti-C3, in the presence of Mg^{2+}.

In contrast, Minta and Lepow[40] used a solid-phase radioimmunoassay, employing polystyrene tubes coated with monospecific anti-human properdin. The tubes fail to bind radiolabeled IgG, C3, or C5. Competitive binding, to the coated tubes, of increasing amounts (10 to 50 ng) of unlabeled properdin with a constant amount (40 ng) of ^{125}I-labeled properdin forms the basis of the assay.

5. ISOLATION OF PROPERDIN FACTOR D (PROENZYME) OR PRO-C3PA*ASE*, OR PRO-GBG*ASE*, AND FACTOR $\overline{D}$

a. ISOLATION OF HUMAN FACTOR D (PROENZYME)[*41]

Factor $\overline{D}$ was identified as a serine esterase. The proenzyme form factor D was isolated chromatographically; by the action of trypsin, D → $\overline{D}$. Factor D has a weight of ~25,000 daltons. The proenzyme is resistant to DFP, but $\overline{D}$ is inactivated. This fact led to a search among 25,000-dalton proteins of human serum from a calibrated Sephadex G-75 column. These were treated with 10^{-3} M DFP at 30° for 30 minutes to inactivate

[40] J. O. Minta, I. Goodkofsky, and I. H. Lepow, *Immunochemistry* **10**, 341 (1973).

* Sections 17.E.5.a and b were contributed by the Editors.

[41] D. T. Fearon, K. F. Austen, and S. Ruddy, *J. Exp. Med.* **139**, 355 (1974).

any factor $\overline{D}$, then dialyzed free of DFP. Upon trypsin activation (10 μg/ml for 0.5 to 2 minutes), terminated by adding soybean trypsin inhibitor (50 μg/ml), factor $\overline{D}$ was demonstrably present.

i. Procedure

Step 1. Chromatography on Quaternary Aminoethyl A-50 Sephadex (QAE-Sephadex). Freshly drawn blood was collected into hexadimethrine (3.6 mg per 10 ml of blood) and EDTA (10 mg per 10 ml of blood). Plasma (80 ml) was dialyzed against 0.035 M phosphate, pH 8.0 at 4°. The precipitate was removed. The supernatant was applied to a 5 × 90 cm column of the anion exchanger in the same buffer. NaCl gradients were used to elute; 15-ml fractions were taken, assays being run on 0.4-ml portions for factor B, factor $\overline{D}$, and trypsin-inducible factor $\overline{D}$. The latter activity eluted at 7.5 mS, $\overline{D}$ at 8.7 mS, and factor B at 10.3 mS. The tubes with proenzyme D were pooled and concentrated to 5 ml.

Step 2. Gel Filtration on Sephadex G-75. The yield from step 1 was applied to a 2.6 × 90 cm column of G-75 equilibrated with 0.05 M barbital-buffered saline, pH 7.5, with 0.025% gelatin, and 0.5 mM Mg^{2+} and 0.15 mM Ca^{2+}. Proenzyme D tubes were located, pooled, and concentrated to 1 ml.

Step 3. Filtration on Calibrated Sephadex G-75. The yield from step 2 was passed through a 0.5 × 90 cm column of G-75 equilibrated with the buffer of step 2, the column being calibrated. Proenzyme D filtered in the same volume as the chymotrypsinogen marker (25,000 daltons); factor $\overline{D}$ was absent.

ii. Assay for Proenzyme Factor D

Factor D samples were treated with 0.45 μg of trypsin in a volume of 0.04 ml of DGVB^{2+} for 30 minutes at 37°, and 4.5 μg of soybean trypsin inhibitor in 0.01 ml of DGVB^{2+} was added. Then 5 μg of CoF and 10 μg of factor B in 0.5 ml of DGVB^{2+} were added, and tubes were incubated at 37° for 30 minutes to generate CoF-dependent C3 convertase. To this, 0.1 ml of GVB–EDTA containing 5 × 10^7 sheep erythrocytes and 0.4 ml 1:4 of guinea pig serum in the same buffer were added, and incubation was carried out at 37° for 60 minutes. (Factor $\overline{D}$ was more efficient in effecting hemolysis than was trypsin-treated proenzyme D.)

b. PREPARATION OF HUMAN PROPERDIN FACTOR $\overline{D}$
(C3-PROACTIVATOR-CONVERTASE, C3PA*ase*, GBG*ase*)[42]

After the purification of factor B proenzyme, it was found that CoF and factor B were insufficient to complex and cleave C3. Two additional

---

[42] L. G. Hunsicker, S. Ruddy, and K. F. Austen, *J. Immunol.* **110**, 128 (1973).

factors, $\overline{D}$ and E, were isolated and found to complete the system. E appears to be a cofactor that increases the enzymatic activity of $\overline{D}$. $\overline{D}$ is separated from euglobulin, with apparent size of 35,000 daltons. It is a serine esterase.

i. Procedure

Step 1. Separation of Euglobulins. Fresh plasma, 300 ml, was dialyzed vs 0.005 M EDTA, pH 5.4. The precipitate was washed, dissolved in 30 ml 0.01 M Tris·HCl, pH 7.5 with 0.3 M NaCl and dialyzed to equilibration. Some insoluble material was removed.

Step 2. Chromatography on DEAE-Cellulose. The yield from step 1 was applied to a 2.5 × 100 cm column of the exchanger in the same buffer. The column was washed and eluted with a shallow NaCl gradient. $\overline{D}$ eluted between 1.8 and 2.3 mS. Fractions were concentrated and equilibrated vs 0.01 M Tris · HCl, pH 7.5, 0.002 M EDTA with NaCl added to conductance of 7.5 mS.

Step 3. Gel Filtration on Sephadex G-200. The yield from step 2 was filtered by upward flow at 40 ml/hour through a 5 × 100 cm column of G-200 in the same buffer. Activity was recovered in postalbumin position.

ii. Assay

(a) Incubation of 4 μg of CoF, 2.5 μg of purified factor B, and the test fraction in DGVB²⁺ (total volume, 0.2 ml) were carried on at 37° for 30 minutes. (b) Sequential additions were made of 0.1 ml of sheep erythrocytes (5 × 10⁷) in GVB–EDTA and 0.4 of ml 1:4 fresh guinea pig serum in GVB–EDTA. Hemolysis was determined after 60 minutes at 37°, and the average number of effective sites per cell (Z) was computed.

c. Purification of Guinea Pig Factor $\overline{D}$[*][43]

Factor $\overline{D}$ (Section 17.A, Fig. 1B) is one of the "properdin" enzymes used in the "alternative pathway" of complement activation. It is a basic protein (pI 9.35), with calculated weight of 22,000 daltons and sedimentation velocity of 2.6 S.

i. Procedure

Step 1. Separation of Pseudoglobulin. Units of 80 ml of guinea pig serum are washed precisely as in step 1 of Section 17.D.3.e.i.

---

* Section 17.E.5.c was contributed by the Editors, in consultation with Manfred M. Mayer.

[43] V. Brade, A. Nicholson, G. D. Lee, and M. M. Mayer, *J. Immunol.* **112**, 1845 (1974).

Step 2. Chromatography on DEAE-Cellulose. The procedure duplicates step 2 of Section 17.D.3.e.i, fractions containing factor D activity being identified (see below).

Step 3. Chromatography on CM-Cellulose. The concentrated pool from 3 units each of 80 ml of serum was diluted with water at 0° and 0.1 M acetic acid to pH 6.0 and to conductivity of 2 mS. A 3.7 × 40 cm column of exchanger was equilibrated with 0.04 M phosphate, pH 6.0, containing 0.001 M EDTA, and the sample was applied. After thorough washing, a linear salt gradient was established (250 ml of limit buffer, 0.2 M NaCl). A second salt gradient was then applied, using 250 ml of the 0.2 M NaCl and 250 ml of limit buffer, 0.6 M NaCl. Fractions containing factor D were pooled, neutralized with 0.5 M Tris-base in water, and concentrated.

Step 4. Gel Filtration on Sephadex G-150. The yield of step 3 was passed through a 1.5 × 90 cm column of G-150 equilibrated with 1% NH_4HCO_3, pH 8.0. Elution rate was 20 ml per hour. Fractions with factor $\bar{D}$ were introduced into a siliconized flask containing 1 ml of 0.01 M phosphate, pH 7.3, with 2% lysine monochloride. The product was lyophilized and redissolved in 0.005 M phosphate pH 7.5.

Step 5. Isoelectric Focusing, pH 8 to 10. The technique follows Section 17.E.6.c.i, excepting for the ampholine used. Fractions (2–2.5 ml) containing factor D were pooled.

Step 6. Filtration on Sephadex G-25. To remove sucrose and ampholines, the yield of step 5 was passed through a 1.5 × 20 cm column of G-25 equilibrated with the NH_4HCO_3 buffer used in step 4 but containing 0.1% lysine monochloride and 0.1% gelatin. Factor $\bar{D}$ fractions were pooled and lyophilized.

ii. Tests for Activity

A special test was developed, based upon assembling the C3-cleaving properdin enzyme on zymosan and allowing it to decay to the point at which activity could be restored only by adding extra factor B *and* factor $\bar{D}$.

(a) Zymosan was boiled for 30 minutes in 0.9% NaCl at 4 mg/ml, then washed with and resuspended in 0.9% NaCl to the same concentration.

(b) The zymosan (Z) was washed twice with GVB^{2+}, sedimented, and drained. Enough warmed 1:10 guinea pig serum was added to suspend Z to 1 mg per milliliter. After 5 minutes at 27°, the tube was chilled to 0°, centrifuged cold, washed twice with GVB^{2+} and once with $DGVB^{2+}$. The product (ZX), which cleaves C3, can be stored for several hours as a moist pellet at 0°.

(c) ZX was resuspended in GVB^{2+} to 2 mg/ml and held at 37° for 120 minutes; the enzyme capability of ZX is lost (ZX^d), but C3b remains bound.

(d) Test: 0.5 mg of ZX^d (pellet), 0.1 ml of factor B (20 U), 0.1 ml of C3 (100 to 150 U), and 0.1 ml of fractions diluted in GVB^{2+}. The 0.4 ml portions were held at 27° for 30 minutes. An amount of factor $\overline{D}$ producing 50% inactivation of C3 was termed 1 unit.

iii. Purity

One band was visible in disc polyacrylamide gel electrophoresis run under special conditions: 7.5% acrylamide, 0.2% bisacrylamide gel; β-alanine acetic acid buffer, pH 4.5; temperature 3 to 6°.

6. PURIFICATION OF PROPERDIN FACTOR B (C3PA, GBG)*

Factor B is the substrate for the action of factor $\overline{D}$ (Section 17.A, Fig. 1B). Identification of human factor B came via two routes. In one, a glycine-rich γ-glycoprotein was detected in human serum, then its proenzyme predecessor form of glycine-rich β-glycoprotein was found. It was later identified with factor B. In the other approach, factor B was isolated from a complex forming with CoF, termed C3PA. As with GBG, purified factor B does not react directly with CoF. For complexing, two cofactors were needed, of which factor $\overline{D}$ presented the necessary enzymatic function (Section 17.E.5.b).

a. PREPARATION I OF HUMAN PROPERDIN FACTOR B (GBG, C3PA, OR C3-PROACTIVATOR)[44,45]

i. Characteristics

Factor B has been identified as glycine-rich β-glycoprotein (GBG), identical with β_2-glycoprotein II. GBG possesses 5.4% hexose, 4.2% acetylhexosamine, 0.9% N-acetylhexosaminic acid, and 0.1% fucose. The sedimentation constant is 6.2 S. GBG exhibits at least 5 bands in polyacrylamide gel electrophoresis. The molecule is a tetramer with 3 or more kinds of subunits.

ii. Procedure

Step 1. Rivanol Precipitation of Euglobulins. Plasma (2 liters) was precipitated at 3% protein concentration with 0.84% Rivanol (6,9-

---

* Sections 17.E.6.a and b were contributed by the Editors and parts of Section 17.E.6.b by Hans J. Müller-Eberhard.

[44] T. Boenisch and C. A. Alper, *Biochim. Biophys. Acta* **221**, 529 (1970).

[45] C. A. Alper, T. Boenisch, and L. Watson, *J. Immunol.* **107**, 323 (1971).

diamino-2-ethoxyacridine lactate, or Ethodin, Winthrop Laboratories, New York) at pH 8.0. Precipitate was removed.

Step 2. Ammonium Sulfate Precipitation. The supernatant from step 1 was adjusted to 1.5%, and ammonium sulfate was added to 2 M and the precipitate was removed. The supernatant was dialyzed against water and then against 0.01 M citrate pH 7.0.

Step 3. Chromatography on CM-Sephadex (C-50). The supernatant was applied to a 2 × 40 cm column of C-50 in the same buffer and the column was washed. A linear citrate gradient was applied (800 ml of limit buffer 0.1 M sodium citrate) and fractions of 12 ml were collected. Fractions reactive with anti-GGG (a degradation product of GBG, isolated previously) were pooled and dialyzed *vs* 0.02 M phosphate, pH 6.4, with conductance adjusted by NaCl to 4 mS.

Step 4. Chromatography on DEAE-Sephadex (A-50). The yield from step 3 was applied to a 2 × 40 cm column of A-50 in the same buffer. Linear gradient elution with NaCl was carried out (800 ml of limit buffer, 0.02 M phosphate, pH 6.4, with salt added to 4.0 mS). Fractions reactive with anti-GGG were pooled and concentrated by ultrafiltration to 3 ml.

Step 5. Gel Filtration on Sephadex G-200. The concentrate from step 4 was filtered through G-200; the slower of the two peaks contained GBG, the other being hemoglobin–haptoglobin complexes. Again reactive fractions were concentrated and tested for purity.

iii. Yield and Purity

The yield was 13%. One arc was seen in IEA on agarose at pH 8.6 *vs* anti-GGG and anti-GBG. The anti-GBG serum could detect spontaneous breakdown of GBG to GGG and GAG upon storage of serum. GBG in serum remained stable when frozen or was stabilized for some weeks by 0.003 M EDTA. Isolated factor B (GBG) is stable. The product migrates in agarose as 4 to 6 discrete, closely spaced bands, suggesting genetic polymorphism. The difficulty in identifying factor B with the protein with which CoF complexes (Section 17.A, Fig. 1B)[46] may be connected with the "cofactors" required in the attachment of CoF.

iv. Assay[47]

Serum, 0.1 ml, freshly depleted of factor B by inactivation (56° for 30 minutes) was mixed with 0.1 ml of the unknown and 0.6 mg of zymosan (washed sediment); similar tubes had no zymosan added; after suspension, mixtures were incubated at 37° for 60 minutes with shaking.

[46] C. A. Alper, I. Goodkowsky, and I. H. Lepow, *J. Exp. Med.* 137, 424 (1973).
[47] I. Goodkowsky and I. H. Lepow, *J. Immunol.* 107, 1200 (1971).

Each tube received 9.8 ml of cold GVB^{2+} and zymosan was sedimented: the 1:50 dilutions of the original reaction mixture were assayed for C6, using C6-deficient rabbit serum (Section 17.D.2.e.iii). Percent inactivation of C6 was calculated from the difference of titers in the tubes with and without zymosan.

b. Preparation II of Human Properdin Factor B, via the C3PA Pathway[48]

i. Characteristics

C3PA* is a heat-labile (50° for 30 minutes) serum protein which has an *s* rate of 5 S, molecular weight of 80,000, the solubility characteristics of a pseudoglobulin and the electrophoretic mobility of a β_1-globulin, with a serum concentration of 100 to 200 μg/ml. It is not sensitive to hydrazine. In the presence of Mg^{2+} it forms an enzymatically active complex with cobra factor (CoF), acquiring the mobility of a γ-globulin and attacking C3 through the "alternative pathway" (Section 17.A, Fig. 1B). C3PA is likewise activated directly through the properdin pathway and its several activating systems; inulin was particularly useful.

ii. Procedure

Step 1. Removal of Euglobulins. One liter of fresh serum is dialyzed overnight against 10 liters of 0.008 *M* EDTA, pH 5.4. The precipitate is removed by centrifugation, and the supernatant is brought to pH 7.0 with 0.1 *N* NaOH.

Step 2. Chromatography on Bio-Rex 70. The pseudoglobulin is equilibrated with 0.03 *M* phosphate buffer pH 7.0 containing 0.002 *M* EDTA at a conductance of 5 mS and applied to a 5.5 × 50 cm column of Bio-Rex 70 (Bio-Rad, Richmond, California) equilibrated with the same buffer. A sodium chloride gradient is applied as far as 50 mS, and the fraction eluted between 15 and 22 mS is collected.

Step 3. Chromatography on CM-Cellulose. The product from step 2 is concentrated and equilibrated with 0.02 *M* phosphate buffer pH 6.0, likewise with 0.002 *M* EDTA, then is applied to a 2.5 × 40 cm column of CM-32 (microgranular) in the same buffer. A sodium chloride gradient is applied up to 25 mS, and C3PA activity is found between 5 and 9 mS.

Step 4. Chromatography on DEAE-Cellulose. The yield from step 3 is concentrated and equilibrated with 0.005 *M* phosphate buffer, pH 7.3,

[48] O. Götze and H. J. Müller-Eberhard, *J. Exp. Med.* 134, No. 3, part 2, 90S (1971).
* C3PA was formerly termed C3-SPI.

containing 0.002 M EDTA, having a conductance of 1 mS. The material is applied to a 1.5×25 cm column of DE-32 (microgranular) in the same buffer. A sodium chloride gradient is applied up to 15 mS. C3PA elutes between 2 and 4.5 mS. The product is concentrated on an Amicon UM-10 membrane (Amicon Corp., Lexington, Massachusetts).

iii. Characterization of the Product and Assay of Activity

The product from step 4 is homogeneous in polyacrylamide disc electrophoresis. A pure preparation of C3PA should not affect native C3. Mixed with an equimolar amount of CoF (Section 17.E.7), the two proteins bind as a complex, which can be visualized by disc electrophoresis. The product yielded a monospecific rabbit antiserum, giving a single precipitin band with C3PA in the region of the β- and α_2-globulins.

iv. Assay of Activity

Of the C3PA-containing sample, 0.05 ml is mixed with 5 μl of a solution of 3×10^{-3} M CaCl$_2$ and 1×10^2 M MgCl$_2$ in saline (buffers 1b and 1c, Section 17.B, Table I) and 5 μg of purified cobra venom factor (Section 17.E.7). After 5 minutes at 37°, 30 μg of purified C3 (Section 17.D.2.d) is added, the total reaction volume not to exceed 0.1 ml. Incubation is continued for 30 minutes at 37°. Then 10 μl of this mixture is applied to an agar slide, and conversion of C3 is determined by immunoelectrophoretic analysis.

c. PURIFICATION OF GUINEA PIG FACTOR B (HLF)[*49]

Heat-labile factor (HLF) appears to be a functional parallel (and antigenically related) to the human factor B, or GBG (Section 17.E.6); it is required for CoF to inactivate C3 by the alternative pathway (Section 17.A, Fig. 1B); but other serum factors are required as well. HLF has a molecular size of $\sim$100,000 daltons.

i. Procedure

Step 1. Separation of Pseudoglobulin. Add 5 ml of 0.1 M EDTA to 50 ml of guinea pig serum at 0° and adjust pH to 7.5 with 1 M acetic acid; dilute with water at 0° to 255 ml (pH 7.5). Collect precipitate after the preparation has stood at 0° for 60 minutes.

Step 2. Chromatography on DEAE-Cellulose. Apply supernatant from step 1 to a 3.7×40 cm column of DEAE-cellulose equilibrated with 0.005 M phosphate, pH 7.5, containing 0.025 M NaCl and wash column thor-

---

* Section 17.E.6.c was contributed by the Editors in consultation with Manfred M. Mayer.

[49] V. Brade, C. T. Cook, H. S. Shin, and M. M. Mayer, *J. Immunol.* **109**, 1174 (1972).

oughly. Establish a linear NaCl gradient (300 ml of limit buffer, 0.15 M NaCl) and maintain a flow rate of 50 ml per hour. To fractions with HLF activity (see Assay), add 3 M NaCl to 0.15 M NaCl, pool and concentrate in collodion bags. Yield is greater than 70%, with 7-fold increase in concentration.

Step 3. Chromatography on CM-Cellulose. Dilute the yield from step 2 with water at 0° and 0.1 M acetic acid to pH 5.75 and 0.86 mS. Any precipitate occurring at this point represents a high loss of HLF. Load a 3.7 × 40 cm column of CM-52 cellulose (Whatman, H. Reeve Angel Inc., Clifton, New Jersey) with a 0.02 M acetate buffer, pH 5.75. Wash the column well, and apply a linear NaCl gradient *vs* 200 ml of limit buffer of 0.2 M NaCl. Then pass 200 ml of straight limit buffer and next 300 ml of 0.4 M NaCl in pH 5.75 acetate buffer. Eluted fractions (6 to 9 mS) during the gradient and later stepwise washings are neutralized immediately with 0.5 M Tris in water. Fractions with HLF activity are pooled and concentrated. Activity is increased 3-fold.

Step 4. Chromatography on QAE-Sephadex. Dialyze the yield from step 3 *vs* 0.05 M Tris·HCl, pH 8.0, at 4°. Load a 2 × 20 cm column of QAE-Sephadex in the same buffer. Wash the column and apply a linear gradient (limit buffer, 200 ml with 0.15 M NaCl). Wash with limit buffer. Locate and pool fractions with **HLF** activity (ca 7 mS), adjust to pH 7.0 concentrate. Activity is increased about 3-fold.

Step 5. Isoelectric Focusing, pH 5 to 8. Arrange a 110-ml LKB column for sucrose density gradient with 1.5% ampholine, pH 5 to 8. Mix the yield from step 4 with the light ampholine solution. Apply anode to the top, initially with 400 V, 2.5 mA, raising voltage to maintain 1 to 1.5 W (about 2 days). Continue 2 days more, then collect fractions 2 to 2.5 ml and pool those possessing HLF activity. Peak activity occurs at pH 6.3 (6 to 6.5 range).

ii. Tests for Activity

Check that normal guinea pig serum inactivated at 56° for 30 minutes does not inactivate C3 when inoculated with CoF. In this system, addition of HLF-containing fractions will cause inactivation; 0.1 ml CoF (28 U)[50] + 0.2 ml 1:5 heated guinea pig serum (~150 U of C3) + 0.1 ml of appropriately diluted HLF are held at 37° for 30 minutes. Isotonic GVB with 0.15 mM Ca^{2+} and 1.0 mM Mg^{2+} is used throughout as diluent. C3 is titrated,[51] and units of HLF concentration are determined: 1 unit is 50% inactivation of C3.

[50] H. S. Shin, H. Gewurz, and R. Snyderman, *Proc. Soc. Exp. Biol. Med.* **131**, 203 (1969).

[51] H. S. Shin and M. M. Mayer, *Biochemistry* **7**, 2997 (1968).

iii. Purity

In disc polyacrylamide electrophoresis, 2 bands are noted close together, perhaps analogous to two different allotypes as described for GBG (Sections 17.E.6.a and b). By IEA *vs* both rabbit anti-HLF and anti-GP serum, one precipitation line of beta-mobility plus a second faint line appeared. The purification appears to remove cofactors which may remain in other products and may allow an apparently "direct" action of CoF on factor B.

7. ISOLATION OF COBRA VENOM FACTOR (CoF) *[52]

a. CHARACTERISTICS

The cobra factor (CoF) is a protein with an s rate of 7 S, a weight of approximately 140,000 daltons, and an electrophoretic mobility at pH 8.6 comparable to that of a serum β-globulin. Per se, this protein has no effect on C3. However, together with the C3PA and other cofactors present in human, rabbit, guinea pig, or mouse serum, it forms an active enzyme that is able to inactivate C3 *in vitro* and *in vivo*. This active enzyme consists of a firm bimolecular complex of the precursors and has an s rate of 9 S and a weight of approximately 220,000 daltons. The effect of the C3A on native C3 in the C3 shunt pathway resembles that of the $\overline{C4,2}$ enzyme (Section 17.A, Fig. 1B). The C3 molecule is cleaved into C3a anaphylatoxin and hemolytically inactive (C3b)i. To deplete a rabbit of its C3, approximately 1 mg of purified cobra factor is required per kilogram of body weight. Injection of cobra factor is followed by formation of active Factor $\overline{B}$ (C3A), having a half-life of 32 hours as judged by plasma disappearance, and by loss of C3 activity from the serum and disappearance of immunologically detectable C3 protein.

b. PROCEDURE

Since cobra factor is one of the most anionic proteins in cobra venom, preparative electrophoresis (step 1) is a convenient method to achieve an approximately 30-fold initial purification. In addition, the various toxic proteins and peptides present in snake venom are eliminated by this procedure. Since cobra factor is considerably larger in molecular size than any of the anionic components with which it migrates together during electrophoresis, complete purification is obtained by Sephadex filtration (step 2).

Step 1. Preparative Block Electrophoresis. One gram of lyophilized

---

* Section 17.E.7 was contributed by Hans J. Müller-Eberhard.

[52] H. J. Müller-Eberhard and K. E. Fjellström, *J. Immunol.* **107**, 1666 (1971).

crude cobra venom is dissolved in approximately 16 ml of electrophoresis buffer G (Section 17.D, Table I). Eight milliliters of crude, dissolved cobra venom* is applied to each of two Pevikon blocks prepared with barbital buffer G (pH 8.6, ionic strength 0.05). Application is made in the middle of each block. Electrophoresis is performed at 3.5 V/cm for 20 hours. Segments (1.25 cm wide) of the blocks are eluted with 5 ml of barbital buffer. The eluates are analyzed for protein and for cobra factor activity as described below. The activity is found in fractions adjacent to the anodal side of the origin. These fractions from both blocks are pooled and concentrated by ultrafiltration to a volume of approximately 3 to 4 ml.

Step 2. Filtration on Sephadex G-100. The density of the concentrated electrophoretic fraction is raised by the addition of sodium chloride so that the material can be layered between the upper surface of the Sephadex column and its supernatant buffer. A 3.5 × 150 cm column containing 1150 ml of packed Sephadex G-100 is used, equilibrated with Tris buffer, pH 8.2, containing 1 M sodium chloride (buffer O, Section 17.D, Table I). The flow rate is adjusted to 15 ml per hour, and 5-ml fractions are collected. The fractions are analyzed for protein and for cobra factor activity. The active principle is retarded slightly and is eluted from the column immediately following the void volume. Fractions exhibiting activity are pooled, concentrated by ultrafiltration, and dialyzed against physiological saline.

c. Assay of Activity

Cobra factor activity can be determined in the following fashion. Dilutions of the protein ranging from 0.5 to 10 μg are incubated with 0.5 ml of human serum diluted 1:20 in a total volume of 0.6 ml for 30 minutes at 37°. Thereafter, 0.4 ml containing 2×10^8 EA (Section 17.B.1.d) is added to measure residual hemolytic activity, allowing 20 minutes at 37°. The amount of cobra factor causing 50% reduction of lysis is thus determined.

d. Yield and Purity Criteria

From 1 gm of crude cobra venom, 3 to 4 mg of highly purified cobra factor are obtained. Purified cobra factor analyzed at 0.5 mg/ml yields a single band upon analytical polyacrylamide gel electrophoresis. Using the above described activity assay, approximately 2 μg of purified cobra factor will abolish 50% of the hemolytic activity of 0.5 ml of human serum at a dilution of 1:20.

* Cobra venom was purchased from the Ross Allen Reptile Farm, Silver Springs, Florida.

8. FORMATION AND ISOLATION OF C3a[*][53]

a. CHARACTERISTICS

C3a (Section 17.A, Fig. 1A) is a physiological cleavage product of C3, and functions as anaphylatoxin and chemotactic agent. As anaphylatoxin, it can cause smooth muscle contraction, an increased capillary permeability, and histamine release from mast cells. As chemotactic agent, it attracts white cells to respond to a gradient of C3. The two functions appear to arise and disappear rather independently. C3a is a very basic peptide with a weight of 7000 daltons and an electrophoretic mobility at pH 8.5 of $+2.1 \times 10^{-5}$ cm^2/V per second. It is produced by treatment of purified C3 with $\overline{C4,2}$ or trypsin.

b. PROCEDURE

Step 1. Formation by Enzymatic Treatments of C3

Method 1. Alteration of C3 by Trypsin. Fifty milligrams of purified human C3 (Section 17.D.2.d) at a concentration of 1 mg/ml is treated with 1% trypsin (w/w) for 60 seconds at 20° and pH 7.6. The reaction is stopped by the addition of soybean trypsin inhibitor in an amount equal to twice that of trypsin present. The mixture is then acidified with 1.0 N HCl to pH 3.5. The solution is cleared by centrifugation and concentrated to 5 ml using an Amicon pressure filtration device and the ultrafilter UM 05.

Method 2. Alteration of C3 by $\overline{C4,2}$. Alternatively, C3a may be formed using the $\overline{C4,2}$ enzyme; 100 μg C4 (Section 17.D.2.c) is mixed at 30° with 500 μg of ^{oxy}C2 (Section 17.D.2.b.v) in VB. After 5 minutes, 50 μg of C1$\overline{s}$ (Section 17.D.2.a.vi) is added, and incubation is continued for 30 minutes at 30°. The total reaction volume should not exceed 2 ml. This material is then added to 50 mg purified C3 at 5 mg/ml (Section 17.D.2.d), and the mixture is incubated for 30 minutes at 37° and pH 7.3. Acidification and concentration are done as above.

Step 2. Isolation of C3a

Method 1. Gel Filtration. A 5-ml sample is layered on a 2.5 × 90 cm column of Sephadex G-100, equilibrated with 0.15 M acetate buffered saline, pH 3.6, prepared from nine parts of 0.01 M acetic acid, one part 0.01 M sodium acetate, and 8.78 gm of NaCl per liter. The flow rate is adjusted to 15 ml per hour, and fractions of 3.5 ml are collected. Aliquots of the fractions are analyzed for protein by the Folin method. The

---

* Section 17.E.8 was contributed by Hans J. Müller-Eberhard.

[53] V. A. Bokish, H. J. Müller-Eberhard, and C. G. Cochrane, *J. Exp. Med.* **129**, 1109 (1969).

C3a fragment is eluted in fractions immediately preceding the internal column volume.

Method 2. Preparative Gel Electrophoresis. Alternatively, a 5-ml sample is separated in a Buchler Fractophor apparatus using a 2.5-cm separating column of 6% polyacrylamide gel concentration, with buffer of pH 4.5 as described by Reisfeld *et al.*[54] A current of 100 mA is applied, the flow rate is adjusted to 10 ml per hour, and 2.5-ml fractions are collected. C3a is completely eluted after 6 hours.

Fractions of either procedure containing C3a are pooled and concentrated using the Amicon ultrafilter UM 05.

c. ASSAY OF ACTIVITY

The activity of C3a anaphylatoxin is assayed by measuring contractions of segments of isolated guinea pig ileum.[55]

d. YIELD AND PURITY CRITERIA

Approximately 2 mg of C3a may be obtained from 50 mg of C3. Isolated C3a represents a well defined protein band on polyacrylamide gel electrophoresis at pH 4.5[54] and on cellulose acetate electrophoresis at pH 8.5. Approximately 1 to 2 μg of protein are sufficient to cause a contraction of smooth muscle in the Schultz–Dale bath.

9. C5a (HUMAN AND GUINEA PIG)*

a. CHARACTERISTICS

C5a (Section 17.A, Fig. 1A) is a cleavage product of C5, produced either by tryptic splitting or as a consequence of incubating EAC1–5 when the amount of C5 offered is sufficiently large. Guinea pig C5a has been shown to be a basic protein, requiring an acid pH[54] for electrophoresis in polyacrylamide gel.[56] Human C5a possesses anaphylatoxic activity (contracts guinea pig ileum),[57] and is chemotactic for polymorphonuclear cells (PMNs). The assigned weight was 10,000 daltons. Guinea pig C5a has been shown to be both anaphylatoxic and chemotactic, attracting equally guinea pig mononuclear leukocytes and rabbit PMNs.[58] The assigned weight was 8500 daltons. Gel filtration and sucrose density gradient examinations of human C5a chemotactic activity showed one com-

[54] R. A. Reisfeld, U. J. Lewis, and D. E. Williams, *Nature (London)* **195**, 281 (1962).

[55] C. G. Cochrane and H. J. Müller-Eberhard, *J. Exp. Med.* **127**, 371 (1968).

* Section 17.E.9 was contributed by the Editors.

[56] R. Snyderman, H. S. Shin, and M. H. Hausman, *Proc. Soc. Exp. Biol. Med.* **138**, 387 (1971).

[57] C. G. Cochrane and H. J. Müller-Eberhard, *J. Exp. Med.* **127**, 371 (1968).

[58] P. A. Ward and L. J. Newman, *J. Immunol.* **102**, 93 (1969).

ponent of major activity and one slightly heavier component of lesser activity.

b. Procedures and Results

Human C5 (Section 17.D.2.d.iii) is treated briefly with trypsin (2% of weight of C5) at pH 7.8, acting for 5 minutes at 32°. Soybean tryptic inhibitor (SBTI) is added to stop the reaction, and the mixture is adjusted to pH 3.5 with 0.5 N HCl. The product from 150 μg of C5 suffices to cause a strong contraction of segments of guinea pig terminal ileum, leading to desensitization. Degradation by trypsin can be followed by IEA with use of rabbit anti-C5^{hu}, by appearance of a long arc of faster-moving material.[58]

The *chemotactic* property has been studied by digesting human C5 with 20% its weight of trypsin at 30°. Nearly optimal activity appears in 10 minutes and diminishes slowly; curiously, anaphylatoxic activity for guinea pig ileum was absent; only skin-bluing activity upon intradermal injection into guinea pigs given a previous intravenous injection of Evans blue persisted.[58]

F. Antisera to Complement Proteins*

1. INTRODUCTION

Monospecific antisera to individual components of complement are of great importance both in research on the pathways of complement utilization and in clinical studies. Clinical applications include determination of inherited deficits in complement components, fluctuation in concentration of components in disease, and search by fluorochrome-coupled antibody for deposition of complement in tissues.

Presently, monospecific antisera to human complement components are available commercially, but these must be validated by each purchaser: exceptionally careful examination of every antiserum is needed. Antibodies to components other than the desired one must be absent, and also antibodies to noncomplement serum proteins. Unless the antiserum is truly monospecific or can be made so, as by use of affinity chromatography to remove contaminants, its use will be seriously limited. It may also be necessary to free the antiserum from complement components of the rabbit antiserum according to the intended purpose. Only as these criteria are met can observations be interpreted unequivocally, for example on the inhibition of reaction of a given component by antibody.[1]

The modes employed for inciting antibody synthesis vary from one

---

* Sections 17.F.1 and 17.F.2 were contributed by Manfred M. Mayer and the Editors.

[1] M. M. Mayer and J. A. Miller, *Immunochemistry* 2, 71 (1965).

laboratory to another. Alum precipitates of a component, or incorporation in complete or incomplete Freund's adjuvant (CFA, IFA), can be useful (Vol. I, Chap. 2.A.2).*

2. ANTISERA TO GUINEA PIG COMPONENTS

Monospecific antisera to guinea pig complement components are now available. Antibodies to guinea pig C2, C3, C5, and C9 are mentioned in Section 17.D.3, and to guinea pig factor B (HLF) in Section 17.E.6.c.

a. PROCEDURE

As an example of general procedures, rabbit-anti-C2^{gp} is presented. The anti-guinea pig C2 was obtained by precipitating the pure antigen with alum (Vol. I, Chap. 2.A.2.i and ii), and giving one to three courses of intravenous inoculations. Each course comprised 12 injections, three per week, with doses increasing from 0.5 to 4 ml; a total of 20 ml of antigen was administered to each rabbit per course. The animals were bled 6 or 7 days, or both, after the last injection of each course.

b. ABSORPTION OF COMPONENTS OF RABBIT COMPLEMENT

C components of the rabbit, especially C1, are removed by five absorptions with an unrelated specific precipitate, made from human serum albumin and its homologous rabbit antibody at equivalence in the presence of 10 mM EDTA, the latter being necessary to prevent absorption of rabbit C1 at this stage. The precipitate is washed twice with isotonic saline, and 2 mg of drained specific precipitate nitrogen are resuspended smoothly in 20 ml of rabbit anti-guinea pig C2 and allowed to react for 30 minutes at 20°. The precipitate is removed by centrifugation at 0°, and the supernatant fluid is absorbed similarly with successive portions of specific precipitate nitrogen—0.4 mg, and three 0.2-mg portions.

c. ASSAY FOR EXTENT OF ABSORPTION

The extent of removal of rabbit C1 may be checked either by directly analyzing for C1 (Section 17.D.3.a.iii), or by measuring the $\overline{CI}$ activity on the specific precipitates in terms of inactivation of C2. In the latter procedure, the specific precipitate collected after exposure to the anti-C2 serum is washed twice with buffer containing 0.15 mM Ca^{2+} and 1.0 mM Mg^{2+} (buffer 1d without gelatin, Section 17.B, Table I) and resuspended in the same diluent to ca. 20 μg of precipitate N/milliliter. This suspension is incubated at 30° with an equal volume of C2 diluted to 10 to 20 units/ml,

---

* With proteins of ~40,000 daltons, we have been surprisingly successful with single injections of small amounts of material (as, 80 to 120 μg adsorbed to alumina), followed by a rest period of 8 weeks and one fluid intravenous reinjection of 100 to 200 μg. Trial bleedings are made 7 days later.—M. W. Chase

samples of the mixture are centrifuged to remove the specific precipitate and immediately analyzed for residual C2. If the specific precipitate is free of $C\overline{1}$, there will be no loss of C2. Once this condition is met, the antiserum is exposed to one additional portion of specific precipitate.

Tests for other rabbit C components show that C2 is usually lost after the first absorption, and C4 after the second.

To establish whether the antiserum contains antibodies to C components other than C2, it is tested for inhibitory action on $EAC\overline{1},4$ (Section 17.C.2.b) and EAC4 cells (Section 17.C.2.c); any antibodies found may be removed by absorption with the appropriate intermediate complexes. Antibody to factors of the C3 complex (C3, C5, C6, C7, or C8) may be detected by measuring residual C2 in a partially neutralized mixture of C2 and anti-C2 in two ways: in one set of tubes, the C-EDTA (buffer 7c, Section 17.B, Table I) is added to the mixture of $EAC\overline{1},4$ + C2 + rabbit anti-C2 directly after incubation at 30.0° C, in the other the cells are first removed by centrifugation and resuspended in fresh diluent. If the antiserum does not interfere with the conversion of $SAC\overline{1,4,2}$ to S*, the results should be the same for both procedures.

3. RABBIT ANTISERA TO HUMAN COMPLEMENT COMPONENTS*

a. Introduction

Owing to clinical usefulness, the greatest effort has gone into obtaining monospecific antisera to human complement components. And for research purposes, antisera have been prepared to human C1q, C1r, C3c, C3d and to the inhibitors $C\overline{1}$-INH and C3b-In. Examples of making specific specific antisera by immunization of rabbits with the purified protein will be cited: to human C1q,[2-5] C1s,[6,7] C2,[8,9] C3[10,11] C4,[12,13] C5,[10]

---

* Section 17.F.3 was contributed by Hans J. Müller-Eberhard and the Editors.

[2] M. A. Calcott and H. J. Müller-Eberhard, *Biochemistry* 11, 3443 (1972).

[3] J. H. Morse and C. L. Christian, *J. Exp. Med.* 119, 195 (1964).

[4] K. Yonemasu and R. Stroud, *J. Immunol.* 107, 309 (1971).

[5] V. Agnello, R. J. Winchester, and H. G. Kunkel, *J. Immunol.* 107, 309 (1971).

[6] A. L. Haines and I. H. Lepow, *J. Immunol.* 92, 479 (1964).

[7] G. Valet and N. R. Cooper, *J. Immunol.* 112, 341 (1974).

[8] M. J. Polley and H. J. Müller-Eberhard, *J. Exp. Med.* 128, 533 (1968).

[9] M. R. Klemperer, *J. Immunol.* 101, 812 (1968).

[10] U. R. Nilsson and H. J. Müller-Eberhard, *J. Exp. Med.* 122, 277 (1965).

[11] C. B. Carpenter, T. J. Gill, J. P. Merrill, and G. J. Dammin, *Amer. J. Med.* 43, 854 (1967).

[12] H. J. Müller-Eberhard and C. E. Biro, *J. Exp. Med.* 118, 447 (1963).

[13] S. Ruddy, C. B. Carpenter, H. J. Müller-Eberhard, and K. F. Austen, *in* "Mechanisms of Inflammation Induced by Immune Reactions" (P. A. Miescher and P. Graber, eds.), p. 231. Schwabe, Basel, 1968.

C6,[14] C8,[15] C9,[16] and C3b-In.[17] It is useful to note that C6-deficient rabbits[18] will produce rabbit anti-rabbit C6.

b. Preparation of Antisera

In our laboratory, rabbits are injected subcutaneously with 10 to 100 μg of purified protein in complete Freund's adjuvant for three or more times at weekly intervals. Two weeks after the last injection, the animals are bled. When only smaller amounts of protein are available, 0.1 ml containing 1 to 10 μg of purified protein in complete Freund's adjuvant is injected into each popliteal lymph node of a rabbit according to Goudie et al.[19] One month later, 0.1 ml of a similar mixture is injected intramuscularly and the animal is bled 6 to 10 days later. Other methods of immunization, such as alum precipitates, can be employed.

To obtain an antiserum suitable to detect C3, an alternative method can be used which does not necessitate prior purification of the protein[20] (see Section 17.F.4.a).

c. Quantitation of Complement Proteins by Radial Immunodiffusion[21]

The general method is described in Vol. II, Chap. 14.C.6. It was introduced by Feinberg[22] although usually called the Mancini test. An optimal amount of antiserum to a complement protein is incorporated at 56° in 1.5% Noble agar in isotonic medium containing 0.1 M NaCl, 0.03 M potassium phosphate buffer at pH 8.0, 0.01 M EDTA, and 0.01% sodium azide. The liquid antiserum–agar mixture is poured on 1×3 inch plastic plates (Hyland Laboratories, Los Angeles, California) or glass slides and allowed to solidify. Then, 12 circular antigen wells, 3 mm in diameter, are cut in the agar. The wells are loaded with 8 μl of test sera and of dilutions of a standard solution containing a known amount of isolated complement protein. (The concentration of antiserum is determined in advance, as described below.) The plates are kept for 72 hours at 4° (in the case of C1q, at room temperature), and the diameter of the rings is measured. Optimal conditions for diffusion of C1q are given in Section

---

[14] C. M. Arroyave and H. J. Müller-Eberhard, *Immunochemistry* **8**, 995 (1971).

[15] J. A. Manni and H. J. Müller-Eberhard, *J. Exp. Med.* **130**, 1145 (1969).

[16] U. Hadding and H. J. Müller-Eberhard, *Immunology* **16**, 719 (1969).

[17] S. Ruddy, L. G. Hunsicker, and K. F. Austen, *J. Immunol.* **108**, 657 (1972).

[18] K. Rother, U. Rother, H. J. Müller-Eberhard, and U. R. Nilsson, *J. Exp. Med.* **124**, 773 (1966).

[19] R. B. Goudie, C. H. W. Horne, and P. C. Wilkinson, *Lancet* **2**, 1224 (1966).

[20] M. R. Mardiney, Jr., and H. J. Müller-Eberhard, *J. Immunol.* **94**, 877 (1964).

[21] P. F. Kohler and H. J. Müller-Eberhard, *J. Immunol.* **99**, 1211 (1967).

[22] J. G. Feinberg, *Int. Arch. Allergy Appl. Immunol.* **11**, 129 (1957).

17.D.2.a.iii. Commercial illuminators with calibrated scales are sold for the purpose. More accurately, in our laboratory precipitin rings are photographed, using dark-field illumination (Vol. III, Chap. 14.E.2.b) either on film or enlarged directly on high-contrast bromide printing paper. The negatives of photographs on film are placed in an enlarger, and the diameter of the projected precipitin ring is measured twice at right angles to compensate for possible ring distortion. The area of the precipitin rings is directly proportional to the concentration of the protein in the standard solution. A standard curve may therefore be obtained from the reference material and the concentration of a complement protein in the test serum is determined by relating the measured area of its precipitin ring to the standard curve.

The optimal concentration of antiserum depends on the relative proportions of antibody and antigen and must be determined by testing various antiserum dilutions. It is emphasized that the immunochemical method quantitates complement protein regardless of its functional status. However, for fresh serum an excellent correlation has been found between immunochemical and hemolytic titration data.[21] The immunochemical quantitation has been applied to C1q,[23] C1s,[24] C2,[25] C3,[21] C4,[21] and C5.[21] The average values obtained are, respectively, 200, 130, 25, 1200, 430, and 75 μg/ml serum. The lowest measurable concentration appears to be approximately 5 μg/ml.

4. DETECTION OF COMPLEMENT IN TISSUES BY FLUOROCHROME-COUPLED ANTI-C3*

The fixation of complement at sites of immunological reaction *in vivo* may be demonstrated by the fluorescent antibody technique.[26] The detection of fixed complement in tissue sections generally may be taken to indicate an underlying antigen–antibody interaction. The accumulation of immune reactants results from antibody combining with antigen in a target tissue, or from antigen–antibody complexes arising elsewhere in the body and subsequently depositing, along with complement, in various tissues. The fluorescent antibody technique therefore demonstrates the participation of complement fixation itself in disease processes. Antisera

[23] P. F. Kohler and H. J. Müller-Eberhard, *Science* **163**, 474 (1969).

[24] M. J. Polley, unpublished observations.

[25] N. R. Cooper, M. J. Polley, and H. J. Müller-Eberhard, *Immunochemistry* **7**, 341 (1970).

* Section 17.F.4. was contributed by Peter M. Henson and the Editors.

[26] P. J. Lachmann, H. J. Müller-Eberhard, H. G. Kunkel, and F. Paronetto, *J. Exp. Med.* **115**, 63 (1962).

directed against the third component (C3) have been generally employed for this procedure as they are easy to prepare and large quantities of C3 become bound to immunologic reactants *in vivo*.

As clinical experience has matured, it has become evident that the complement components remaining at a particular site will vary according to the age of the lesion. Consequently, parallel examinations of each tissue are made with fluorescein-coupled monospecific anti-C3 and with monospecific anti-C1q.[28] On an experimental basis, anti-C3c and anti-C3d, also, are being used in parallel studies.[27]

a. PREPARATION OF ANTISERUM TO "C3"

Purified C3 protein may be used to prepare the antiserum, the purification procedure being time-consuming. A simpler method is to employ a crude C3b adsorbed [along with properdin (Section 17.E.4) and one or two other factors] onto the surface of zymosan particles. Fresh normal serum (or fresh serum preserved by storage at −70°) is absorbed with 10 mg/ml of zymosan (Fleischmann type A) which has been previously boiled for 30 minutes and washed three times with saline. The boiled, washed zymosan is sedimented and the sediment is resuspended in the serum sample; the mixture is shaken or stirred constantly for 30 minutes at room temperature. The zymosan is centrifuged at 2500 rpm for 20 minutes. Serum proteins that have not been adsorbed to the yeast cell walls are removed by washing six times with large volumes of saline. The zymosan is then suspended in saline (about 1 ml of saline for each 25 mg of zymosan) and incorporated into an equal volume of incomplete Freund's adjuvant. Rabbits (2.5 kg) are injected *once*, both subcutaneously and in the footpads with 120 mg of the zymosan complex. Test bleed after 3 weeks, and if anti-C3 antibody is found by immunoelectrophoretic analysis (see below), the rabbits should be exsanguinated. [If necessary, one can wait another few days and test again for anti-C3 levels, but continued immunization leads to the development of a number of contaminating antibodies.]

Antibodies to rabbit C3 may be obtained by immunizing 400 gm of guinea pigs in a similar manner using 20 mg of serum-treated zymosan per guinea pig.

b. CHARACTERIZATION AND PURIFICATION OF THE ANTISERUM

Upon immunoelectrophoresis of fresh normal serum a strong C3 line should be produced after development with the antiserum (Fig. 1). Confirmation that this is C3 may be obtained by parallel examination of

---

[27] H. Kunkel, personal communication, 1974.

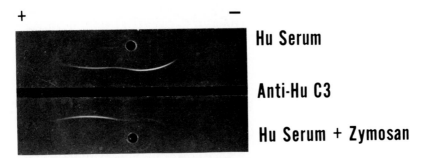

Fig. 1. Immunoelectrophoretic analysis of rabbit antiserum to human C3. Electrophoresis of normal human serum (Hu) and serum absorbed with zymosan (10 mg/ml) was performed in agar, with anti-human C3 antiserum placed in the trough. The unabsorbed serum shows both active and inactive C3. After absorption of the serum with zymosan, conversion of C3 to the inactive form, which does not bind to zymosan, is shown by the change in electrophoretic mobility.

serum which has been absorbed with zymosan (10 mg/ml) or with immune precipitates, procedures which convert the C3 protein to inactive C3. Inactive human C3, which does not bind to the adsorbent, has a different electrophoretic mobility (inactive *rabbit* C3 is an exception). The immunoelectrophoretic patterns of human C3 before and after absorption with immune reactants are shown in Fig. 1. In other species such as the guinea pig or mouse, the change in electrophoretic mobility is in the other direction; rabbit C3 does not exhibit such altered mobility.

Immunoelectrophoresis will also reveal antibodies against other serum proteins. Antibody to γ-globulin is commonly present, and this may be removed by absorption of the antiserum with purified γ-globulin. Commercial γ-globulin (Cohn fraction II) often contains some C3 protein and should be further purified by DEAE-cellulose chromatography. Only that fraction issuing in the void volume from a column of DEAE-cellulose equilibrated with 0.01 M phosphate buffer, pH 8.0, should be used for the absorption. Antibodies against an α_2-globulin are sometimes observed, but the identify of this protein is not yet certain. Removal of these contaminating antibodies requires isolation of the antigen and appropriate absorption of the antiserum. In all cases, the purity of the preparation must be established by IEA *vs* whole serum and dilutions of the serum.

c. Conjugation of the Antiserum and Examination
   of Tissue Sections for Fixed C3

After absorption of unwanted antibodies, the immunoglobulins may be precipitated with ammonium sulfate or separated by DEAE-cellulose chromatography prior to conjugation with fluorescein isothiocyanate by methods described in Volume V.

Frozen sections of tissue may be examined directly using the fluorescent anti-C3 antiserum (see Volume V). Kidney sections from various human nephritides,[27] especially from disease associated with systemic lupus erythematosus (SLE), often show C3 fixed in the glomeruli. Securing known positive control sections of human origin may provide some difficulty.

In laboratory animals, 1-hour-old Arthus reactions or glomeruli examined 2 hours after injection of nephrotoxic antibody (mammalian in origin) are found to contain C3 abundantly.[28] Alternatively, an *in vitro* system may be used. Frozen sections of normal kidney or liver are allowed to react with serum (heated at 56° for 30 minutes) containing complement-fixing antibodies against the cells or tissues [for example, anti-nuclear antibodies from cases of systemic lupus erythematosus (SLE)]. Subsequent addition of fresh normal human serum to the section, incubation for 30 minutes at 37°, followed by washing, will yield sections that will react with the C3 antiserum. A negative control for this *in vitro* complement fixation test is provided by parallel tests made with normal serum heated at 56° for 30 minutes.

[28] W. D. Linscott and C. G. Cochrane, *J. Immunol.* **93,** 972 (1964).

CHAPTER 18

Neutralization Reactions

A. Toxin–Antitoxin Systems

1. INTRODUCTION*

The ability of antitoxin to neutralize diphtheria toxin was recognized well before the turn of the century, but the puzzling quantitative relationships between antigen and antibody have become understood only slowly over the last several decades. As for the antigen, crude toxic culture filtrates of *Corynebacterium diphtheriae* contain not only toxin,† but its breakdown product toxoid and other bacillary antigens. Both toxin and toxoid bind alike to antitoxin. Accordingly, antitoxin constitutes the stable standard, for which Ehrlich's original antitoxic unit (AU) has been adopted. International and National Standard Antitoxins result from long immunization schedules with toxoid in horses. In brief, neutral mixtures of toxin and Standard Antitoxin are found by *in vivo* testing, and then the particular preparation of toxin is mixed in the same amount with dilutions of other antitoxic sera to locate neutral mixtures once again, and so these sera are calibrated to become working stocks based on the International Standard.

In determining neutral mixtures, anomalous relationships were found‡:

---

* Section 18.A.1 was contributed by Merrill W. Chase.

† Diphtheria toxin appears to be an enzyme of bacteriophage origin, synthesized by phage-infected *Corynebacterium diphtheriae*. Its toxicity is attributed to splitting nicotinamide adenine dinucleotide (NAD^+), releasing nicotinamide and transferring adenosine diphosphate ribose to form the enzymatically inactive ADP riboside of transferase II. The net effect is to block protein synthesis [T. Honjo, Y. Nishizuka, O. Hayashi, and I. Kato, *J. Biol. Chem.* **243**, 3553 (1968); D. Gill, A. M. Pappenheimer, Jr., R. Brown, and J. Kurnick, *J. Exp. Med.* **129**, 1 (1969); R. J. Collier and J. Kandel, *J. Biol. Chem.* **246**, 1496 (1971)].

‡ A comprehensive discussion on the development of the various "units" and their relationship is given by G. S. Wilson and A. A. Miles *in* "Topley and Wilson's Principles of Bacteriology and Immunity," 5th ed., pp. 278–283 and 1698–1702. Williams & Wilkins, Baltimore, Maryland, 1964. Units of measurement of diphtheria toxin applicable to *in vivo* experiments are the MLD (minimal lethal dose), the L_0 (Limes nul) dose, and the L+ (Limes tod) dose. The MLD is the smallest amount of a toxic filtrate that, injected subcutaneously, will kill most guinea pigs of 250 gm

exactly prepared, neutral mixtures might, by increase in total volume or change in holding temperature, be found toxic.[1, 2] Such findings are explained by differences in *avidity* (*affinity*) among antitoxins, i.e., the firmness of binding. Some working stocks are of less avidity than the highly avid International and National Standard Antitoxins. Jerne[3] worked out methods for measuring avidity, elaborated from basic studies of Glenny and Barr.[4] The latter workers used a "dilution ratio" method [Section 18.A.3.b.iii(a) and 18.C.2.c.i] in which antitoxins of lesser avidity revealed themselves by the requirement for more antitoxin to neutralize a unit amount of toxin when the reaction volume was large. Jerne's solid contribution was to devise a method for plotting curves of neutralization and from these to calculate "avidity constants" [Section 18.A.3.b.iii(b)]. (The constant that Jerne developed is not described here.) Evidently, parameters of both "antitoxic units" (AU/ml) and "avidity" are needed to properly and fully describe an antitoxic serum.

Because both toxin and antitoxin are combined at high dilution, the problem of stability deserves mention. Toxins are *relatively* stable in concentrated form after aging for some months, and especially when purified. They must be kept in the dark at 0 to 4°. Either immediate dilutions of concentrate can be used as in the Ramon test (Section 18.A.2.a.i) or toxin will remain stable if diluted in 0.5% peptone solution, as for *in vivo* work. Even high-titered International or National Standard Antitoxins (horse) become subject to surface denaturation if diluted in saline media to 0.01 AU/ml (dilutions of 1:60,000 to 1:95,000)[5]; whenever such dilution would give less than about 5 μg of protein per milliliter, diluent containing peptone or other suitable protein must be used. This type of denaturation holds as well for diphtheria toxin and many enzymes and phages.[6]

Toxoid not only arises spontaneously in toxic culture filtrates, but toxic filtrates may be converted wholly to toxoid by incubation with 0.4% for-

---

body weight within 96 hours. The L_0 dose of toxin is the largest amount that, when mixed with 1 unit of antitoxin and injected subcutaneously into 250-gm guinea pigs, produce a minimal edema at the site of inoculation. The L+ dose is the smallest amount of toxin that, mixed with 1 unit of antitoxin and injected subcutaneously, will kill within 96 hours. The difference between the L+ and the L_0 doses is *not* 1 MLD, but varies widely (10 to 100 MLD) owing to differences in avidity of immunoglobulins and to complexing of antigen with antibody in various proportions. Other units of measurement, Lf and Lr, are described later.

[1] A. T. Glenny and M. Llewellyn-Jones, *J. Pathol. Bacteriol.* 34, 143 (1931).
[2] A. T. Glenny, M. Barr, and M. F. Stevens, *J. Pathol. Bacteriol.* 35, 495 (1932).
[3] N. K. Jerne, *Acta Pathol. Microbiol. Scand.,* Suppl. 87 (1951).
[4] A. T. Glenny and M. Barr, *J. Pathol. Bacteriol.* 35, 91 (1932).
[5] M. W. Chase, *Bacteriol. Proc.,* Abstract M-63 (1953).
[6] M. H. Adams, *J. Gen. Physiol.* 31, 417 (1948).

malin at 37° for several weeks ("formol toxoid"). The exact mechanism is not established.[7] Formol toxoid is the basis of the prophylactic preparation used for immunization, often adsorbed to alumina.

Early studies conducted with horse diphtheria antitoxin indicated neutralization of toxin without any visible reaction *in vitro*. Finally Ramon discovered a narrow range of concentrations in which flocculation would occur. This flocculation reaction is discussed in Section 18.A.2.a.i and also in Volume III, Chap. 13.A.1.b. Flocculation measures the sum of toxin plus toxoid in the sample of toxin.

The horse immunoglobulin which gives the narrow-zone flocculation is a γ_1-globulin, formerly called β_2-globulin or T-component. A precipitating (and antitoxic) γ_2-globulin can also be present in samples of horse antitoxin.[8] Guinea pig antitoxin appears to be IgG_1, serving to prepare dermal sites for PCA reactions. Rabbit antitoxin belongs chiefly in the γ_2-globulins and yields typical precipitin curves with diphtheria toxin.

The introduction of *in vitro* methods for neutralization represented a great forward stride, although problems have remained (see footnote to paragraph 2 of this Section). Section 18.A.2 deals with such assay methods.

In vivo methods for studying toxin–antitoxin interactions are presented in Section 18.A.3. Only *in vivo* methods will reveal how much toxin is represented by a given number of flocculating units (Lf) in a given crude toxin filtrate. And *in vivo* methods will readily determine the concentration of antitoxin within 10% of its actual value, and, with slightly more effort, to 5% or even still closer to true value. Accordingly, toxin–antitoxin neutralization *in vivo* is one of the more favorable methods for approximating actual antibody concentrations.

Some of the techniques given here are also to be found in "La Pharmacopée Européenne," Vol. 2, Maisonneuve S. A. Sainte Ruffine, Ars sur Moselle, France.

[7] W. E. van Heyningen, "Bacterial Toxins," p. 13. Thomas, Springfield, Illinois, 1950.
[8] E. H. Relyveld, O. Girard, R. Corvazier, and M. Raynaud, *Ann. Inst. Pasteur (Paris)* **92**, 631 (1957).

2. METHODS FOR TOXIN AND ANTITOXIN ASSAY
"IN VITRO"

a. TITRATION OF DIPHTHERIA TOXIN AND ANTITOXIN*

Flocculation tests between toxin and antitoxin may be carried out in three different ways: (1) the Ramon or so-called β-technique,[1] in which

* Sections 18.A.2a.i and ii were contributed by E. H. Relyveld and M. Raynaud†

† Deceased.
[1] G. Ramon, *C. R. Soc. Biol.* **86**, 166 (1922).

a constant amount of toxin is employed with varying amounts of antitoxin; the total volume usually varies, although the volume can be kept
constant amount of antitoxin is used with varying amounts of toxin, the
constant; (2) the Dean and Webb or so-called α-technique,[2] in which a
Wyman or so-called γ-technique, in which the total concentration of toxin
total volume being either constant or variable;* (3) the Bowen and
and antitoxin remains constant, the ratio of antitoxin to toxin being
variable.[3, 4]

The flocculation titers may or may not be the same when determined
by the Ramon[1] or the Dean and Webb methods,[2] depending on the serum
under study. The discrepancies observed have been the subject of many
controversies, but in our opinion they disappear upon using the method
of Bowen and Wyman.[3, 4] With certain sera rich in γ_2-antitoxin (IgG), it
may be useful to employ the technique of Bowen and Wyman.[3-5]

In practice, for therapeutic horse sera the Ramon flocculation test,
which will be described here, gives titers identical with those obtained
by the more complex technique of Bowen and Wyman.

i. The Ramon Flocculation Method

(a) *Reagents.* In the Ramon flocculation test, one determines the
amount of antitoxin that gives the most rapid flocculation with a constant
amount of toxin.

Three reagent solutions are required.

A reference standard, namely, the International Standard for the Flocculation Test provided by the State Serum Institute (Copenhagen), containing 1800 Lf(A) units† per ampoule of freeze dried serum.

A concentrated toxin solution, 1000 to 5000 Lf(T)‡ per milliliter. We
recommend the use of a pure toxin preparation made according to one
of several techniques.[6-9] The toxin has to be standardized frequently
against the International Standard for the Flocculation Test.

[2] H. R. Dean and R. A. Webb, *J. Pathol. Bacteriol.* **29**, 473 (1926).
* This order of addition, the total volume being variable, was applied specifically
to the flocculation of diphtheria toxin by A. T. Glenny and U. Wallace, *J. Pathol.
Bacteriol.* **28**, 317 (1925).—Eds.
[3] H. E. Bowen and L. Wyman, *J. Immunol.* **70**, 235 (1953).
[4] H. E. Bowen and L. Wyman, *J. Immunol.* **71**, 86 (1953).
[5] M. Raynaud and E. H. Relyveld, *Ann. Inst. Pasteur Paris* **97**, 636 (1959).
† Lf(A): Lf unit of antitoxin.
‡ Lf(T): Lf unit of pure toxin, corresponding to 1 antitoxic unit (AU) for some
hyperimmune sera. The *flocculating* unit termed Lf was introduced by A. T. Glenny
and C. C. Okell, *J. Pathol. Bacteriol.* **27**, 187 (1924).
[6] I. Kato, H. Nakamura, T. Uchida, J. Koyama, and T. Katsura, *Jap. J. Exp. Med.*
30, 129 (1960).

A laboratory standard of antitoxin, available in quantity, for use in the actual testing; this standard is sometimes an official national standard. Otherwise, it can be prepared by peptic digestion* of serum obtained from hyperimmunized horses, immunization having been carried out by injecting a preparation of pure toxoid or by digestion of a specific precipitate obtained by flocculating purified toxin with a commercial serum as used by Relyveld *et al.*[10,11] and Relyveld.[8] The laboratory standard must be checked carefully against the standardized toxin preparation.

(*b*) *Procedure*

(*i*) *Standardization of the toxin preparation.* The International Standard Serum for the flocculation test is diluted to 100 Lf units per milliliter (Lf/ml) in 0.9% sodium chloride solution buffered at pH 6.8 to 7.0 with $M/15$ KH_2PO_4–K_2HPO_4, containing Merthiolate 1:10,000.† From this dilution, volumes ranging by 0.1-ml increments from 0.20 ml to 0.80 ml are added to a series of tubes (10 mm i.d.). The concentrated toxin solution is then diluted to about 50 Lf/ml; 1 ml is added to each tube as quickly as possible in order to minimize differences in the "zero" times among the several tubes. Alternatively 0.5 ml of toxin having a titer of about 100 Lf/ml can be employed.

---

[7] C. G. Pope and M. F. Stevens, *Brit. J. Exp. Pathol.* **39**, 139 (1958).

[8] E. H. Relyveld, "Toxine et antitoxine diphtériques. Etude immunologique." Hermann, Paris, 1959.

[9] E. H. Relyveld and M. Raynaud, *Ann. Inst. Pasteur Paris* **107**, 618 (1964).

* Partial peptic digestion was introduced I. A. Parfentjev [U.S. Patent 2,065,196 (1936)] to secure a marked impairment of species specificity for the purpose of preparing safer therapeutic horse antitoxin. Digestion is conducted at pH 4 to 4.5 for 4 to 24 hours at 37° and stopped when 70 to 80% of the protein is no longer coagulable by heat. The solution is subjected to dialysis, precipitation at 50% saturated ammonium sulfate, and treatment with finely subdivided calcium phosphate to remove any residual pepsin [A. J. Weil, I. A. Parfentjev, and K. L. Bowman, *J. Immunol.* **35**, 399 (1938)].—Eds.

[10] E. H. Relyveld, P. Grabar, M. Raynaud, and C. A. Williams, Jr., *Ann. Inst. Pasteur Paris* **90**, 688 (1956).

[11] E. H. Relyveld, O. Girard, R. Corvazier, and M. Raynaud, *Ann. Inst. Pasteur Paris* **92**, 631 (1957).

† The phosphate buffer is essentially represented by buffer 28 in Vol. II, Appendix II, prepared at pH 6.9 but with substitution of $M/15$ K_2HPO_4 for $M/15$ Na_2HPO_4; to it is added, per liter, 9 gm of NaCl and 100 mg of Merthiolate (thiomerosal). It is to be noted that this buffer is hypertonic; 4.5 mg of NaCl results in an isotonic solution (Vol. II, Appendix II, buffer 35). The authors store a 3.5 M stock phosphate buffer at room temperature, made by mixing 952 gm of KH_2PO_4 with 875 ml of 4 N KOH and bringing the volume to 2 liters. The working buffer contains, per liter, 20 ml of this stock with added NaCl and Merthiolate. The pH should fall between 6.8 and 7.0.

Preliminary titration. The tubes are swirled to mix the reagents and placed in a water bath at 45° with only the bottom two-thirds immersed, in order to facilitate formation of convection currents. The tubes are read from time to time by inspection against a black screen with the aid of a magnifying glass. As soon as one tube (or perhaps more) shows flocculation at this magnified scale, the whole rack is brought to room temperature. In this way the rate of reaction is decreased in the tubes that have not yet flocculated, so that these tubes will stay opalescent or even clear for a longer time. An abundant precipitate will settle more or less rapidly in the tube than first showed flocculation.

Final titration. A second titration based on the first is carried out in the same way with serum quantities increasing by only 0.05 ml in order to determine the exact flocculation titer of the diluted toxin solution. "Flocculating units" of toxin and antitoxin are mathematically equal in the tube showing the most rapid flocculation. If two or three tubes flocculate at the same time, the arithmetic mean of the corresponding titers is calculated. Flocculation reactions carried out with pure toxin and purified serum can take place very rapidly and several tubes can flocculate simultaneously. Hence it is advisable to carry out tests with purified reagents at room temperature. The same technique may be used for the determination of any unknown toxin or toxoid.

(*ii*) *Standardization of the working antiserum.* Since the International Flocculation Standard is available only in limited supply, for routine purposes a laboratory standard serum must be used. Standardization is carried out with the stock toxin solution diluted to exactly 80 Lf/ml.*

Preliminary titration. For most therapeutic sera the preliminary test may be carried out with 2 ml of toxin solution at 80 Lf/ml added to various volumes of serum. The serum dilutions (1:1, 1:2, 1:4, . . .) are each tested in increments of 0.1 ml (0.1 to 1 ml). This test leads to an approximate value for flocculating units of the antiserum, which is next diluted to about 100 Lf(A) per milliliter.

Final test. This is carried out as under (*i*) by adding 1-ml portions of diluted toxin (80 Lf/ml) to amounts of the diluted serum ranging from 0.6 to 1.0 ml in increments of 0.05 ml.

(*iii*) *Titration of unknown antitoxin samples.* Routine titrations are carried in the same way. Antitoxin titers lower than 100 units per milli-

---

* For accurate dilution, it is helpful to use pipettes calibrated "to contain" rather than "to deliver." Such pipettes can be clamped vertically in a ring-stand and controlled by a rubber tube passing to a 5-ml syringe clamped horizontally; a T tube introduced into the tubing between pipette and syringe is fitted with a short length of rubber on the open port and is closed by a clamp: this device allows rinsing out, with full drainage from the pipette as desired.—Eds.

liter are determined by using 1 ml of toxin solution diluted to 20 Lf/ml and samples of undiluted antiserum in volumes of 0.2, 0.25, 0.30, 0.40, 0.50, 0.60, 0.80, and 1 and 2 ml.

Analogous procedures may be used for the Dean and Webb method with constant amounts of serum and a constant final volume.

Many variations are possible in the techniques described and are practiced in different laboratories. We recommend against using in manuscripts for publication the simple phrase "flocculation titers have been determined by the Ramon flocculation method." Instead, one should indicate *the manner of testing* (varying amounts of toxin or antitoxin, variable or constant volume); the *total amount* of toxin and serum used; the *total volume* of the mixtures. In this way, it will be easy to reconcile differences commonly observed between results secured in different laboratories.

ii. Determination of Diphtheria Antitoxin by Immunodiffusion in Agar

Serum titers are determined by double diffusion in gel in comparison with a known standard of antitoxin which has been found to have an *in vivo/in vitro* value* close to 1. A stock 2-fold concentration of agar (1.5%) with sodium chloride (2.0%) and Merthiolate (1:5000) is prepared. The agar is melted at 100° and cooled to 45° in a water bath; an equal volume of pure toxin at 20 Lf/ml, also at 45°, is mixed with the agar; and 0.5 ml-quantities are dispensed into tubes of 9 mm i.d. by means of a Pasteur pipette, to provide pure diphtheria toxin at a concentration of 10 Lf/ml. A layer of plain agar is poured over the first.

Dilutions of some standard serum in phosphate-saline buffer are then added in 0.5-ml amounts over the agar layer at concentrations of approximately 30, 20, 10, 5, and 2.5 Lf/ml, and 0.5-ml volumes of unknown sera (from the same species of animal) are added to other tubes. After 6–12 days at 37°, the position and intensity of the bands of the unknown sera are compared with those given by dilutions of the known serum. The band of each unknown which corresponds with some known antibody concentration is taken as the titer of the unknown.

This method gives only an approximate value for the serum titers. It must be kept in mind that precipitating but nonneutralizing antibodies have been described[8, 12–13] as well as neutralizing antibodies of only low

---

* The *"in vivo/in vitro"* value represents the ratio of antitoxic units (determined by the L+ or Lr methods) and flocculating units (Lf) of the serum. This is expressed as the L+/Lf or Lr/Lf ratio of the antitoxin.

[12] M. Raynaud, E. H. Relyveld, O. Girard, and R. Corvazier, *Ann. Inst. Pasteur Paris* **96**, 129 (1959).

[13] E. H. Relyveld and M. Raynaud, *Ann. Inst. Pasteur Paris* **96**, 537 (1959).

precipitation titers.[14-15] Precipitation bands are in no wise a measure of neutralizing antibody titers, even if *in vivo/in vitro* values of serum titers are close to 1.0 for some hyperimmune preparations.

The method is useful, however, for testing sera of low titers, as in bleedings taken at the beginning of hyperimmunization or when only small quantities of serum are available.

iii. Determination of Diphtheria Antitoxin by Indirect (Passive) Hemagglutination*

Another method for detecting the presence of antitoxin consists in determining its ability to agglutinate erythrocytes bearing fixed diphtheria toxoid as by use of tanned red cells.[16] The method is discussed in Chap. 16.B.2. Tanned erythrocytes were exposed at pH 6.4 to 130 Lf/ml of toxoid, or tanned formalinized cells were exposed to 13 Lf/ml of the same toxoid. The toxoids used included highly purified preparations containing ~2600 Lf/mg protein nitrogen. The sensitivity of the method is indicated by ability to detect about 0.001 to 0.002 μg of antitoxin: a rabbit antitoxin with 0.39 mg of antibody/ml gave an HA titer of 1:326,000, and a horse antitoxin with 0.8 mg of antibody per milliliter also showed the same HA titer. Less than 0.005 AU/ml, approximating the limit of the *in vivo* neutralization reaction,[17, 18] was detected with both horse and rabbit antitoxin. Among horse antitoxins of high avidity, a specimen having 500 AU/ml agglutinated at 1:20,000,000, while horse antitoxins of low avidity were weaker—a specimen rated at 250 AU/ml agglutinated at 1:2,500,000. Assurance that antitoxin is being measured depends upon the state of purity of the original toxin used as source of the toxoid employed for coating the red cells. Impure toxoid could lead to agglutination by antibodies to corynebacterial proteins other than toxin/toxoid.

Agglutination vs doubled dilutions of serum indicate at best differences of 1 tube in antibody concentration. Yet for research purposes, a sensitive detection of antibody, with some approximation to its actual concentration, can be highly useful, and can well precede a much more accurate determination of antibody concentration by *in vivo* neutralization meth-

[14] E. H. Relyveld, A. J. van Triet, and M. Raynaud, *Antonie van Leeuwenhoek J. Microbiol. Serol.* **25**, 369 (1959).

[15] E. H. Relyveld, A. J. van Triet, and M. Raynaud, *Antonie van Leeuwenhoek J. Microbiol. Serol.* **26**, 349 (1960).

* Section 18.A.2.a.iii was contributed by Merrill W. Chase.

[16] A. B. Stavitsky, *J. Immunol.* **72**, 368 (1954b).

[17] A. B. Stavitsky, *J. Immunol.* **72**, 360 (1954a).

[18] D. T. Fraser, *Trans. Roy. Soc. Can. Sect. V* **25**, 175 (1931).

ods and determinations of avidity (Sections 18.A.3.a and 18.A.3.b.iii).

Hemagglutination inhibition (HAI) offers a sensitive method for detecting minute amounts of antigen, by incubating suitable dilutions of antiserum both with and without suspected antigen, and later adding presensitized red cells (Chap. 16.B.2).

b. TITRATION OF TETANUS TOXIN, TOXOID, AND ANTITOXIN[*][†]

i. The Ramon Flocculation Method

Titration by the Ramon flocculation test is essentially the same as described for the diphtheria system. It must be kept in mind, however, that false zones are very often seen in the tetanus flocculation test. Therefore it is advisable for laboratories which practice this method repeatedly to prepare the following two standards. (1) A purified tetanus toxin,[19, 20] giving only one major brand when tested by immunodiffusion against a complex serum containing many antibodies against the constituents of the crude toxin. The use of such a purified tetanus toxin will avoid or minimize "false" flocculating zones in the determination of the flocculating titer of any complex antitetanal serum. (2) An antitetanal horse serum prepared by immunizing horses with a purified toxoid and toxin, and found to give only one zone when tested with a crude toxin as described by Raynaud et al.[21] When a serum of this type is employed to determine the flocculation titer of a crude toxin, one does not observe any false zone, and the titer of the toxin may be determined unequivocally. It is recognized that preparation of a "one-zone tetanus flocculating serum" is presently restricted to only a few specialized laboratories.

[Fortunately, a new "Second International Standard Tetanus Antitoxin" (TE6/66/2) has been introduced which presents no multiple flocculating zones and is suitable for in vitro assays by flocculation.[22] One antitoxic unit is the activity contained in 0.03384 mg. The in vivo/in vitro ratio is 1.4, since the "Lf equivalent" is 1.4 times less than the antitoxin unitage.—Ed.]

---

* Section 18.A.2.b was contributed by E. H. Relyveld and M. Raynaud‡

† For neutralization in vivo, see Section 18.A.3.c.
‡ Deceased.
[19] M. Raynaud and A. Turpin, C. R. Acad. Sci. **242**, 574 (1956).
[20] A. Turpin and M. Raynaud, Ann. Inst. Pasteur Paris **97**, 718 (1959).
[21] M. Raynaud, A. Turpin, E. H. Relyveld, R. Corvazier, and O. Girard, Ann. Inst. Pasteur Paris **96**, 649 (1959).
[22] J. Spaun and J. Lyng, Bull. W. H. O. **42**, 523 (1970).

ii. The Problem of Multiple Zones

If one does not have access to a "one-zone antitetanal serum," multiple zones will be found in general. Different methods have been proposed for identifying the true zone and have been discussed by several workers.[22a, 23, 23a]

The first of the proposed methods is based on the assumption that the true zone corresponds with a neutral mixture. In the Ramon test (constant amounts of toxin and increasing amounts of antitoxin), the mixture just before the true zone is reached contains an excess of toxin, whereas the mixture just after the zone is nontoxic. By injecting animals with the total mixture or the supernatant corresponding to these three successive tubes, it is easy to recognize which one represents the neutral mixture.

In the second proposed method, it is assumed that the particular flocculating tube which contains the real toxin with its homologous antibody is the one that will be able to absorb more added antitoxin than will tubes containing floccules that correspond to other antigens than the toxin itself. Accordingly, to washed floccules prepared from tubes just before and just after the zone under study, one adds a known amount of antitoxin. After 1 hour of incubation at room temperature and centrifugation, the antitoxin remaining in the supernatant is measured by an *in vivo* test.[22a–24]

The third method, rarely employed, consists in digesting the specific floccule with pepsin and measuring the amount of liberated antitoxin by an *in vivo* test. The yield of antitoxin upon peptic digestion may vary between 10 and 50%.

Certain false zones may be identified as such by the use of special preparations of antigens. Suspensions of young cultures of *Clostridium tetani*, for example, absorb antibodies corresponding to the heat-labile H-antigens.* Flocculation reactions carried out with such absorbed antiserum are devoid of false zones due to these antibodies.[25]

According to Cinader, the second method listed above is the only one that gives reliable results, yet none of these methods is able to solve the problem for all antitetanal sera, especially for certain nonavid sera of

---

[22a] P. J. Moloney and J. N. Hennessy, *J. Immunol.* **48**, 345 (1944).

[23] B. Cinader and B. Weitz, *J. Hyg.* **51**, 293 (1953).

[23a] B. Cinader, "The Interaction of Tetanus Toxin and Antitoxin." Thesis, Univ. of London, 1948.

[24] B. Cinader and B. Weitz, *Nature (London)* **166**, 785 (1950).

* Such procedures must be carried out only in isolation facilities by persons with competent microbiological training.

[25] A. R. Prévot and J. Pochon, *C. R. Soc. Biol.* **128**, 152 (1938).

very low L+:Lf value which are able to flocculate toxin without neutralizing it appreciably. It can be stated, however, that (1) the flocculation titer of a serum can be unequivocally determined by the use of pure tetanus toxin, which can be prepared by any laboratory engaged in the production of tetanus toxoid, and (2) the flocculation titer of a crude toxin can be determined unequivocally only by the use of a "one-zone serum," which is not easy to prepare, but is represented by the new International Standard Antitoxin.

c. Titration of Streptolysin O and Anti-Streptolysin

i. Introduction*

Streptolysin O (SLO) is one of the soluble hemolysins produced by streptococci of groups A, C, and G. Antistreptolysin O (anti-SLO) is antibody that appears, or increases in titer, because of recent infection with group A streptococci. (The incidence of cases in which titers rise in response to infections with groups C or G is low and does not affect the usefulness of the test in any important way.)

Streptolysin O, oxidizable and heat labile, is present in young culture filtrates of group A streptococci but is oxidized and inactive; further, it is often accompanied by streptolysin S. For use, SLO is reduced by hydrosulfite or cysteine; if stored for periods of 6 weeks or longer in the cold, streptolysin S disappears. Commercial preparations of lyophilized, reduced SLO are available, but the adequacy of titration is questioned by several experts, who continue to use their own reagents. SLO also contains antigenic material that is not capable of activation by reduction and serves in effect like a toxoid.

Anti-SLO specifically inhibits the hemolytic action of activated SLO on mammalian erythrocytes. Since both oxidized and reduced forms of SLO combine with the antibody, only the antibody can serve as a standard, just as is the case with diphtheria antitoxin and the toxin/toxoid mixture (Section 18.A). The standard is based on the original antiserum of Todd, and reduced SLO is titrated against it to determine "combining units."

In principle, a standardized immune serum is employed to define, by neutralization of hemolytic activity, some unit of SLO [chiefly the Todd unit in this country or the Lh unit described in Section 18.A.2.c.iv.(b)]. Various dilutions of patient's serum are incubated with a constant amount of fully reduced SLO, rabbit erythrocytes are added to the tubes, incubation at 37° is carried out for 45 minutes, and the titer of the patient's serum is expressed as a fixed end point: in the Todd system, the highest

* Sections 18.A.2.c.i through iii were contributed by Merrill W. Chase.

dilution that inhibits lysis *completely;* in the Lh system, the highest dilution that restricts the degree of hemolysis to 50% (HD_{50}). Narrow dilution increments of patient's serum (see below) are used in these tests, not the 2-fold serial dilutions customarily employed in serological tests.

ii. The Clinical Problem

As McCarty[26] has written:

> The pattern of the antistreptolysin O response following streptococcal infection has been well established. A rise in titer of the antibody is usually first detectable in the second week after onset of the infection; a rapid increase then ensues with the titer reaching a maximum in most cases at about four weeks. The period during which this maximum is sustained and the rate of subsequent fall in titer are variable but, in general, a return to the initial antibody level requires at least several months.
>
> In the case of rheumatic fever, because of the "latent interval" which follows the streptococcal infection, the onset of rheumatic symptoms usually occurs during the period of rapidly rising antistreptolysin titer just prior to the time when the maximum is reached. Thus, it is possible to demonstrate a rising titer only in those patients who are first seen early in the course of the disease.

Accordingly, several or many serial samples from each patient are examined, and the test has become routine for hospital laboratories. Here, we shall present only the broad outlines of the Todd test; the concentration of indicator rabbit red cells varies from 3% to 5% in different laboratories, a circumstance which affects the "titers" read. In one research center, new patients are screened at serum dilutions of 1:25, 1:100, 1:500 and 1:1000; the proper range is then examined in final titrations using appropriate sections from the following dilutions, expressed as reciprocals: 25, 50, 75, 100, 150, 200, 250, 300, 400, 500, 600, 700, 800, 900, 1000, 1200, 1400, 1600, 1800, 2000, 3000, 4000, 5000. On subsequent visits, significant dilutions can be chosen for the titration.

The basic Todd procedure is outlined here,[26] with dilutions of a positive serum of known titer made in saline, and controls consisting of erythrocytes in isotonic saline and erythrocytes mixed with one combining unit of reduced SLO.

1. Varying dilutions of the serum to be tested, in a volume of 1 ml., are mixed with 1 combining unit of streptolysin O in 0.5 ml. and incubated in a water bath at 37°C. for 15 minutes.
2. 0.5 ml. of a 5% suspension of washed rabbit erythrocytes are added to each tube and incubation continued for 45 minutes.
3. The tubes are read for lysis after being allowed to stand at room temperature for 30 minutes (or alternatively after brief centrifugation). The reciprocal of the highest serum dilution which effects *complete* inhibition of lysis represents

[26] M. McCarty, *Bull. Rheum. Dis.* **7**, Suppl. on Diagnostic Procedures, p. **23** (1957).

the antistreptolysin O titer in units per ml. Titrations of standard sera of known titer are run in parallel as controls.

Because of the lability of streptolysin, not more than 12 sera and the control serum are assigned to one worker. The most significant range of dilutions is 1:100 to 1:400. The lysin is kept at 0° after dilution in 0° saline to 1 combining unit per 0.5 ml as determined by previous titrations on the lot of lysin.

In other laboratories, saline heavily buffered at pH 6.5 (0.067 M phosphate) is often used,[27] whereas in the procedure given in Section 18.A.2.c. iv, 0.1% bovine serum albumin is added to such buffer.

In contrast to the clinically useful Todd method, the procedure described in Section 18.A.2.c.iv presents a polished research tool.

iii. Preparation of Streptolysin

The classic medium has been the Todd-Hewitt[28] beef heart infusion broth as modified by Swift and Hodge,[29] finally subjected to sterile filtration. Medium at 37° was inoculated, per liter, with 25 ml of young culture of the "Richards strain" (group A streptococcus) and incubated for 16 hours. Other steps are listed here without detail: sterile filtration, reduction by adding 1 gm of finely ground sodium hydrosulfite per liter, deaeration on the vacuum pump, filling of 100-ml Florence flasks to the neck, sealing with warm yellow petroleum jelly, and storage in the cold room for at least 6 weeks. Amounts of 10 ml and 20 ml are then transferred for use to potato tubes and again sealed and refrigerated.

This complex filtrate has served well as standard SLO, 0.15 ml to 0.18 ml per 0.5 ml total volume usually representing one combining unit. Diluted samples are held at 0° and are stable for a few hours.

A simple medium yielding much higher titers of SLO in the absence of streptolysin S, has been described by Alouf and Raynaud.[30] It is based on yeast extract and on special pancreatic and peptic peptones. A subculture of Kalbak's strain S-84 (known as Institut Pasteur strain A78), avirulent for mice and appearing to lack M-protein, is inoculated in the logarithmic phase of growth, incubation being stopped after 8 hours. Titration, made in DH_{50} units per milliliter and in LhT units per milliliter, as in Section 18.A.2.c.iv, shows about 7-fold increase in DH_{50} over SLO prepared in Todd–Hewitt broth, and a 3.5-fold increase in LhT units. The great advantage of the semisynthetic medium is the ease of handling

[27] L. A. Rantz and E. Randall, *Proc. Soc. Exp. Biol. Med.* **59**, 22 (1949).
[28] E. W. Todd and L. F. Hewitt, *J. Pathol. Bacteriol.* **35**, 973 (1932).
[29] H. F. Swift and B. E. Hodge, *Proc. Soc. Exp. Biol. Med.* **30**, 1022 (1933).
[30] J. E. Alouf and M. Raynaud, *Ann. Inst. Pasteur Paris* **108**, 759 (1965).

very large volumes for purification; one step of ultrafiltration is required, employing the apparatus of Relyveld.[8]

iv. *Titration of Streptolysin O (SLO) and Anti-SLO by the Method of Alouf et al.*[*][30, 31]

(a) *Determination of the Hemolytic Activity of Streptolysin O.* One hemolytic dose (HD_{50}) of streptolysin O may be defined as the amount of activated toxin causing lysis of 50% of a given amount of rabbit red cells, conveniently 1.25×10^8 cells contained in 0.5 ml. Lysis is measured after centrifugation by reading hemoglobin absorption at 541 nm in comparison with the reading secured following complete lysis of this number of erythrocytes.

Rabbit erythrocytes are collected by cardiac puncture with a syringe containing a few drops of heparin solution (2500 IU/ml). Cells are washed 3 times with phosphate-buffered saline (PBS) at pH 6.5 containing serum albumin‡ (also used for other operations), and centrifuged at 2000 rpm.

A 2.25% solution of cells is made up, which after dilution to 1:100 exhibits an absorbancy at 650 nm of about 0.340. The suspension is standardized to obtain an optical density of 0.200 at 541 nm when 0.5 ml of the suspension is lysed, by adding 14.5 ml of 0.1% sodium carbonate solution and centrifuging. The standardized suspension contains $2.5 \pm 0.35 \times 10^8$ cells per milliliter and liberates 7 mg of oxyhemoglobin after lysis.

Activation of SLO is made by reduction at room temperature for 10 minutes by adding neutralized cysteine or β-mercaptoethanol solution in 0.05 M final concentration, just prior to the titration.

Titration of SLO is then carried out in two steps.

Step 1. One milliliter of successively doubled dilutions of the streptolysin solution starting with 1:2 is added to a series of tubes. Then 0.50 ml of the standardized red cell solution is quickly added to each tube. The tubes are mixed and held for 45 minutes in a water bath at 37°. After centrifugation, optical densities of the supernatant liquids are measured and the HD_{50} value is determined by plotting the data on a log-probit scale.

---

* Section 18.A.2.c.iv was contributed by E. H. Relyveld and M. Raynaud.†

† Deceased.

[31] J. E. Alouf, M. Viette, R. Corvazier, and M. Raynaud, *Ann. Inst. Pasteur* **108**, 476 (1965).

‡ Buffered saline with 0.079 M phosphate at pH 6.5 is prepared by dissolving 7.47 gm of $NaH_2PO_4 \cdot H_2O$, 8.91 gm of $Na_2HPO_4 \cdot 12\ H_2O$, and 4.5 gm of NaCl per liter. Bovine serum albumin is added to provide 0.1%. This solution should also be used for all dilutions of SLO and anti-SLO serum.

Step 2. A second more precise determination is carried out after diluting the streptolysin O solution to about 4 HD_{50} units/ml and adding decreasing amounts to a row of 11 tubes: the first tube receives 0.5 ml, and each later tube receives 0.05 ml less, so that the final tube receives none. Buffer solution is then added up to a final volume of 1 ml. Titration is carried out as above.

(*b*) *Determination of the Combining Power of Streptolysin and Its Antiserum.* Because a part of the streptolysin O is inactive, being present in the form of toxoid, determination of the HD_{50} is not a very precise method. It is therefore recommended to measure simultaneously the combining power of toxin and toxoid with the corresponding antibody.

Determination of the Lh dose of SLO. One Lh* dose of streptolysin, termed Lh(T) for toxin, may be defined as the quantity of SLO giving 50% hemolysis after combination with 1 IU of anti-streptolysin O, termed Lh(A) for antibody.

Determination of Lh. The reaction will be conducted in 2.5-ml total volumes, using the phosphate buffer containing 0.1% BSA, fresh rabbit red cells standardized at 1.25×10^8 cells in 0.5 ml, and antiserum that is diluted just before titration. Have all solutions cooled to 0 to 4°. In a series of tubes place amounts of streptolysin O starting with 1.50 ml and decreasing successively by 0.05 ml, down to 1.00 ml; add buffers to bring the volumes of all tubes to 1.5 ml. Add to each tube 0.5 ml of antiserum diluted to 2 IU/ml. Hold the tubes at 37° for 15 minutes; then add to each tube 0.5 ml of the red cell suspension to deliver 1.25×10^8 cells; hold at 37% for 45 minutes; centrifuge, dilute the supernatants in 0.1% Na_2CO_3 solution, read absorbancy at 541 nm. The 50% end point is determined, and Lh values are calculated.

Determination of antiserum titers. Antibody titers in patient's serum or animals are determined similarly as follows: Serum must be inactivated by heating at 56° for 30 minutes, dilutions are made as above and all reagents are cooled to 0° to 4°. Streptolysin O is diluted up to 5 units/ml, and 0.2 ml is mixed with various amounts of serum.

d. STAPHYLOCOCCAL TOXIN‡§

i. *Titration of α-Hemolysin, Toxoid, and Antitoxin*

While flocculation reactions can be carried out in the manner described for diphtheria and tetanus toxins, this method is only rarely employed

---

* Lh, hemolytic unit of toxin.

† Section 18.A.2.d was contributed by E. H. Relyveld and M. Raynaud.‡

‡ Deceased.

§ For titration *in vivo,* see Section 18.A.3.d.

because of the absence of well defined standard flocculation sera. Instead, the capacity of the toxin to hemolyze rabbit erythrocytes is determined. One can use as a unit either total or 50% lysis of rabbit red blood corpuscles.

(a) *Hemolytic Activity of Staphylococcal Toxin.* The smallest quantity of toxin giving *total* lysis of a standardized amount of cells is the minimal hemolytic dose of toxin (MHD). According to Kayser and Raynaud,[32] determination of the dose which hemolyses 50% of the cells (HD_{50}) is a more accurate method.

Rabbit blood is taken by cardiac puncture with oxalate (one-tenth volume of 2% sodium oxalate),* and the cells are centrifuged and washed three times with phosphate-buffered saline (0.079 M phosphate), pH 7.0.† The washed cells are suspended to the original volume of blood.

(i) *The minimal hemolytic dose.* This dose is determined by mixing 2 ml of toxin at various doubled dilutions starting with 1:100 and 0.1 ml of the standardized red cell suspension. The tubes are incubated at 37° for 30 minutes and examined for complete lysis.

(ii) *The HD_{50} value.* This value is more accurate[32] and is determined as follows. The buffered saline, described above, has 1% of gelatin dissolved in it, and 1 volume of the suspension of washed erythrocytes is diluted with 3 volumes of gelatin–PBS. The suspension is standardized by hemolyzing one part with 99 parts of 0.1% Na_2CO_3 solution and measuring absorbancy at 541 nm. The original suspension is then adjusted to yield to an optical density of 2.1 after lysis, what means approximately a 1:20 dilution, i.e., 1.1×10^8 cells/ml.

One milliliter of the diluted suspension is mixed with 1 ml of the gelatin-buffer solution and 1 ml of toxin at various doubled dilutions starting with 1:100. The tubes are centrifuged after incubation at 37° for 30 minutes, and optical densities of the supernatant fluids are measured and expressed as percentage of lysis. The 50% end point is determined on a log-probit scale.

(b) *Determination of the Combining Power of Toxin and Toxoid with Antitoxin.* One hemolytic dose of toxin (LhT) may be defined either as the smallest quantity of toxin which, in the presence of 1 unit of antitoxin, gives either *total* hemolysis or gives *50%* hemolysis of a standardized red cell suspension.

---

[32] A. Kayser and M. Raynaud, *Ann. Inst. Pasteur Paris* **108**, 215 (1965).

* One-tenth volume of a mixture of 1.2% ammonium oxalate and 0.8% potassium oxalate is recommended in Vol. 1, Chap. 2.C.2.b.

† Very strongly buffered saline at pH 7.0 (0.079 M phosphate), approximating buffer 35E (Vol. II, Appendix II.8) is used by the present authors: 126 ml of 0.2 M NaH_2PO_4 and 268 ml of 0.2 M Na_2HPO_4 plus 4.5 gm of NaCl is brought to 1 liter.

TABLE I

PROTOCOL FOR DETERMINING THE COMBINING POWER OF
Staphylococcus α-HEMOLYSIN[a]

	Tube No.				
	1	2	3	4	5
Antitoxin at 1 unit per ml (ml)	1	1	1	1	1
Toxin (ml)	0.1	0.15	0.20	0.25	0.30
Saline (ml)	0.9	0.85	0.80	0.75	0.70
Red cell suspension[b] (drops per tube)	1	1	1	1	1

[a] Contents are mixed and held in the water bath at 37°C for 1 hour.

[b] Rabbit cells washed 3 times, resuspended to original volume, and then diluted 1:3 can be used. Tubes are left for 10 minutes in the room, then one drop of cell suspension is added to each.

(*i*) *End points by complete hemolysis.* A simple method of carrying out titrations is presented in Table I.

The combining power is expressed in terms of the smallest amount of toxin giving complete hemolysis.

Staphylococcal toxoid is titrated in a similar way.[33] One milliliter of antitoxin corresponding to 2 units is mixed with graduated quantities of toxoid (0.075, 0.10, 0.125, . . . ml), and the volume is brought to 2 ml. The tubes are incubated at 37° for 30 minutes, and an amount of toxin, slightly less than 1 Lh, e.g., 95%, is added. The tubes are left in the room for 10 minutes, then one drop of the rabbit red cell suspension is added. Thrice-washed rabbit cells resuspended to original volume and then diluted 1:3 can be used. The tubes are then incubated for 1 hour at 37°. Titers are expressed in terms of the mixture containing the smallest amount of toxoid which shows complete hemolysis.

Serum titers are determined in a reversed way, by adding graduated quantities of antitoxin to a series of hemolysis tubes, followed by 1 Lh of toxin solution and saline. Serum titers are expressed in terms of the largest quantity of serum giving complete hemolysis.

(*ii*) HD_{50} *values as end points.* Determination of 50% hemolysis may be used for titration. The simplest instance is represented by toxin titration. Antitoxin corresponding to 1 uint is introduced into each of a series of hemolysis tubes, followed by decreasing quantities of diluted toxin, e.g., 1, 0.9, 0.8, . . . ml, and the volume is brought to 2 ml with the buffer solution. After 5 minutes at laboratory temperature, 1 ml of the standardized red cell suspension is added. Optical density is determined after 30 minutes' incubation at 37° and centrifugation; 50% hemolysis is determined from a log-probit scale.

[33] P. Mercier and J. Pillet, *Bull. W. H. O.* **2**, 45 (1949).

Again, the Lh unit (LhT) of toxin can be redefined as that amount which, in the presence of 1 unit of antitoxin, is capable of hemolyzing 50% of the erythrocytes, i.e., the mixture contains 1 HD_{50} of free toxin.

The measurement of antitoxin is carried out in the reverse way, against the Lh unit as determined as just described. Dilutions of antitoxin are mixed with 1 Lh unit of toxin (total volume, 2 ml) to determine the amount which leaves 1 HD_{50} of toxin free. After 5 minutes' contact between serum and toxin, red blood cells are added; this is followed by incubation, centrifuging, and measurements of optical densities. The quantity of serum corresponding to 1 HD_{50} of toxin left free in the mixture contains 1 Lh unit of anti-alpha antibodies (LhA).

ii. Titration of Staphylococcal β-, γ-, and δ-Hemolysins

Methods described for α-toxin can be used, but in the titration of β-hemolysin sheep red blood cells must be employed. γ-Hemolysin lyses rabbit and sheep red cells most effectively; δ-hemolysin lyses rabbit and horse cells more effectively than sheep cells.[32]

e. Titration of Clostridium welchii (C. perfringens) Type A α-Toxin, Toxoid, and Antitoxin by the Egg-Yolk Reaction[*][†]

The α-toxin of C. welchii type A is responsible for the lethal, dermonecrotic, and hemolytic effects of culture filtrate. It is a lecithinase with phosphatase activity, splitting egg yolk lecithovitellin in the presence of Ca^{2+} into phosphocholine and stearyloleylglyceride. The α-toxin is inhibited by its antitoxin.

The Le unit[§] is that amount of toxin which, in the presence of one unit of antitoxin, will just cause a faint opalescence to appear in egg yolk solution.[34]

The yolk of one egg (18.5 gm) is washed and beaten up with 500 ml of 0.9% NaCl. Then 0.4 gm of calcium acetate and 20 gm of kaolin are added followed by filtration through paper and finally through a sterile filter (Seitz pad). The filtrate is stored in the cold.

A borate buffer is used at pH 6.77 to 6.8,[**] with addition of 2.925 gm

---

* Section 18.A.2.e was contributed by E. H. Relyveld and M. Raynaud.‡

† For titration in vivo, see Section 18.A.3.e.

‡ Deceased.

§ The Le unit indicates egg as the test substance. The unit has also been termed Lb (for binding) or Lv (for vitellin).

[34] W. E. van Heyningen, "Bacterial Toxins," p. 27. Blackwell, Oxford and Thomas, Springfield, Illinois, 1950.

** The buffer is based on buffer 14, Volume II, Appendix II.8, but uses 970 ml of 0.2 M boric acid and 30 ml of 0.05 M sodium tetraborate per liter, and accordingly lies on the toe of the titration curve.

of NaCl per liter. The toxin solution is stabilized by addition of peptone or gelatin to 1%.

The test consists of mixing constant amounts of antitoxin with various amounts of toxin (Table II) and holding at room temperature for 30

TABLE II

PROTOCOL FOR DETERMINING NEUTRAL MIXTURES OF *Clostridium welchii*
TOXIN AND ITS ANTITOXIN[a]

	Tube No.										
Additions	1	2	3	4	5	6	7	8	9	10	11
Buffer (ml)	0.9	0.8	0.7	0.6	0.5	0.4	0.3	0.2	0.1	0	1
Antitoxin at 1 unit/ml (ml)	1	1	1	1	1	1	1	1	1	1	1
Toxin solution (ml)	0.1	0.2	0.3	0.4	0.5	0.6	0.7	0.8	0.9	1	0

[a] Contents are mixed and held for 30 minutes at room temperature. Then add 0.5 ml of the egg yolk emulsion is added and the preparation is incubated at 38° for 1 hour.

minutes. Then 0.5 ml of the egg yolk emulsion is added. After incubation at 38° for 1 hour, the tubes are read for development of turbidity, which indicates enzymatic activity of free α-toxin.

Antitoxin is titrated in the same way by adding various quantities to one combining unit of toxin (LeT).

3. NEUTRALIZATION OF TOXIN *IN VIVO*

a. INTRODUCTION*

Neutralization of diphtheria toxin by antiserum raised against it ("antitoxin") was originally measured by subcutaneous injection of mixtures into guinea pigs of 250–270 gm weight.† Römer[1] in 1909 showed that intense reddening or even dermonecrosis resulted when very small, nonlethal amounts of toxin were injected intradermally into guinea pigs. His observation was later developed by Glenny and Allen[2] into a titration system, by making multiple intradermal injections of varying toxin–antitoxin mixtures into normal guinea pigs to find neutral mixtures. Still an-

---

* Section 18.A.3.a was contributed by Merrill W. Chase.

† The units that came into use—minimum lethal dose (MLD), antitoxic unit (AU), Lo and L+ doses, are described in Section 18.A.1, footnote to paragraph 2.

[1] P. H. Römer and T. Sames, *Z. Immunitaetsforsch. Exp. Ther.* 3, 344 (1909).

[2] A. T. Glenny and K. Allen, *J. Pathol. Bacteriol.* 24, 61 (1921).

other unit, the minimal reacting dose (MRD), was introduced, equal to
ca 1:500 of the MLD dose. Fraser[3, 4] transferred the test system to rabbits, in which the larger skin area permitted from 16 to 60 mixtures to
be tested simultaneously by intradermal testing. Readings of toxicity
were made at 36 hours.

In such *in vivo* titration, whether one chose guinea pig or rabbit as
test subject, "nonavid" antitoxins were encountered. Glenny and Barr[5]
devised a system, the "dilution ratio," for expressing the degree of avidity
(Section 18.A.3.b.iii). In this system various amounts of antitoxic sera
were used to neutralize 1 Lr dose of toxin* in two different volumes—2 ml
and 200 ml. Such mixtures were kept 15 minutes in the room and injected
in 0.2-ml volumes intradermally into guinea pigs. The results were of
great utilitarian value, but the procedure is superseded by methods introduced by Jerne[6] [Section 18.A.3.b.iii.(b)].

It is to be emphasized once again that the content of toxin in a culture
filtrate can be measured only by *in vivo* methods, since *in vitro* methods
register the sum of toxin and (naturally occurring) toxoid in the filtrate.

b. Diphtheria Antitoxin†

i. Titration by the Intracutaneous Neutralization Technique

(a) *Determination of the Lr/10 Dose of Toxin.* Male white albino rabbits of 6 lb or more are used.§ Animals are shaved with an electric clipper.

---

[3] D. T. Fraser and H. E. Wigham, *J. Amer. Med. Assoc.* **82**, 1114 (1924).
[4] D. T. Fraser, *Trans. Roy. Soc. Can. Sect. V* **25**, 175 (1931).
[5] A. T. Glenny and M. Barr, *J. Pathol. Bacteriol.* **35**, 91 (1932).
* Mixtures giving minimal (but not negative) skin reactions in the presence of 1
AU define the Lr dose of toxin. The Lr dose closely approaches the L_0 dose as
defined previously (Section 18.A.3.a.). Skin tests are performed on the Lr/10 and
Lr/100 level and allow the use of many sites without additive toxic effects of unneutralized mixtures.
[6] N. K. Jerne, *Acta Pathol. Microbiol. Scand.,* Suppl. **87** (1931).

† Sections 18.A.3.b.i.(a) and (b) were contributed by M. Raynaud‡ and E. H. Relyveld.

‡ Deceased.
§ Large albino rabbits or rabbits with nonpigmented skin which are in stationary
hair phase are best employed, a circumstance chiefly encountered in winter months
in the colder climates. Such rabbits, if clipped free of hair, do not experience further
growth of hair for some weeks; when hormonal stimulation for hair growth resumes,
either normally or as consequence of injections of only partially neutralized dipth-
theria toxin, patches of skin ("islands") become sharply elevated and vigorous hair
growth occurs; by peripheral extensions, the rabbit grows its new coat. In the
stationary hair phase, use of dipilatory is not recommended since the skin becomes
"brittle" and harder to inject. If depilatory *must* be used, because the rabbit is not
in the stationary hair phase, the commercial product, Nair cream (Carter-Wallace,

An Oster Model A-2 clipper* provided with an Ang-Ra No. 2 or a size 30 blade can be used.

On each side of the spine, 2 ranks of 4 to 6 squares (4 × 4 cm) are drawn with an eyebrow pencil or a wetted indelible pencil. The shaved area is first sponged with 70% alcohol.

Crude diphtheria toxin is used for titration, the sterile stock solution being kept at 0° to 4°. Portions of 100 ml are withdrawn when needed, Merthiolate is added to a 1:10,000 dilution. Standardization of the toxin is carried out against the International Standard of Diphtheria Antitoxin (Statens Serum Institute, Copenhagen, Denmark), which is distributed as a solution containing, in 66% glycerol, 10 International Antitoxic Units (IAU) per milliliter. Dilutions are made in a sterile solution prepared from 9 gm of NaCl and 10 gm of peptone per liter of water at pH 7.4.

Antitoxin is diluted to 1 AU/ml for titration on the Lr/10 level (i.e., 0.1 IAU) and mixed with equal volumes of various toxin dilutions. After *2 hours' incubation at room temperature* each mixture is injected (0.2 ml) by the intradermal route. Tuberculin-type syringes (1 ml), fitted with needles of gauges 26, 27, or 30 and ⅜ to ⅝ inch in length, are used. Titrations are carried out in 2 rabbits as shown in Table III.

Alternatively, one can mix 0.5 ml of a solution containing 2 AU/ml with 0.5 ml of toxin dilution and inject 0.1 ml of the mixtures. The absolute amount is the same: 0.1 International AU (Lr/10 level), but the *concentration* (which, in our opinion, is the most important factor) is 1 AU/ml as half-volume.

(*b*) *Titration of Unknown Sera against Toxin at Lr/10 Dosage.* Different dilutions of unknown sera are mixed in equal volumes with the toxin (standardized as in Table III) diluted to contain 10 Lr/10 doses of toxin per milliliter (or 20 Lr/10 doses per milliliter in the alternative method).

Titrations are carried out in the same way by determining the serum dilution giving a reaction of 13 mm in diameter. The reciprocal value of the dilution gives the serum titer in AU/ml determined on the Lr/10 level.

It may be observed that the "level of titration" refers to the *absolute amount* of antitoxin (or toxin) injected. In the technique recommended

---

Inc., New York, based on calcium thioglycolate) is recommended for 4- or 5-minute contact, after careful clipping with a No. 0000 blade, rather than the various barium sulfide preparations. Prompt removal of depilatory is required, with avoidance of the cream penetrating into standing hair. Rabbits can be used only once. Individual rabbits vary in responsiveness to unneutralized toxin (Fig. 1), hence a method for evaluating the individual rabbit is given in Section 18.A.3.b.iii(b). [Editors].

* John Oster Manufacturing Company, Milwaukee, Wisconsin. Model 50, with detachable blades, is also satisfactory for animal clipping.

TABLE III

Titration of Diphtheria Toxin–Antitoxin Mixtures in Rabbit Skin

Toxin dilution, 1 ml	Antitoxin solution,[a] 1 ml (AU)	No. of the squares	Diameter of the reaction after 48 hours (mm)[b]	
			Rabbit No. 1	Rabbit No. 2
1:30	1	1	9	26, 22	26, 20
1:32.5	1	2	10	23, 22	26, 20
1:35	1	3	11	20, 20	19, 20
1:37.5	1	4	12	18, 19	19, 17
1:40[c]	1	5	13	13, 17	13, 11
1:42.5	1	6	14	0, 0	0, 0
1:45	1	7	15	0, 0	0, 0
1:47.5	1	8	16	0, 0	0, 0

[a] Equivalent to the International Antitoxic Unit.

[b] The 2 values represent readings at the duplicate test sites ("squares").

[c] In this example, Lr/10 = 1:40 toxin dilution, tested in 0.2 ml of the final mixture; average diameter of reaction is 13 mm. The 1:40 dilution of the toxin solution contains 10 Lr/10 doses per milliliter.

by the W.H.O.,[7] the absolute level is 0.01 IAU (Lr/100 level), but the *final concentration* of antitoxin in the mixture is 0.05 IAU/ml.

It is recommended, when recording results of antitoxin measurements for publication, to specify the concentration of antitoxin in the final mixtures; time and temperature of incubation of the mixtures of toxin and antitoxin before injection to animals; total volume injected.

Titers lower than 1 unit/ml (corresponding to undiluted serum) cannot be determined on the Lr/10 level. For this reason toxin is also standardized on the Lr/100 or Lr/1000 level, and titrations are carried out as described just above.

The same titration method can also be carried out in the albino guinea pig, by the intradermal route of injection as described by Glenny and Llewellyn-Jones (1931).[8]

(c) *Titration at the "Neutral Point."** The neutral point, found by incubating toxin–antitoxin mixtures with Standard Antitoxin present at a final concentration of 0.005 AU/ml, is a valid parameter and possesses advantages over methods that are based on subneutral mixtures as standards. When the Standard Antitoxin is replaced by an experimental anti-

[7] *Bull. W. H. O.*, Suppl. 2, "International Pharmacopoeia" 1st ed, Vol. 1 (1951).

[8] A. T. Glenny and M. Llewellyn-Jones, *J. Pathol. Bacteriol.* 34, 143 (1931).

* Section 18.A.3.b.i.(c) was contributed by Merrill W. Chase.

toxin, the "titer" determined in these secondary tests is often, as Jerne has stressed, only an approximation unless avidity differences are taken into account (Section 18.A.3.b.iii).

The principle underlying titration at the neutral point consists of mixing equal volumes of Standard Antitoxin at 0.01 AU/ml as half-volume (hv)* and a half-volume containing varied amounts of toxin to find how much toxin is neutralized when these mixtures are held at 37° for 3 or 4 hours and are then injected into rabbit skin in 0.1-ml (or 0.15-ml) volumes. The amount of toxin so found then becomes the standard for comparing other antitoxins under similar conditions. In principle, this test approximates results using toxin at the "Lr/1000 level" [Section 18.A.3.b.i.(a)], excepting that *neutral* mixtures are sought; both these tests will evaluate very low concentrations of antitoxin such as may be encountered in research situations (see Table III).

Buffered peptone diluent. The diluent recommended by Jerne[6] conserves toxin and antitoxin even during incubation at 37° for several weeks; it affords superior stability over diluents based on gelatin. Phosphate-buffered saline (1.65 gm of KH_2PO_4, 6.06 gm of Na_2HPO_4, and 4.75 gm of NaCl per liter) with 0.5% peptone, such as Difco proteose peptone, at 7.38, $\Gamma/2 = 0.22$, and preserved with thimerosal at 1:30,000 (0.3% of 1% stock) is used to dilute both toxin and antitoxin. Thimerosal at this concentration does not affect reactions in rabbit skin, but it cannot be used for intradermal injections of guinea pigs.

Toxin. The preparation of toxin can be crude or purified; its minimal lethal dose (MLD) must be determined carefully.† Only when crude toxin has become stabilized so that toxoid is no longer being generated spontaneously can the preparation serve to compare antitoxins. Accordingly, the MLD must be checked again at suitable intervals.

The largest amount of toxin that will be completely neutralized by addition of an exactly equal volume of Standard Antitoxin at a concentration of 0.01 AU/ml must be determined. This amount of toxin then serves for testing all unknown antitoxins.

In the author's studies, it was possible to use a purified toxin prepared in the laboratory of A. M. Pappenheimer, Jr. Very little if any toxoid was present in the preparation [for details see Section 18.A.3.b.iii.(b)

---

* Since equal volumes of doubled concentrations of toxin and antitoxin are mixed, it is useful to adopt the terms *half-volume* (hv) for the doubled concentrations and *final concentration* (fc) for the resulting mixture (see Table IV).

† The quantity MLD, described in Section 18.A.1 is the smallest amount of toxin which will kill guinea pigs of 250-gm body weight within 96 hours. A series of accurate dilutions is made and injected subcutaneously near the sternum. Groups of 3 to 6 animals, in excellent health, are used for each dilution.

and Fig. 1]. With this preparation, 1 volume of 0.25 Lf/liter, giving reactions of 14 to 20 mm prior to addition of antitoxin, was just neutralized by 1 volume of 0.01 AU/ml, i.e., the tests are made at AU/200.

Standard antitoxin. Such standards are obtainable (in limited supply) from various national and international sources, such as the Division of Biologic Standards, Bethesda, Maryland. These are horse antitoxins of high avidity, adjusted to some fixed number of AU/ml containing 66% glycerol. Dilution is made with extreme precision in the buffered peptone diluent to secure 0.01 AU/ml. Pipettes calibrated to "contain" are best, and external control of the pipette, which should be fixed rigid and vertical, is advisable. The dilution is dispensed into suitable vials and sealed against evaporation. It is well to wipe the caps with 70% alcohol, allow to dry, and overseal with Parafilm.

Working antitoxin. Standard Antitoxin is not available in working quantities. Accordingly, the laboratory must prepare its own antitoxin and standardize it against the Standard Antitoxin. The working antitoxin is usually prepared in rabbits by giving spaced subcutaneous injections of alum-precipitated diphtheria toxoid (such as 25 Lf) over several months and bleeding on day 7 after the last injection, providing that previous tests during the immunization have shown good titers, say 80 to 200 AU/ml (peak titers in rabbits approximate 300 AU/ml). Such titers can be determined directly by *in vivo* neutralization or approximated by *in vitro* tests (Sections 18.A.2 and 16.B.2). For final testing, *in vivo* neutralization is requisite.

The proper dilution of *working antitoxin* is determined which provides exactly 0.01 AU/ml, by standardization against the proper dose of toxin, and sufficient vials are prepared in the peptone diluent for the expected work load over a period of some months. It is particularly necessary to know that the avidity of the *working antitoxin* is sufficiently high (Section 18.A.3.b.iii).

Rabbits. The choice and preparation of rabbits is described in Sections 18.A.3.b.i.(a) and 18.A.3.b.iii.(b). According to Jerne,[6] the most accurate results are secured when injections are made within a rectangle of 8 × 4 inches (10 × 20 cm) just below the scapula and above the crest of the ileum; 36 sites are then available. But a well-grown rabbit can provide up to 72 sites; those sites of lesser desirability [see Section 18.A.3.b.iii.(b)] are highly useful in first approximations of antitoxin content.

Dilutions of antitoxins. Logarithmically spaced dilutions are prepared as *hv* dilutions, starting with neat serum undiluted and three master dilutions of 1:10, 1:20, and 1:100. The appropriate dilutions are selected from the dilution series shown in Table IV. Irregular amounts smaller than 1 ml are easily delivered by means of a micrometer-actuated

TABLE IV
LOGARITHMIC DILUTION SERIES FOR ANTITOXIN[a]

Ml/liter	Dilution (hv)[b]	Log (fc)[c]	Ml/liter	Dilution (hv)[b]	Log (fc)[c]
125	1:4	2.1	0.625	1:800	−0.2
100	1:5	2.0	0.5	1:1000	−0.3
83	1:6.3	1.9	0.4	1:1250	−0.4
62.5	1:8	1.8	0.312	1:1600	−0.5
50	1:10	1.7	0.25	1:2000	−0.6
40	1:12.5	1.6	0.2	1:2500	−0.7
31.2	1:16	1.5	0.16	1:3150	−0.8
25	1:20	1.4	0.125	1:4000	−0.7
20	1:25	1.3	0.1	1:5000	−1.0
16	1:31.25	1.2	0.08	1:6250	−1.1
12.5	1:40	1.1	0.0625	1:8000	−1.2
10	1:50	1.0	0.05	1:10000	−1.3
8	1:63	0.9	0.04	1:12500	−1.4
6.25	1:80	0.8	0.0312	1:16000	−1.5
5	1:100	0.7	0.025	1:20000	−1.6
4	1:125	0.6	0.02	1:25000	−1.7
3.12	1:160	0.5	0.016	1:31500	−1.8
2.5	1:200	0.4	0.0125	1:40000	−1.9
2	1:250	0.3	0.01	1:50000	−2.
1.6	1:315	0.2	0.008	1:62500	−2.1
1.25	1:400	0.1	0.006	1:80000	−2.2
1	1:500	0	0.005	1:10000	−2.3
0.83	1:625	−0.1			

[a] Undiluted (neat) serum and accurate master dilutions of 1:10, 1:20, and 1:100 (and so on) allow ready calculation of the series of logarithmic dilutions.

[b] hv, half-volume to which an equal volume of toxin is to be added.

[c] fc, final concentration of the reactants, i.e. $2 \times hv$.

"Agla"[*] syringe. Used as half-volumes (hv) with an equal volume of the proper dose of toxin (that which is neutralized by 1 volume of 0.01 AU/ml), a neutralizing dilution of 1:1.25 would represent 0.0125 AU/ml; 1:2000 would represent 20 AU/ml. Very fine gradings can therefore be made.

For a completely unknown antitoxic serum, it is best to make one or two estimates, such as 20 AU/ml (1:2000) and 50 AU/ml (1:5000), and to test these on the less desirable flank sites on one rabbit serving to test other toxin–antitoxin mixtures; closer estimates are then secured on a second rabbit, and finally a proper dilution series can be run. This

[*] Wellcome "Agla" Micrometer Syringe Apparatus (Burroughs Wellcome and Company, London, England).

procedure is economical whenever repeated tests are being run in the laboratory, either antitoxic titers or avidity determinations (Subsection b.iii). Initial estimates can be secured by injecting the skin of albino guinea pigs providing Merthiolate is omitted and buffer is sterile, or by passive hemagglutination (Section 18.A.2.a.iii).

Titration of unknown antitoxins. Although a rather large number of potential skin sites are available on a mature rabbit, one should not squander rabbits, particularly those in the resting hair stage, by injecting many dilutions of an unknown antiserum or a large number of sites with potentially unneutralized toxin.

One volume (as little as 0.2 ml) of toxin at the known concentration is mixed with 1 volume of each of the chosen dilutions of antitoxin(s). Besides this series, the toxin is set up against 1 volume of standard antitoxin at 0.01 AU/ml, and expediently also with 90%, 82%, and 75% of this dose (0.009, 0.0082, and 0.0075 AU/ml) to provide *mixtures that are not fully neutral.* The responses to known nonneutral mixtures tell us much about the sensitiveness of the particular rabbit to toxin (Table V; Fig. 1)—narrow or broad—and also they provide standard lesions for comparison with other nearly neutral mixtures of unknown antitoxin(s) on the same rabbit. Later, test mixtures can then be planned much more appropriately, allowing reduction in the number of mixtures needed.

The mixtures are stoppered and placed in the 37° water bath for 3 hours and then are loaded into syringes, to be injected into carefully randomized sites on the grid inscribed on the back [see Section 18.A.3.b.iii.(b)].

Readings are made after 1, 2, and 3 days, scoring the diameters of reactions (in millimeters) and their intensity (Table V). Redness may be slight (r) or marked (R). Induration may be slight (i) or marked (I). There may be slight central necrosis (n) or greater necrosis (N). The reaction maximum is usually at 72 hours.

Practical examples are given in Table V, data being drawn from tests with bleedings of quite low titers preparatory to making avidity determinations. By using 2 rabbits and only a few sites (those on rabbit 5L were tested in duplicate), we find the titer to fall between 0.8 and 1.6 AU/ml. But in view of the reaction given by 75% neutralized toxin, a closer approximation would probably yield a value close to 1.0 AU/ml for No. 1380 and 1.6 AU/ml for No. 1378. The principle holds for sera of any titer. For example, a rabbit antitoxin, tested first at only 1:700, was found to neutralize. Later tests with 1:1000, 1:3000, and 1:5000 also neutralized. Third-stage testing with 1:4000, 1:4500, 1:5000, 1:5500, and 1:6000 showed the actual neutral point to be 1:5000, or 50 AU/ml.

TABLE V
DETERMINATION OF ANTITOXIN TITERS[a]

| Readings (hours) | Rabbit 5 H | | | | Rabbit 5 L | | | |

No. 1380, 12-day bleeding

Readings (hours)	1:10[b]	1:40	1:80	1:160
24	x[c]	x	x	7r
48	0	(5)[d]	(5)	9r
72	0	0	0	13r+

No. 1378, 12-day bleeding

Readings (hours)	1:50	1:80	1:125	1:160	1:250	1:400	1:625
24	x	x	x	x	12r	14ri −	17ri +
48	0	0	0	0	14-1/2 Ri	18-1/2 Rin	21RIn+
72	0	0	0	0?	16Ri+	21RI −n	26Ri+ N+

Standard antitoxin

Readings (hours)	0.01	0.009	0.0082	0.0075	0.01	0.009	0.0082	0.0075
72	0	5r	7r	12r	0	0?	9r	11-1/2r

[a] All mixtures contained toxin just neutralized by an equal volume of 0.01 AU/ml Standard Antitoxin. Scoring of diameter, redness, induration and necrosis as given in text.

[b] Serum dilution used as half-volume.

[c] x indicates irritative redness, with no definite reaction.

[d] Parentheses indicate uncertain reading.

*ii. Titration of Diphtheria Antitoxin by the L+ Method[7]**

(a) *Preliminary Test for Determination of the L+ Dose of Toxin.*
Mixtures are prepared in 0.9% NaCl to contain 1 IAU of antitoxin and various amounts of toxin. The total volume, to be injected by the subcutaneous route, is 4 ml. These mixtures are incubated at room temperature. Our own recommendation is for an incubation period of 2 hours although the Pharmacopoeia[7] specified at least 15 minutes but not more than 60 minutes. The mixtures (4ml‡ each) are injected subcutaneously into healthy guinea pigs weighing 250 to 270 gm. At least 3 animals are to be used per dose. Animals are observed for 5 days.

One L+ dose of the toxin represents the minimal amount which, mixed with one International Antitoxin Unit, will cause the death of all the animals of the group within 4 days. From a theoretical point of view, it

* Section 18.A.3.b.ii.(a) was contributed by M. Raynaud† and E. H. Relyveld.

† Deceased.

‡ Some laboratories prefer to prepare the mixtures in total volumes of 2 or 3 ml.

would be better to use 6 animals per dose and choose as the end point the death of 50% of the animals of the group.

(b) *Determination of the Titer of an Unknown Serum.* Using the L+ dose of toxin determined in this way, one prepares similar mixtures containing increasing amounts of the serum under study, also in total volumes of 4 ml.

After incubation at room temperature under the exact condition of incubation used to determine the L+ dose, groups of 3 to 6 guinea pigs are injected with each mixture. The mixture that contains the largest amount of antiserum yet kills all the animals in 4 days is taken as containing 1 AU.

The precision varies with the number of animals used: for 2 animals, 96 to 104%; 4 animals, 97 to 103%; 6 animals, 97.5 to 102.5% (for $p = 0.99$).[7]

The rabbit intracutaneous method is preferable for these reasons: (1) several sera can be titrated on the same animal; (2) control, with the same dose of toxin and different amounts of the standard (as in Subsection b.i) can be repeated on the same animal as the unknown. In this way individual variation in response is minimized, namely variations among animals in the size of the cutaneous lesion produced by a given amount of free toxin.

One has to take care not to inject mixtures containing a too large excess of underneutralized toxin. The general intoxication by diphtheria toxin, even if it does not kill the rabbit within 2 days, may inhibit the local skin reactions overall.

iii. Avidity Determinations

(a) *Dilution Ratio as an Indirect Measure of Avidity.** For all antitoxins, especially those against diphtheria and tetanus, it is important to have some indication of the avidity ("quality") of the neutralizing antibodies, a parameter that defines the firmness of combination of toxin with antitoxin and determines the therapeutic effectiveness of the particular antitoxin.‡

* Section 18.A.3.b.iii. (a) was contributed by M. Raynaud† and E. H. Relyveld.

† Deceased.

‡ Differences in "avidity" or affinity have now been recognized as a general property of less "mature" antibodies (Vol. III, Chap. 13.A.2.a.x(a), 13.A.3.a.v, 13.C.1.d, 13.C.2) and are easily apparent in studying anti-hapten antibody (Vol. III, Chap. 15.C. and 15.D.). High "avidity" or affinity of antitoxin for toxin is rather easily secured if the immunization schedule has been carried on for a sufficiently long time; 3 well spaced injections of 25 Lf of toxoid of alum-precipitated toxoid suffice for rabbits, 5 or 6 for guinea pigs, a larger dose and number of injections for horses, and so on. Therapeutic sera should always be of high avidity. [Editors]

Since the problem exists equally with tetanus antitoxin, the latter is described here along with diphtheria antitoxin. In 1932, Glenny and Barr[5] introduced the "dilution ratio" to describe the binding affinity of diphtheria antitoxins, and Cinader[9] and Cinader and Weitz[10, 11] made independent studies with the tetanus system. The "nonavid" antitoxins are characterized by the fact that their ability to neutralize toxin is low when measurements are made against a "low level of antitoxin," yet is higher if measured at a "high level of antitoxin." The Glenny and Barr system is described in Section 18.A.1.

Accordingly, it is recommended that one determine the neutralizing titer of any serum at different concentrations (see Subsection ii). For diphtheria antitoxin, it is easy to use the Lr/10, Lr/100, Lr/1000 levels.

The dilution ratio for anti-diphtheria sera, according to the Cinader and Weitz notation,[10, 11] is the ratio of the titers, calculated for undiluted serum, as determined at the Lr/10 and Lr/1000 levels. For tetanal antitoxin, titers can be determined in mice at the L+/5 and L+/250 levels. The dilution ratio will be the ratio of titers determined at these levels.

For *avid sera* the dilution ratio is *equal to or less than unity*. With sera of this type, the apparently higher value observed at low antibody concentrations depends on the use of an end point (Lr or L+) which differs from the neutral L_0 end point, and corresponds to a toxin–antitoxin mixture containing a given fixed amount of *free toxin;* for details see Cinader and Weitz.[10] This effect may be of a significant numerical value; indeed the dilution ratios may be as low as 0.45 for certain antitetanal sera.

For *nonavid sera*, the dilution ratio is greater than 1.0. Ratios of the order of 1.5, 2, 4, 6, and even larger may be encountered. The reduction in titer at low concentrations of antibodies is attributed to a dissociation of the neutral or just-neutral mixtures by dilution.

One must note that the dilution ratio of Glenny and Barr,[5] as defined for diphtheria antitoxin, is the inverse of the dilution ratio introduced by Cinader and Weitz[10, 11] for tetanus antitoxin.

(b) *Determination of Avidity by Jerne's Methods.** The dilution ratio method, as emphasized in the important studies of Jerne,[6] gives different values in tests made with various toxin concentrations and nonavid antisera; i.e., curves describing neutralization are not parallel. To draw such curves, it was necessary to measure free toxin as the neutral point was

[9] B. Cinader, "The Interaction of Tetanus Toxin and Antitoxin," Thesis, Univ. of London, 1948.
[10] B. Cinader and B. Weitz, *J. Hyg.* **51**, 293 (1953).
[11] B. Cinader and B. Weitz, *Nature (London)* **166**, 785 (1950).

* Section 18.A.3.b.iii.(b) was contributed by Merrill W. Chase.

approached. For this purpose, rabbits were injected intradermally with graded doses of one crude, stable preparation of toxin, and measurement was made at 44 hours of the diameter of dermonecrosis or reddening. Jerne's scale is shown on the left ordinate of Fig. 1, and his findings

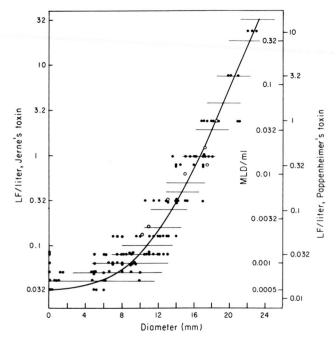

Fɪɢ. 1. Reactions produced by graded doses of diphtheria toxin upon intradermal injection into rabbits. The curve and left-hand scale (1550 reactions on 54 rabbits) are constructed from data of N. K. Jerne [*Acta Pathol. Microbiol. Scand.*, Suppl. 87 (1951)] and represent data secured with a stable, crude toxin. The *experimental* points were found when a purified toxin was used, confirming the general validity of the curve. Right scale and points: tentative results with purified toxin.

served to construct the solid-line curve of Fig. 1, the final horizontal lines indicating the spread in his values. The present writer, employing a rather highly purified toxin of Cohn and Pappenheimer,* duplicated the Jerne curve in 109 trials (experimental points plotted vs the right-hand scale of Fig. 1). The purified toxin contained about 3 times more toxin per ml than Jerne's crude toxin–toxoid mixture; e.g., essentially all of the

* The particular toxin contained 99,200 MLD/ml, an estimated 2060 Lf/ml, 1350 μg of TCA-precipitable N per milliliter, and 1140 μg of toxin-N per milliliter. See M. Cohn and A. M. Pappenheimer, Jr., *J. Immunol.* **63**, 291 (1949). [Preparations of toxin of this degree of purity are described by A. M. Pappenheimer, Jr., *J. Biol. Chem.* **120**, 543 (1937); **125**, 201 (1938).]

flocculating activity of the purified toxin was represented by toxin. It is also evident from Fig. 1 that individual rabbits vary considerably in their response to very small amounts of toxin, necessitating determination of multiple experimental points near the toe of the curve.

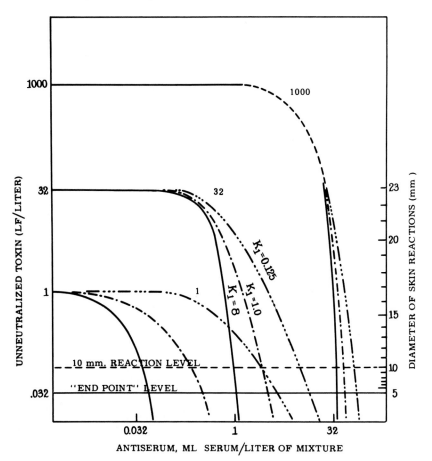

Fig. 2. Neutralization of toxin by antisera of various avidities. ——, $K_1 = 8$, hyperimmune sera; – • –, $K_1 = 1$, typical of rabbit and second stimulus sera of other animals, – • • • – • • •, $K_1 = $ ca 0.125, typical of first antibody produced by horse, human, guinea pig, ferret. Adapted from data of N. K. Jerne, *Acta Pathol. Microbiol. Scand.*, Suppl. 87 (1951).

Employing this basic curve and testing for free toxin in mixtures of various antitoxins incubated with his toxin, Jerne epitomized sera of different avidities (Fig. 2); for calculations of values for constant K_1, the reader is referred to the original monograph.[6] Figure 2 represents experiments with toxin and antitoxin at 1, 32, and 1000 Lf/liter (Jerne's toxin) made with sera of widely different avidities; the "end point" concentration is the limit of detectability of free toxin by intradermal injection. Diameters of observed dermonecrosis or redness are given by the right-hand scale. Where the initial concentration of reactants is very high (the "1000" curve), hardly any difference is observed among the various toxins. But upon further dilution (the "32" and "1" curves), great and nonparallel differences appear with antitoxin specimens of lower avidity.

(i) *Principles of tests for avidity.* For use as a practical research tool, we adapted Jerne's "variant method" to our purposes[12] and found it to be well suited. It exploits the differences between the neutralization curves at Jerne's "1 Lf/liter" and higher concentrations, such as at Jerne's "32 Lf/liter" (Fig. 2, examples with avidities of $K_1 = 1.0$; also see Fig. 20A of Jerne's monograph[6]). We have generally used a 50:1 difference rather than the 32:1 shown in these examples. Two series of mixtures are prepared, one employing nearly optimal conditions for neutralization and the other suboptimal conditions for neutralization. For optimal conditions, we chose the Q_{50} procedure, or method B, in which a high initial concentration of toxin (50×0.4 Lf/liter of our toxin) is allowed to react with high initial concentrations of antitoxin, and incubated for 4 hours at 37°. Then, just before injecting the rabbit, each mixture is diluted 1:50 to provide tests based on toxin at 0.4 Lf/liter. In the second series, termed method A, the toxin is used directly at 0.4 Lf/liter with various concentrations of antitoxin, and mixtures are incubated for only 5 minutes at 37° before injection into the same rabbit.

Two examples of the method are presented (Fig. 3). The left-hand column gives the logarithm of the final concentration (fc)* of standard antitoxin in each injection mixture (see AU per liter), or, for experimental sera, the final concentration in terms of milliliters per liter. The *working concentrations* of both antitoxins used for method A are shown. The *working concentrations* for use in method B are 50 times greater (the toxin also is 50 times greater) during incubation, but final 1:50 dilution gives the final concentration of antitoxin as injected. Entries in the various columns are readings of reaction diameters (millimeters) at 72 hours. These values are plotted in Fig. 4, curves then being constructed to pass through the "end point." With International Standard Antitoxin, there is at best only a 4-fold difference between the efficient Q_{50} method B and the inefficient method A. But with the first bleeding of rabbit No. 4967 (Figs. 3 and 4), the story is quite different: curves secured with

[12] M. W. Chase and O. A. Wager, *Fed. Proc., Fed. Amer. Soc. Exp. Biol.* **16**, 638 (1957).

* See footnote to Section 18.A.3.b.i.(c).

Log fc AU/liter or Ml serum/liter	International Standard Antitoxin (horse)		Experimental Rabbit Antitoxin Tx IV b, No. 4967, 13th day	
	A	B	A	B
1.4			0, 0, 0 ——	
1.3			0, 0, 12 ?	
1.2.			5, 5, 8, 8	
1.1			6, 8, 12	
1.0			6, 9, 11, 13	
0.9			11, 12	
0.8			12, 16. 17	
0.7	0			
0.6	0, 0		11, 16, 18	
0.5	0			
0.4	0, 0		13, 17	
0.3	0			
0.2	0, 0		19	—0, 0, 5 ——
0.1	0, 0, 0 ——	0		5, 5
0	0, 0, 0, 0 ?5, 8, 8	0	17	0, 5, 5, 5
- 0.1	0, 10, 12, 12, 13	0, 0		5, 7, 8, 8
- 0.2	0? 0? 13, 13	0, 0, 0, 0	15	5, 6, 6. 10
- 0.3		0, 0, 0, 0		9, 10
- 0.4	11, 15	0, 0, 0, 0, 0 ——		11, 14, 14, 15
- 0.5		0, 0? 12		
- 0.6		5, 8, 12, 12, 13, 14, 14		15
- 0.7		11, 12, 13, 13		
- 0.8		14, 14		
- 0.9		14, 15		
- 1.0		12, 13, 17		
- 1.1				
- 1.2		14, 16		

FIG. 3. Avidity determined by differences in neutralization between procedures A and B. The tests were made with the purified Cohn–Pappenheimer toxin described in the text, here used at 0.4 Lf/ liter *fc*.

this serum of low avidity (milliliters of serum per liter *fc*) cross the "end point" at widely different places: the inefficient method A requires approximately sixteen times as much antitoxin to neutralize the same amount of toxin as by the Q_{50} method B.

For research purposes, we could very well determine 3 or 4 characteristically different curves of neutralization with guinea pig antitoxins during the course of immunizing injections.

(*ii*) *Planning utilization of the rabbit.* For maximal utilization of skin on a rabbit in resting hair phase (or in practical absence of "hair islands"), 36 squares may be used on each side by drawing four lines from neck to pelvic girdle on each half of the back with a wetted indelible pencil, and also 13 crosslines. Not all of these are to be regarded as *prime sites* which are required for studying neutralization (see p. 298), but the extra sites have utilitarian value. The *prime* sites are 40 squares on the back; the cephalad 4 and the caudal 4 are second grade; the 24 *flank* squares are apt to be overly responsive.

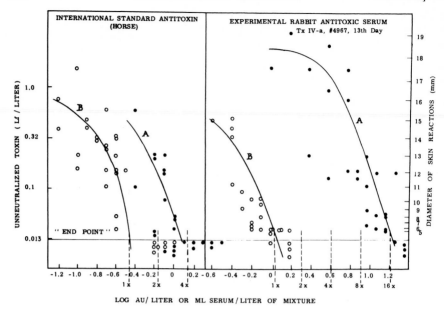

Fig. 4. Graphic representation of antitoxins of high and low avidity. Plots are of data shown in Fig. 3.

Mixtures of toxin and antitoxin are randomized carefully over the grid to isolate the expected stronger toxic reactions in nonprime sites.

For practical purposes, the rabbit must not be subjected to a large number of hardly neutralized toxin sites, hence the prime areas should be used for almost-neutral mixtures. Obviously suitable concentrations can be known only from prior experience. Accordingly, the flank sites and sites *above* the caudal margin of the scapulae and *below* the ileal crests (p. 307) are useful in preliminary tests where information is wanting regarding the approximate titer of a particular antitoxin.

(*iii*) *Avidity determinations (Jerne's Variant Method)*. To carry out the procedure, it is necessary to dilute a particular toxin to equal the reactions given by "1 LF" of Jerne's toxin-toxoid preparation (Fig. 1), i.e., to produce direct reactions in rabbit skin which fall within the range of 8 to 13 mm at 72 hours. In the case of the particular toxin which we used (see footnote on p. 304) it was necessary to dilute the dose which was just neutralized by one volume of 0.01 AU/ml of standard antitoxin to 1:7.75 to serve as half-volume. For Q_{50} mixtures, the hv dose was 50 times greater.

To plan dilutions of an antitoxic serum, we proceeded as follows. The AU/ml of the serum, ascertained previously by the method of Section 18.A.3.b.i(c) was diluted to 0.01 AU/ml as usual and then by an additional 1:7.75. (Obviously, toxins containing toxoid would be adjusted to give the stated range of dermonecrosis, and the neutralizing dose of anti-toxin would be adjusted accordingly.) This value is adequate for planning the hv of the Q_{50} series: say that it is 1:13,400. Turning to Table IV, take the next lowest log-scale dilution (1:16,000) and plan further hv dilutions down to 1:100,000; after 6 log dilutions have been planned, one dilution can be skipped. Multiply these concentrations of serum by 50; then the actual dilutions to be made, expressed as reciprocals, are 315, (400), 500, 625, 800, 1000, (1600), 2000. The dilutions near the top and bottom of the series (those within parentheses) can be omitted.

For tubes of the A series, where only the dilute toxin will be used, choose the *next* lower log dilution, here 1:16,000, and lay out 13 *higher* concentrations (Table IV) expressed as reciprocals, namely 1000, (1250), 1600, (2000), 2500, (3150), 4000, (5000), 6250, (8000), 10,000, (12,500), and 16,000. On the first rabbit to be tested, the alternate dilutions (within parentheses) can be omitted.

Thirteen sectors on the grid will be needed. Also, a toxin "asymptotic value" is required, in which two sites receive, respectively (a) the amount of toxin that is used directly in the dilute series A and (b) a 50-fold dilution of concentrated toxin which has been incubated with an equal volume of buffer and then has been held at 37° with the Q_{50} series and finally similarly diluted 1:50. Further, we recommend that the individual rabbit's capacity to discriminate various amounts of free toxin be tested by using the regular amount of toxin with antitoxin at 0.01, 0.009, 0.082, and 0.0075 AU/ml described in Section 18.A.3.b.i.(c) (Titration of Unknown Antitoxins). Accordingly, 19 of the 44 to 48 sectors are committed. The remaining spaces can be used for testing other antitoxins. We often have secured preliminary curves on 4 antitoxins by using the flank rows for the mixtures having the *most* and the *least* antitoxin in each series. As one example of proper utilization, of 60 available squares injected on one rabbit, only 13 sites (including the toxin asymptotes) gave the stronger reactions, and all other sites also gave useful results. (Employing such a large number of sites is practicable only when avidity determinations are being run with dilute toxin.) With preliminary curves at hand, closer planning and the testing of dilutions in duplicate or triplicate on single rabbits will rapidly accumulate the data required to round out the curves and particularly to provide a multiplicity of values near the toe of the curve for method A. This is in fact the general procedure from which the data of Figs. 3 and 4 were obtained, for which several rabbits were used.

After the planned dilutions have been set up, they are placed in two series of carefully labeled tubes. The Q_{50} series has the 50-fold amount of toxin added and mixed well, after which the tubes are stoppered and placed in the 37° water bath for 4 hours. To the tubes of the other series, the dilute toxin is added sequentially, so that syringes can be loaded and injections made after exactly 5 minutes of contact at room temperature. These injections are timed to be finished just prior to the 4-hour incubation of the Q_{50} series. Then tubes of the Q_{50} series are removed singly from the bath, diluted 1:50, and injected. Teams of three persons are highly useful: one to dilute, one to fill syringes, and one to make injections (0.1-ml volumes).

In this way, the approximate AU/ml titer [Section 18.A.3.b.i.(c)] and a close estimate of avidity of the antitoxin can be secured readily. Empirical curve can be drawn, or one can calculate the Jerne K_1 constants.[6]

c. TITRATION OF TETANUS ANTITOXIN*†

The titration of tetanus antitoxin may be carried out in guinea pigs or mice. The results may be identical or different, depending on the serum. The mouse:guinea pig ratio (M:G) has been used as an indicator of the avidity of the sera.[10, 13]

i. Titration in Mice

(a) *Preliminary Determination of the L+/10 Dose of Tetanal Toxin in Mice.* Mixtures are prepared which contain, in a total volume of 0.5 ml,§ 0.1 International Antitoxin Unit and various amounts of tetanal toxin. The mixtures are incubated at room temperature for 1 hour. They are injected by the intramuscular route into albino Swiss mice weighing 17 to 20 gm. One uses at least 3 mice per mixture. Animals are observed for 5 days. One L+/10 dose of toxin represents the minimal amount which, mixed with 0.1 IAU, will cause the death in 4 days of all the animals of the group. (A 50% end point would be preferable from a statistical point of view.)

The International Standard tetanus antitoxic serum is a freeze dried preparation containing 1400 IAU per ampoule. The IAU of 1950 is twice the former (1928) unit and now corresponds to the American Unit.

(b) *Titration of an Unknown Serum.* Mixtures are prepared as in subsection (a) containing one L+/10 dose of tetanal toxin and various amounts of the unknown sera in a total volume of 0.5 ml.

---

* Sections 18.A.3.c through 18.A.3.f were contributed by M. Raynaud‡ and E. H. Relyveld.

‡ Deceased.

† For *in vitro* tests, see Section 18.A.2. The method given here follows *Bull. W. H. O.* Suppl. 2, p. 338 (1951) but uses L+/10 rather than L+/5.

[13] G. F. Petrie, *League Nat. Bull. Health Organ.* **10**, 113 (1943).

§ *Bull. W. H. O.* Suppl. 2, (1951) indicates volumes of 0.4 to 0.6 ml, with titration on the L+/5 level. Some laboratories employ total volumes of 1 ml or even 2 ml.

Incubation, injection, and period of observation of mice follows the routine of subsection (a). The mixture that contains the largest amount of antiserum yet will cause the death with symptoms of tetanus of all the mice of the group within 4 days contains 0.1 IAU. Some workers prefer to inject the mixtures by intraperitoneal route, but if so, the injection routine of subsection (a) must be altered likewise.

ii. Titration in Guinea Pigs

(a) Preliminary Determination of the L+/10 Dose of Toxin. The method is carried out as in mice, but the mixtures containing 0.1 IAU and various amounts of toxin are prepared in a total volume of 4 ml (certain laboratories prefer 2-ml volumes) incubated at room temperature for 1 hour and injected by the intramuscular route in the hind leg of guinea pigs weighing 340 to 370 gm. Three animals at least are used per mixture. The L+/dose (guinea pig) represents the minimal amount of toxin that will cause the death, with tetanal symptoms, of all the animals of the group in 4 days.

(b) Titration of an Unknown Serum. Mixtures are prepared containing 1 L+/10 dose of toxin [as determined in subsection ii.(a)] and various amounts of the unknown serum in a total volume of 4 ml. Incubation and injection are made in the same way. The mixture that contains the largest amount of antiserum yet causes the death of all the animals of the group in 4 days contains 0.1 IAU.

iii. Titration at L+/100 and L+/500 Levels

Titration of antitoxin in mice may be carried out at lower levels: L+/100, L+/500. Mixtures are prepared that contain 1/10 of a L+/10 dose of toxin (L+/100 level) and 1/50 of a L+/10 dose of toxin (L+/500 level) and various amounts of antitoxin, but it is recommended to determine the L+/100 or L+/500 dose of toxin as in Subsection i.(a) above. Incubation, injections, observation of animals are as in Subsection i.(b).

d. In Vivo TITRATION OF STAPHYLOCOCCAL TOXIN AND ANTITOXIN*

Activity of toxin is determined by intraperitoneal or intravenous injection in various dilutions. The minimal lethal dose (MLD) of toxin in the least amount that will, on the average, kill a mouse of 18–20 gm within 96 hours after injection.

The necrotic activity of toxin can also be determined by intradermal injection in rabbits or guinea pigs.

Antitoxin can be titrated as described for the diphtheria system, by

* For titration in vitro, see Section 18.A.2.d.

inoculating toxin–antitoxin mixtures intracutaneously into guinea pigs or rabbits.

Titrations are carried out in mice by inoculating 0.5-ml toxin–antitoxin mixtures intravenously or intraperitoneally. The test dose of toxin is the quantity that, mixed with 1 unit of antitoxin, causes death of the mice within 96 hours, or half the mice within 3 days.

e. Titration of Gas-Gangrene Antitoxins*†

Antitoxins are prepared by hyperimmunization of animals with toxoids obtained by formalin treatment of toxins of the following pathogenic species: *Clostridium perfringens* (*welchii*) types A, B, and C; *C. septicum*, *C. oedematiens*, *C. histolyticum*, and *C. sordellii*.

International standards of antitoxins are used for titration, titers are expressed in international antitoxic units (IAU) per milliliter. Titrations are carried out in albino Swiss mice weighing 19 ± 1 gm; injections of the toxin–antitoxin mixtures are made intravenously, with exception of *C. oedematiens* antitoxin titrations, which are carried out by the subcutaneous route.

Mixtures are made to contain, per milliliter, 2 IAU of antitoxin and various quantities of toxin in order to determine the L+ dose of toxin. Injections of 0.5 ml of each mixture into at least 4 mice are made after incubation at 37° for 45 minutes. One L+ dose of toxin represents the minimal amount which, mixed with 1 IAU of antitoxin, will cause the death of 50% of the animals in 48 hours in case of *C. perfringens* (*welchii*) type A toxin, in 96 hours in the case of *C. sordellii* toxin and in 72 hours in the case of the other toxins. Titrations of antitoxin preparations are carried out in the reverse manner: 1 ml of toxin containing 5 L+ units is mixed with 1 ml of various antitoxin dilutions (e.g., 1:20, 1:30, 1:40, etc.) and the volume of each mixture is adjusted to 2.5 ml. Injections are carried out as described after 45 minutes at 37°. The mixture giving 50% protection of the animals after 48, 72, or 96 hours contains 1 IAU of antitoxin in 0.5 ml.

f. Titration of Botulinus Antitoxins*

Antitoxins are prepared by hyperimmunization of animals with toxoids corresponding to toxins of types A, B, C, and E. Titrations of antitoxin are carried out in albino Swiss mice weighing 20 gm, the test dose being

---

* The methods given here follow the "Pharmacopée Française," 8th ed., Maison-Neuve, S. A., Sainte-Ruffine, Moselle, France, 1965.

† For titration *in vitro* of *Clostridium perfringens* (*C. welchii*) toxin and toxoid, see Section 18.A.2.e.

100 lethal doses of toxin.* One unit of antitoxin corresponds to the
est quantity which neutralizes the test dose of toxin completely. Bo
toxins are very stable and can be used for years if kept in the cold.
tion is carried out by determining the quantity that kills a mouse w
3 days and causes complete paralysis. Serum titrations are carrie
by mixing 5 test doses of toxin in 2.5 ml with the same volume of va
serum dilutions. Intramuscular injection of 1 ml of the mixture is car
out after incubation for 1 hour at 37°. Neutralization of botulinus to
by its corresponding antitoxin is the only useful method for showing
presence of the toxin in food. Neutralization tests are carried out on
tracts of foods made with saline or after suspected materials have be
cultured anaerobically. Tests are carried out in two steps: the lethal do
of the extract or the anaerobic culture fluid is first determined as de
scribed above. Mixtures of 2 to 10 lethal doses of toxin and 1:10 units
of *each* of the five type-specific antitoxins are then injected into mice.

Only one group of animals, namely, those receiving mixtures in which
the toxin is neutralized completely by the antitoxin, will survive. This
"typing" of the toxin is very important in selecting the appropriate
antitoxin.

* It would be preferable to employ an L+ dose of toxin, defined by a corresponding
International Standard.

B. Enzyme–Antibody Interactions*†

The common mechanisms that result in antibody-mediated modification of enzyme activity are now understood and can be used as powerful
tools in immunodiagnosis (e.g., genetic defects, viral leukemias) and in
the analysis of biological phenomena (e.g., genetics of antibody formation, evolution of macromolecules). In this section, we shall regard the
functional consequences of the enzyme–antibody reaction in terms of interaction between two sets of gene products; one set controlling antibody
specificity, the other set specifying enzyme structure.

1. CHARACTERIZATION OF ENZYME–ANTIBODY INTERACTION

Interaction between antibody, enzyme, and substrate is studied to investigate (i) mechanisms by which antibody modifies the activity of bio-

* Section 18.B was contributed by B. Cinader.

† The support of the Medical Research Council, particularly through Grant MT832,
of the National Cancer Institute of Canada, and of the Ontario Heart Foundation
is acknowledged. Thanks are due to Mr. L. Horvath for technical assistance with
the manuscript and to Dr. R. K. Murray and Dr. Sheinin, who have rewritten
and improved portions of Section 18.B.3.c.

logically active molecules (i.e., neutralization), (ii) structural features of enzyme molecules, including their immunochemical relation to precursors, (iii) differences between enzymes of different species to assess evolutionary relationships, (iv) polymorphisms, by examining the antigenic relationships between genetic variants of an enzyme, including those which are catalytically inert, (v) conformational aspects of allosteric enzymes, (vi) the nature of the lesions in inborn errors of metabolism, (vii) the relation between tumor viruses in terms of enzyme markers, such as reverse transcriptase, (viii) the relation between enzymes and derivatives prepared from them, and (ix) localization and quantitation of enzymes or of other antigens in or on cells. The value of studies, listed under (ii) to (ix), depends on the extent to which experimental design is based on the available analysis of the mechanism of antibody-mediated modification of the activity of enzyme action and the variables that affect this modification. For this reason, a major part of this chapter will deal with neutralization. Antibody specificity will be defined in terms of enzyme determinants that have direct or indirect functional relationships with the catalytic space. Antibody-mediated modification of enzyme activity depends on the specificities of the heterogeneous assembly of antibodies in a given antiserum. Factors that determine this heterogeneity must be taken into account in designing a strategy, appropriate for formulation of a particular problem. This aspect of enzyme immunology will form a second major component of this chapter. Applications of enzyme immunology to the solution of fundamental questions of biology and to immunodiagnosis depend on immunoenzymological comparisons. These are based on a common core of methods and strategies, but also require individual approaches that are peculiar to the goals of each type of comparison. In the third part of this chapter a selective guide to appropriate strategies and literature will be provided.

a. ACTIVITY OF PREINCUBATED COMPLEXES OF
   ANTIGEN AND ANTIBODY

The catalytic activity of antigen–antibody complexes is most conveniently determined by mixing constant quantities of enzymes with varying amounts of antibody; volume and protein concentration are kept constant by adding buffer and either normal serum or normal immunoglobulin.* After incubation, excess substrate is added to each tube

* Normal serum can have activating or inhibiting effects on enzymes, exemplified in the case of neuraminidase acting on small substrates [S. Fazekas de St. Groth, *Ann. N. Y. Acad. Sci.* **103**, 674 (1963)]. Similarly, normal γ-globulin was found to enhance the esterolytic activity of CĪ esterase [A. L. Haines and I. H. Lepow, *J. Immunol.* **92**, 479 (1964); I. H. Lepow, *Ann. N. Y. Acad. Sci.* **103**, 829 (1963)]; and normal serum enhanced the activity of glutamate dehydrogenase [B. J. Johnson and D. H. Klemper, *J. Pharm. Sci.* **62**, 1887 (1973)].

and the enzyme activity is measured. The activity is plotted as a function of the quantity of antibody in the system. The enzyme activity generally decreases rapidly at first as antibody increases, and reaches a constant value at higher antibody concentrations (Fig. 1). The magnitude of the residual activity in antibody excess is of practical and theoretical importance in characterizing the interactions between antigen, antibody,

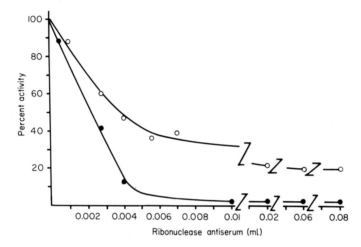

FIG. 1. A comparison of the effect of antibody on ribonuclease in the presence of nucleic acid and cyclic cytidylic acid as substrates. Assays were carried out manometrically. All mixtures contained the same amount of enzyme and various amounts of antibody. The mixtures were incubated at 37° for 30 minutes before the addition of substrate. O——O, cyclic cytidylic acid as substrate; ●——●, nucleic acid as substrate. After M. Branster and B. Cinader, *J. Immunol.* **87**, 18 (1961).

and substrate (Table I). Antisera obtained from an individual animal at various stages in the course of prolonged immunization, differ from one another in inhibitory capacity (Section 18.B.1.d). The residual activity in antibody excess depends also on the molecular size of the substrate, as originally demonstrated in the case of ribonuclease and later confirmed with many other enzymes, such as neuraminidase, C1-esterase, trypsin (Section 18.B.2.b).[1-4] It is essential to determine the residual level of activity with considerable precision, and to determine whether this level of activity is constant by measuring it, in antibody excess, over a 5- or

---

[1] M. Branster and B. Cinader, *J. Immunol.* **87**, 18 (1961).
[2] S. Fazekas de St. Groth, *Ann. N. Y. Acad. Sci.* **103**, 674 (1963).
[3] I. H. Lepow, *Ann. N. Y. Acad. Sci.* **103**, 829 (1963).
[4] R. Arnon, *in* "Antibodies to Biologically Active Molecules" (B. Cinader, ed.), Vol. 1, p. 153. Pergamon, Oxford, 1967.

TABLE I

DEGREE OF INHIBITION BY EXCESS ANTIBODY AND MOLECULAR WEIGHT OF SUBSTRATE

Enzyme			Substrate		Inhibition (%)	Reference[c]
EC No.[a]	Name	Source	Designation	Molecular weight[b]		
1.1.1.27	Lactic dehydrogenase	Rat muscle	NADH	664	45–75	1
		Rabbit muscle	Pyruvic acid	88	60, 73	2
		Schistosoma mansoni			66	3, 4
1.2.1.12	D-Glyceraldehyde-3 phosphate dehydrogenase	Yeast	NAD / 3-Phosphoglyceraldehyde	663 / 170	90–95	5
		Rabbit, rat skeletal muscle	NADH / 3-Phosphoglyceraldehyde	664 / 170	20–60	6
1.2.3.2	Xanthine oxidase	Mammalian	Xanthine	152	65	7, 8
1.4.1.2	l-Glutamic dehydrogenase	Beef liver	NAD / Glutamic acid	663 / 147	>70	9
1.11.1.6	Catalase	Beef liver	Hydrogen peroxide	34	6–3 (precipitate 27–63)	10
					None	11
					35–60	12, 13
1.13.11.11	Tryptophanase	*Escherichia coli*	Tryptophan / Pyridoxal phosphate	204 / 247	100	14, 15
1.14.18.1	Tyrosinase	*Psalliota campestris* / *Neurospora* / *Glomerella cingulata* / *Russula*	Tyrosine	181	None, 100 / None / 50–80 / 100	16, 17 / 18 / 19 / 20
2.4.1.1	α-Glucan phosphorylase	Dog liver	Glucose 1-phosphate	260	100	21
		Cock breast muscle	Glycogen		100	22
		Rabbit skeletal muscle			100	23

EC number	Enzyme	Source	Substrate		%	Reference
2.7.1.1	Hexokinase	Yeast	Glucose	180	100	24
			ATP	507	100	
2.7.3.2	Creatine-ATP phospho-transferase	Rabbit muscle	Creatine	131	100	25
			ATP	507	100	
2.7.7.6	RNA polymerase	Escherichia coli	DNA	—	~100	26
			ATP	507	—	
			GTP	523	—	
			UTP	484	—	
			CTP	483	—	
	RNA polymerase, form II	Calf thymus	Ditto for five substrates		94	27
	Reverse transcriptase (RNA-dependent DNA polymerase)	Murine leukemia virus	Poly(rA)oligo(dT)(12–18)			
			dATP	491	99	28
			dGTP	507		
			dCTP	467	95	29
			dTTP	482		
3.1.1.3	Lipase	Mycobacterium phlei	Tributyrate glycerol	302	100	30
3.1.1.4	Lecithinase (phospholipase A)	Crotalus terrificus	Lecithin (emulsion)	—	100	31
		Bee	Egg yolk	—	≥80	32
3.1.3.1	Alkaline phosphatase	Dog intestine	β-Glycerophosphoric acid	172	None	33, 34
		Mouse (20–25-day-old) duodenum	Phenylphosphoric acid	174	None	35
3.1.3.21	α-Glycerolphosphatase (glycerol-1-phosphatase)	Yeast	Ca-α-glycerophosphate	210	100	36
3.1.4.3	Lecithinase (phospholipase C)	Clostridium welchii	Lecithin (emulsion)	—	100	31, 37–39
3.1.4.5	Deoxyribonuclease	Streptococcus	Deoxyribonucleic acid	—	100	40
		Beef pancreas		—	~100	41
		Bothrops jararaca		—	≥87	42
3.1.4.7	Nuclease	Staphylococcus aureus	Denatured DNA	—	~100	43–47

(continued)

TABLE I (Continued)

EC No.[a]	Name	Source	Substrate Designation	Molecular weight[b]	Inhibition (%)	Reference[c]
3.1.4.22	D-Ribonuclease	Beef pancreas	Ribonucleic acid	—	20–30, up to 98	48–50
		Bothrops jararaca			2–3 × Acty[n]	51–54
					100	55
		Beef pancreas	Cytidine 2′:3′-cyclic phosphate	306	20–50, 200	48, 49, 51–54
	CĪ-esterase	Human	N-Acetyl-L-tyrosine ethyl ester	237	15–53	56, 57
			C4	—	100	
3.2.1.1	Amylase	Barley			95	58
		Hog pancreas			≥95	59, 60
		Human saliva	Starch		≥84	61
		Bacillus subtilis			90	62, 63
		Aspergillus oryzae			90, 94	64–66
3.2.1.17	Lysozyme	Avian	Penta-N-acetylglucosamine	1028	~50	67–71
		Micrococcus lysodeikticus			~100	72–75
3.2.1.18	Neuraminidase	Influenza virus	Sialyl lactose	633	0	76
			Sialyl glycoproteins	>10^5	100	76
3.2.1.20	Acid-α-glucosidase (α-D-glucoside glucohydrolase)	Human placenta	Maltose	342	50	77
			Methyl umbelliferyl Glucopyranoside	338	50	
			Glycogen		98	
		Rat liver	Maltose	342	2	
			Glycogen		95	

EC No.	Enzyme	Source	Substrate			Ref.
3.2.1.23	β-Galactosidase	Escherichia coli	Lactose	342	None	78–82
3.2.1.35	Hyaluronidase	Clostridium welchii	Mucoprotein (umbilical cord)		100	83
	Carbohydrase	Bee			~100	32
		Bacillus palustris	Pneumococcus type III, type VIII, polysaccharides		~100	84
3.4.22.4	Bromelain	Pineapple stem	α-N-Benzoyl-L-arginine ethyl ester	305	~60	85
			Casein		~100	
3.4.12.2	Carboxypeptidase	Beef	Carbobenzoxyglycyl-L-tryptophan	365	≥70	86–89
3.4.21.4	Trypsin	Bovine	Benzoyl-arginine-p-nitroanilide	398	23	90
			Casein		87	
3.4.21.11	Elastase	Pig pancreas	Orcein-elastin		100	91
3.4.22.2	Papain	Carica papaya latex	Benzoylarginine-p-nitroanilide	398	70	90, 92
			Gelatin		72–200	93, 94
			Casein		58–95	90, 92, 93, 95
	Tropomyosinase	η-Antigen; Clostridium oedematiens	Tropomyosin		~100	96
3.4.23.2	Gelatinase	Clostridium tetani	Gelatin		100	97
3.4.23.7.	Streptococcus peptidase A	Group A type 3 hemolytic streptococcus	Protein extract from muscle; diazotized skin proteins		100	98
3.4.24.3	Collagenase	Clostridium welchii	Collagen		100	99
		Clostridium histolyticum			40	100
3.5.1.1	L-Asparaginase	Mycobacterium bovis (BCG strain) E. coli	L-Asparagine	133	60–150	100a
3.5.1.5	Urease	Jack bean	Urea	60	50	101
					66, 78.5	102, 103

(continued)

TABLE I (Continued)

Enzyme			Substrate		Inhibition (%)	Reference[c]
Designation		Source	Designation	Molecular weight[b]		
EC No.[a]	Name					
3.5.2.6	Penicillinase	B. cereus Strain 569 Strain 5/H B. subtilis, strain 749 B. licheniformis strain 749	Penicillin	254–366	98–100 40 90	104, 105 105, 106 107, 108
			Benzylpenicillin	—	50	109
			Methicillin	—	$10 \times$ Acty[n]	
			Cephalosporin	415	~25	
			Benzylcephalosporin	390	~25	
3.5.4.6	5'-Adenylic acid deaminase	—	AMP	347	100	110
3.6.1.3	Adenosinetriphosphatase	Chicken leg muscle Micrococcus lysodeikticus	ATP	507	None 100	110 111, 112
4.1.1.15	Glutamic acid decarboxylase	Mouse brain	L-Glutamic acid	146	50	113
4.2.1.20	Tryptophan synthetase	Neurospora crassa	Indole Serine Pyridoxal phosphate	117 105 247	100	114, 115 116–118 119
5.3.1.9	Phosphoglucose isomerase	Schistosoma mansoni Dog liver	Fructose 6-phosphate Glucose 6-phosphate	260 260	≥ 53 > 68	120 121
6.4.1.1	Pyruvate carboxylase	Yeast	Pyruvic acid	88	100	122

[a] Enzyme numbers are taken from "Enzyme Nomenclature," Recommendations (1972) of the International Union of Pure and Applied Chemistry and the International Union of Biochemistry. Elsevier, Amsterdam, 1973.

[b] No value is given for macromolecules (molecular weight in excess of 10,000).

*Key to references:

1. F. Kubowitz and P. Ott, *Biochem. Z.* **314**, 94 (1943).
2. T. E. Mansour, E. Bueding, and A. B. Stavitsky, *Brit. J. Pharmacol.* **9**, 182 (1954).
3. K. F. Gregory and F. Wróblewski, *J. Immunol.* **81**, 359 (1958).
4. W. F. Henion, T. E. Mansour, and E. Bueding, *Exp. Parasitol.* **4**, 40 (1955).
5. E. G. Krebs and V. A. Najjar, *J. Exp. Med.* **88**, 569 (1948).
6. N. G. Nagradova and I. D. Grozdova, *Biochim. Biophys. Acta* **342**, 105 (1974).
7. J. E. Ultmann, P. Feigelson, and S. Harris, *J. Immunol.* **88**, 113 (1962).
8. J. E. Ultmann and P. Feigelson, *Ann. N. Y. Acad. Sci.* **103**, 724 (1963).
9. A. J. Bollet, J. S. Davis, 4th, and J. O. Hurt, *J. Exp. Med.* **116**, 109 (1962).
10. D. H. Campbell and L. Fourt, *J. Biol. Chem.* **129**, 385 (1939).
11. M. G. Sevag and M. Zacco, *Riv. Ist. Sieroterap. Ital.* **28**, 181 (1953).
12. H. F. Deutsch and A. Saebra, *J. Biol. Chem.* **214**, 455 (1955).
13. R. N. Feinstein, B. N. Jaroslow, J. B. Howard, and J. T. Faulhaber, *J. Immunol.* **106**, 1316 (1971).
14. D. E. Dolby, D. A. Hall, and F. C. Happold, *Brit. J. Exp. Pathol.* **33**, 304 (1952).
15. W. Kümmerling, *Z. Immunitaesforsch.* **103**, 425 (1943).
16. M. H. Adams, *J. Exp. Med.* **76**, 175 (1942).
17. I. W. Sizer, *Science* **116**, 275 (1952).
18. H. Gershowitz, R. D. Owen, and N. H. Horowitz, unpublished data.
19. R. D. Owen and C. L. Markert, *J. Immunol.* **74**, 257 (1955).
20. C. Gessard, *C. R. Soc. Biol.* **54**, 551 (1902).
21. W. F. Henion and E. W. Sutherland, *J. Biol. Chem.* **224**, 477 (1957).
22. I. Jokay, G. Bot, and T. Szilagyi, *Acta Physiol. Acad. Sci. Hung.* **14**, 155 (1958).
23. M. C. Michaelides, R. Sherman, and E. Helmreich, *J. Biol. Chem.* **239**, 4171 (1964).
24. R. E. Miller, V. Z. Pasternak, and M. G. Sevag, *J. Bacteriol.* **58**, 621 (1949).
25. A. J. Samuels, *Biophys. J.* **1**, 437 (1961).
26. J. M. Dubert, B. Hermier, and C. Babinet, *Biochimie* **53**, 185 (1971).
27. C. J. Ingles, *Biochem. Biophys. Res. Commun.* **55**, 364 (1973).
28. E. M. Scolnick, W. P. Parks, G. J. Todaro, and S. A. Aaronson, *Nature (London) (New Biol.)* **235**, 35 (1972).
29. W. P. Parks, E. M. Scolnick, J. Ross, G. J. Todaro, and S. A. Aaronson, *J. Virol.* **9**, 110 (1972).
30. A. Sartory and J. Meyer, *C. R. Soc. Biol.* **225**, 79 (1947).
31. P. C. Zamecnik and F. Lipmann, *J. Exp. Med.* **85**, 395 (1947).
32. E. Habermann and M. M. A. El Karemi, *Nature (London)* **178**, 1349 (1956).

33. M. Schlamowitz, *J. Biol. Chem.* **206**, 361 (1954).

34. L. Korngold, *Int. Arch. Allergy Appl. Immunol.* **37**, 366 (1970).

35. F. Moog and P. U. Angeletti, *Biochim. Biophys. Acta* **60**, 440 (1962).

36. M. G. Sevag, M. D. Newcomb, and R. E. Miller, *J. Immunol.* **72**, 1 (1954).

37. B. Cinader, *Biochem. Soc. Symp.* **10**, 16 (1953).

38. B. Cinader, *Bull. Soc. Chim. Biol.* **37**, 761 (1955).

39. M. G. MacFarlane and B. C. J. G. Knight, *Biochem. J.* **35**, 884 (1941).

40. M. McCarty, *J. Exp. Med.* **90**, 543 (1949).

41. M. McCarty, *J. Gen. Physiol.* **29**, 123 (1946).

42. A. R. Taborda, L. C. Taborda, J. N. Williams, Jr., and C. A. Elvehjem, *J. Biol. Chem.* **195**, 207 (1952).

43. S. Fuchs, P. Cuatrecasas, D. A. Ontjes, and C. B. Anfinsen, *J. Biol. Chem.* **244**, 943 (1969).

44. D. H. Sachs, A. N. Schechter, A. Eastlake, and C. B. Anfinsen, *J. Immunol.* **109**, 1300 (1972).

45. D. H. Sachs, A. N. Schechter, A. Eastlake, and C. B. Anfinsen, *Biochemistry* **11**, 4268 (1972).

46. G. S. Omenn, D. A. Ontjes, and C. B. Anfinsen, *Biochemistry* **9**, 304 (1970).

47. G. S. Omenn, D. A. Ontjes, and C. B. Anfinsen, *Biochemistry* **9**, 313 (1970).

48. M. Branster and B. Cinader, *J. Immunol.* **87**, 18 (1961).

49. R. K. Brown, R. Delaney, L. Levine, and H. Van Vunakis, *J. Biol. Chem.* **234**, 2043 (1959).

50. J. Smolens and M. G. Sevag, *J. Gen. Physiol.* **26**, 11 (1942).

51. B. Cinader, *in* "Antibodies to Biologically Active Molecules" (B. Cinader, ed.), Vol. 1, p. 85. Pergamon, Oxford, 1967.

52. T. Suzuki, H. Pelichová, and B. Cinader, *J. Immunol.* **103**, 1366 (1969).

53. H. Pelichová, T. Suzuki, and B. Cinader, *J. Immunol.* **104**, 195 (1970).

54. B. Cinader, T. Suzuki, and H. Pelichová, *J. Immunol.* **106**, 1381 (1971).

55. A. R. Taborda, L. C. Taborda, J. N. Williams, Jr., and C. A. Elvehjem, *J. Biol. Chem.* **194**, 227 (1952).

56. A. L. Haines and I. H. Lepow, *J. Immunol.* **92**, 479 (1964).

57. I. H. Lepow, *Ann. N. Y. Acad. Sci.* **103**, 829 (1963).

58. H. Lüers and F. Albrecht, *Fermentforschung* **8**, 52 (1924).

59. R. L. McGeachin and J. M. Reynolds, *Biochim. Biophys. Acta* **39**, 531 (1960).

60. R. L. McGeachin and J. M. Reynolds, *Ann. N. Y. Acad. Sci.* **94**, 996 (1961).

61. R. L. McGeachin, J. M. Reynolds, and J. I. Huddleston, Jr., *Arch. Biochem. Biophys.* **93**, 387 (1961).

62. M. Nomura and T. Wada, *J. Biochem. (Tokyo)* **45**, 629 (1958).

63. T. Wada and M. Nomura, *J. Biochem. (Tokyo)* **45**, 639 (1958).

64. T. Amano, H. Fujio, S. Kishiguchi, Y. Noma, S. Shinka, and Y. Saiki, *Med. J. Osaka Univ.* **7**, 593 (1956).

65. T. Wada, *J. Biochem. (Tokyo)* **46**, 329 (1959).
66. T. Wada, *J. Biochem. (Tokyo)* **47**, 528 (1960).
67. R. Arnon, *Eur. J. Biochem.* **5**, 583 (1968).
68. S. Shinka, M. Imanishi, O. Kuwahara, H. Fujio, and T. Amano, *Biken J.* **5**, 181 (1962).
69. M. Imanishi, H. Fujio, M. Sakahoshi, and T. Amano, *2nd Symp. Immunochem.*, Abstract p. 45 *Tokyo, 1968*.
70. H. Fujio, M. Imanishi, K. Nishioka, and T. Amano, *Biken J.* **11**, 207 (1968).
71. H. Fujio, M. Imanishi, K. Nishioka, and T. Amano, *Biken J.* **11**, 219 (1968).
72. H. Fujio, S. Kishiguchi, S. Shinka, Y. Saiki, and T. Amano, *Biken J.* **2**, 56 (1959).
73. E. A. H. Robert, *Quart. J. Exp. Physiol.* **27**, 89 (1937).
74. J. Smolens and J. Charney, *J. Bacteriol.* **54**, 101 (1947).
75. L. R. Wetter and H. F. Deutsch, *J. Biol. Chem.* **192**, 237 (1951).
76. S. Fazekas De St. Groth, *Ann. N. Y. Acad. Sci.* **103**, 674 (1963).
77. T. De Barsy, P. Jaquemin, P. Devos, and H.-G. Hers, *Eur. J. Biochem.* **31**, 156 (1972).
78. M. Cohn and J. Monod, *Biochim. Biophys. Acta* **7**, 153 (1951).
79. M. Cohn and A. M. Torriani, *J. Immunol.* **69**, 471 (1952).
80. M. Cohn and A. M. Torriani, *Biochim. Biophys. Acta* **10**, 280 (1953).
81. W. Messer and F. Melchers, *in* "The Lactose Operon" (J. R. Backwith and D. Zipser, eds.), p. 305. Cold Spring Harbor Laboratory, Cold Spring Harbor, New York, 1969.
82. F. Celada, J. Ellis, K. Bodlund, and B. Rotman, *J. Exp. Med.* **134**, 751 (1971).
83. D. McClean and C. W. Hale, *Biochem. J.* **35**, 159 (1941).
84. G. M. Sickles and M. Shaw, *J. Immunol.* **64**, 21 (1950).
85. M. Sasaki, S. Iida, and T. Murachi, *Biochem. J. (Tokyo)* **73**, 367 (1973).
86. E. L. Smith, B. V. Jager, R. Lumry, and R. R. Glantz, *J. Biol. Chem.* **199**, 789 (1952).
87. H. I. Lehrer and H. Van Vunakis, *Immunochemistry* **2**, 255 (1965).
88. H. N. Beaty, *Biochim. Biophys. Acta* **124**, 362 (1966).
89. K. Amiraian and T. H. Plummer, Jr., *J. Immunol.* **107**, 547 (1971).
90. R. Arnon, *in* "Antibodies to Biologically Active Molecules" (B. Cinader, ed.), Vol. 1, p. 153. Pergamon, Oxford, 1967.
91. B. C. McIvor and H. D. Moon, *J. Immunol.* **88**, 274 (1962).
92. E. Shapira and R. Arnon, *Biochemistry* **6**, 3951 (1967).
93. R. Haas, *Biochem. Z.* **305**, 280 (1940).
94. G. Ramon, *Rev. Immunol.* **9**, 134 (1944–1945).
95. Y. Okada, S. Nakashima, M. Asahi, and Y. Yamamura, *J. Biochem. (Tokyo)* **56**, 190 (1964).

96. M. G. MacFarlane, *Biochem. J.* **61**, 308 (1955).
97. G. Ramon, *Rev. Immunol.* **9**, 139 (1944–1945).
98. E. W. Todd, *J. Exp. Med.* **85**, 591 (1947).
99. C. L. Oakley, G. H. Warrack, and W. E. Van Heyningen, *J. Pathol. Bacteriol.* **58**, 229 (1946).
100. E. Soru and O. Zaharia, *Mol. Cell. Biochem.* **4**, 131 (1974).
100a. E. Soru and O. Zaharia, *Immunochemistry* **11**, 791 (1974).
101. S. Baechtel and M. D. Prager, *Cancer Res.* **33**, 1966 (1973).
102. J. S. Kirk and J. B. Sumner, *J. Biol. Chem.* **94**, 21 (1931).
103. A. A. Marucci and M. M. Mayer, *Arch. Biochem. Biophys.* **54**, 330 (1955).
104. R. D. Housewright and R. J. Henry, *J. Bacteriol.* **53**, 241 (1947).
105. M. R. Pollock, *J. Gen. Microbiol.* **14**, 90 (1956).
106. M. R. Pollock, *Ann. N. Y. Acad. Sci.* **103**, 989 (1963).
107. D. J. Kushner, *J. Gen. Microbiol.* **23**, 381 (1960).
108. M. R. Pollock, J. Fleming, and S. Petrie, *in* "Antibodies to Biologically Active Molecules" (B. Cinader, ed.), p. 139. Pergamon, Oxford, 1967.
109. M. R. Pollock, *Immunology* **7**, 707 (1964).
110. A. Samuels, *Arch. Biochem. Biophys.* **92**, 497 (1961).
111. T. L. Whiteside, A. J. De Siervo, and M. R. J. Salton, *J. Bacteriol.* **105**, 957 (1971).
112. V. Stewart, *in* "Progress in Immunology" (B. Amos, ed.), p. 1199. Academic Press, New York, 1971.
113. T. Matsuda, J.-Y. Wu, and E. Roberts, *J. Neurochem.* **21**, 159 (1973).
114. M. Rachmeler and C. Yanofsky, *J. Bacteriol.* **81**, 955 (1961).
115. C. J. Wust, *Biochim. Biophys. Acta* **54**, 172 (1961).
116. M. D. Garrick, and S. R. Suskind, *Ann. N. Y. Acad. Sci.* **103**, 793 (1963).
117. C. Yanofsky, *Ann. N. Y. Acad. Sci.* **103**, 1067 (1963).
118. C. Yanofsky and J. Stadler, *Proc. Nat. Acad. Sci. U.S.* **44**, 245 (1958).
119. S. R. Suskind, M. L. Wickham, and M. Carsiotis, *Ann. N. Y. Acad. Sci.* **103**, 1106 (1963).
120. E. Bueding and J. A. MacKinnon, *J. Biol. Chem.* **215**, 507 (1955).
121. M. N. Lipsett, R. B. Reisberg, and O. Bodansky, *Arch. Biochem. Biophys.* **84**, 171 (1959).
122. V. Z. Pasternak, M. G. Sevac, and R. E. Miller, *J. Bacteriol.* **61**, 189 (1951).

10-fold range of antibody concentration. This is not always possible, particularly with "early" antibody of low potency, in which event it is often useful to reverse the experimental conditions, i.e., to keep the amount of antibody constant and vary the amount of enzyme. Activities of these mixtures are then compared with those of different quantities of enzyme mixed with normal serum or normal immunoglobulin. When it is intended to correlate enzymatic activities with precipitable nitrogen from enzyme–antibody mixtures, the insoluble complexes, isolated from reaction mixtures, are tested for enzymatic activity by isolating and washing the precipitates in the same way as in the quantitative precipitin test. Care is needed in transferring the resuspended precipitate; this is best carried out by drawing up the precipitate repeatedly in a capillary pipette, until it is extremely well dispersed, before transferring aliquots of the resuspended precipitates. Second aliquots of the same mixtures are transferred after another dispersal, to show that sampling has been adequate. If the quantitative precipitin curve is based on experiments in which the antibody is kept constant and the antigen varied, these results can be converted very easily to plot total nitrogen precipitated for conditions in which the enzyme is constant and the antibody varied.

Comparison of the quantitative precipitin curve (nitrogen values) with corresponding curves based on activity determinations shows that antigen–antibody mixtures in *antigen* excess retain enzyme activity irrespective of the level of residual activity in *antibody* excess (Section 18.B.2.c.iii). Consequently, a series of enzyme–antibody precipitates, constituting a quantitative precipitin test, will *always* include precipitates showing some enzyme activity. Similarly, when antigen and antibody interact in agar, that part of the zone which is in antigen (enzyme) excess will *always* retain some enzyme activity.

Since products of enzyme action often can be converted into colored products, the enzymes precipitated by antibody in double diffusion, single diffusion, or immunoelectrophoresis can be localized as colored reaction products, this procedure being applicable to all enzyme–antibody reactions in agar.[5-11] This type of immunoenzymological procedure is applic-

[5] J. Uriel and J. J. Scheidegger, *Bull. Soc. Chim. Biol.* **37**, 165 (1955).

[6] J. Uriel, *Bull. Soc. Chim. Biol.* **39**, 105, Suppl. 1 (1957).

[7] J. Uriel, *Nature (London)* **188**, 853 (1960).

[8] J. Uriel, in "Analyse Immuno- électrophorétique, ses Applications aux Liquides Biologiques Humains" (P. Grabar and P. Burtin, eds.), pp. 33–56. Masson, Paris, 1960.

[9] J. Uriel, *Ann. Inst. Pasteur* **101**, (1961).

[10] J. Uriel, *Ann. N. Y. Acad. Sci.* **103**, 956 (1963).

[11] J. Uriel, T. Webb, and C. Lapresle, *Bull. Soc. Chim. Biol.* **42**, 1285 (1960).

able to the study of antigenic cellular constituents.[12-14] Antibodies conjugated with horseradish peroxidase, *Escherichia coli* alkaline phosphatase and *Aspergillus niger* glucose oxidase have been used for light microscopy; and antibodies conjugated with peroxidase, for electron microscopy. Enzymes can be coupled with antibodies by means of p,p'-difluoro-m,m'-dinitrophenyl sulfone, carbodiimide, glutaraldehyde, metaxylylene diisocyanate or by various types of antibody–sandwich techniques.[14-18] These techniques have been satisfactory for the ultrastructural localization of surface antigens. For intracellular detection of antigens, it has been found preferable to conjugate peroxidase, cytochrome c or a heme octapeptide with Fab.[19-22] Since the quantity of enzyme can be accurately determined colorimetrically, the quantity of enzyme-labeled antibodies can also be determined accurately and a measure of cellular antigen concentration can be deduced. This potential for sensitive quantitation of cellular antigens is the main advantage of the immunoenzyme techniques over other immunocytological techniques,[23] and may have some advantages over quantitation based on intensity of immunofluorescence.[24, 25]

The neutralization curve for enzyme–antibody complexes (Fig. 1) is the one encountered with most enzyme–antibody systems. However, another type of "neutralization curve" may be encountered in which antibody *activates* rather than inhibits enzyme activity, as is seen in the interaction between ribonuclease and an antiserum elicited with poly-

[12] S. Avrameas, *Histochem. J.* **4**, 321 (1972).

[13] G. A. Andres, K. G. Hsu, and B. C. Seegal, *in* "Handbook of Experimental Immunology, Immunologic Techniques for the Identification of Antigens or Antibodies by Electron Microscopy" (D. M. Weir, ed.), Vol. 2, p. 34. Alden & Mowbray, Oxford, 1973.

[14] L. D. Sternberger, ed., "Immunochemistry." Prentice-Hall, Englewood Cliffs, New Jersey, 1974.

[15] S. Avrameas, *Immunochemistry* **6**, 825 (1969).

[16] E. T. Mason, R. F. Phifer, S. S. Spicer, R. A. Swallow, and R. B. Dreslein, *J. Histochem. Cytochem.* **17**, 563 (1969).

[17] D. H. Clyne, S. H. Norris, R. R. Modesto, A. J. Pesce, and V. E. Pollack, *J. Histochem. Cytochem.* **21**, 233 (1973).

[18] I. Nagatsu, *Acta Histochem. Cytochem.* **7**, 147 (1974).

[19] T. Ternynck and S. Avrameas, *Biochem. J.* **125**, 297 (1971).

[20] J. P. Kraehenbuhl, P. D. De Grandi, and M. A. Lampiche, *J. Cell Biol.* **50**, 432 (1971).

[21] J. P. Kraehenbuhl, R. E. Gallardy, and J. D. Jamieson, *J. Exp. Med.* **139**, 208 (1974).

[22] W. D. Kühlmann, S. Avrameas, and T. Ternynck, *J. Immunol. Methods* **5**, 33 (1974).

[23] S. Avrameas and B. Guilbert, *Eur. J. Immunol.* **1**, 394 (1971).

[24] S. Avrameas, *in* "Immunological Approaches to Fertility Control" (E. Diczfalusy, ed.) *Karolinska Symp. Res. Methods Reprod. Endocrinol. 7th Symp.* Karolinska Institutet, p. 37. Stockholm, 1975.

[25] J. S. Haskill and M. J. Raymond, *J. Nat. Cancer Inst.* **51**, 159 (1973).

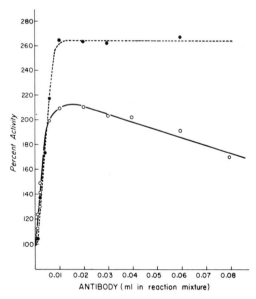

FIG. 2. A comparison of the effect of *activating* antibody on ribonuclease in the presence of nucleic acid and of cyclic cytidylic acid as substrates. Antibody was raised in a rabbit by immunization with polyalanine polytyrosine ribonuclease. Assays were carried out manometrically. All mixtures contained the same amount of native ribonuclease and various amounts of antibody, which were incubated at 37° for 30 minutes before the addition of substrate. ●---●, Cyclic cytidylic acid as substrate; ○——○, nucleic acid as substrate. After B. Cinader, *in* "Antibodies to Biologically Active Molecules" (B. Cinader, ed.), Pergamon, Oxford, 1967.

alanyl-polytyrosyl-ribonuclease,[26] between ribonuclease and selected antibody fractions,[27, 28] and in the interaction between penicillinase and its antibody.[29, 30] This antibody-imposed change of catalytic properties of the enzyme is not the same for each substrate.[27, 29, 30] For instance, activation of penicillinase was found with benzylpenicillin, 6-aminopenicillanic acid, and methicillin, while normal inhibition curves were found with cephalosporin C and benzylcephalosporin C. Complexing of enzyme with antibody lowered not only the maximum rate of substrate conversion (V_{max}), but also the affinity of the enzyme for substrate.[30] An activating effect of antibody has also been observed with ribonuclease as antigen. One rabbit, immunized with ribonuclease conjugated with alanine and

[26] B. Cinader, *in* "Antibodies to Biologically Active Molecules" (B. Cinader, ed.), Vol. 1, p. 85. Pergamon, Oxford, 1967.
[27] T. Suzuki, H. Pelichová, and B. Cinader, *J. Immunol.* **103,** 1366 (1969).
[28] H. Pelichová, T. Suzuki, and B. Cinader, *J. Immunol.* **104,** 195 (1970).
[29] M. R. Pollock, *Immunology* **7,** 707, 1964.
[30] M. Pollock, J. Fleming, and S. Petrie, *in* "Antibodies to Biologically Active Molecules" (B. Cinader, ed.), Vol. 1, p. 139. Pergamon, Oxford, 1967.

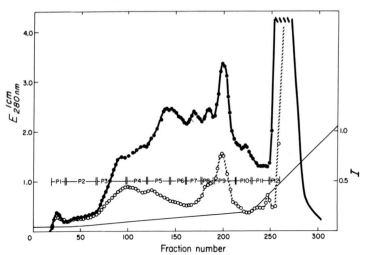

FIG. 3. Elution from DEAE-Sephadex A-50 of rabbit serum directed against bovine pancreatic ribonuclease. Antisera against ribonuclease A were obtained from 16 rabbits on the 255th day after the start of immunization. Normal rabbit sera were obtained from 10 rabbits. All sera were of allotypic specificity A(1+4+). ●——●, pool of ribonuclease (rabbit) antisera; ○···○, pool of normal rabbit sera. After T. Suzuki, H. Pelichová, and B. Cinader, *J. Immunol.* **103**, 1366 (1969).

tyrosine, consistently produced antibody showing this property. The relation between the amount of antibody added and enzyme activity is shown in Fig. 2, as is the effect of the molecular weight of substrate on these "neutralizing" curves[26] (Section 18.B.2.c.i). Antisera raised by immunization with native bovine ribonuclease contain largely inhibitory antibody, but also some antibody molecules that distort the substrate specificity of the enzyme.[27] Fractionation of antisera on DEAE-Sephadex A-50 (Fig. 3) results in separation of distinctive antibody mixtures. Some of them activate the catalytic action on cytidylic acid (P1, Fig. 4), while others inhibit in slight antibody excess, but inhibit less effectively in extreme antibody excess (P6, Fig. 4). Even though this type of activation is exceptional, neutralizing capacity cannot and must not be equated with the total binding capacity of antibody. This may be illustrated by the properties of fractions of lactate dehydrogenase antisera that were obtained by zonal ultracentrifugation in sucrose gradients or by elution from DEAE-cellulose. Some of the fractions gave high titers in passive agglutination but little enzyme inhibition, while others exercised a profound inhibitory effect, but no hemagglutinating capacity.[31] It is clear that en-

[31] C. W. Ng and K. F. Gregory, *Biochim. Biophys. Acta* **192**, 258 (1969).

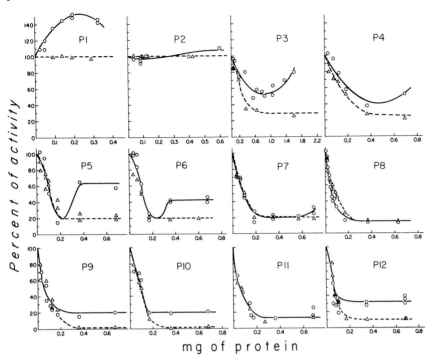

FIG. 4. Modification of enzyme-activity by chromatographic fractions of antiserum. A pool of antisera from 16 hyperimmunized rabbits was obtained on day 245 after the start of immunization. It was fractionated by chromatography over DEAE-Sephadex A-50 (see Fig. 3). The effect on enzyme activity of individual fractions was measured, using yeast ribonucleic acid (--△--) and cyclic cytidylic acid (—○—) as substrates. After T. Suzuki, H. Pelichová, and B. Cinader, *J. Immunol.* **103**, 1366 (1969).

zyme neutralization is a useful biological parameter only when it is linked with a measurement of total combining antibody by a technique that is independent of enzyme neutralization. This is particularly important in situations in which a correlation between titers of enzyme–antibody and a biological effect is to be established, as, for instance, in attempts to reduce fertility by immunization of females with the sperm-specific isozyme of lactate dehydrogenase.[32] In fact, there is much better correlation between fertility reduction and total antibody than there is between fertility reduction and enzyme-inhibiting antibody.[33]

---

[32] E. Goldberg, *in* "Immunological Approaches to Fertility Control" (E. Diczfalusy, ed.), Suppl. 194 *Karolinska Symp. Res. Methods in Reprod. Endocrinol. 7th Symp.* p. 202. Karolinska Institutet, Stockholm, 1975.

[33] E. Goldberg, personal communication.

b. INHIBITORY EFFECT OF ANTIBODY UNDER CONDITIONS
   OF SIMULTANEOUS ADDITION

We have so far dealt with the characterization of enzyme–antibody interactions by measuring the enzyme activity of an incubated mixture of enzyme and antibody, added to substrate. Alternatively, the reactivity can be measured when enzyme and antibody are not preincubated but are mixed in the presence of substrate (simultaneous addition). With most systems the same antibody shows less inhibitory capacity under conditions of simultaneous addition than it displays when combining with enzyme in the absence of substrate. The "protection of enzyme by substrate" has been found with amylase,[34] penicillinase,[35] lecithinase,[36, 37] carboxypeptidase,[38] old yellow enzyme,[39–41] 5'-adenylic acid deaminase,[42] tyrosinase,[43] phosphorylase,[44] and alcohol dehydrogenase.[45] Exceptions to the "protection by substrate" are lactic dehydrogenase[46] and creatine kinase[42] (for discussion, see reference 47). In this connection, it is important to note that the immunological reactivity of glutamic dehydrogenase is altered by regulator molecules, such as ADP or diethylstilbestrol.[48] It seems reasonable to assume that substrates or regulatory molecules may induce conformational changes and thus render some determinants unavailable for combination with antibody. This is the "revers de la médaille" of the situation, to be discussed in a subsequent section, in which antibody changes the conformation of the site which accommodates the substrate.

In dealing with four components, i.e., apoenzyme, antibody, coenzyme, and substrate, the system becomes somewhat more cumbersome to assay, since the effect of the simultaneous addition of apoenzyme and coenzyme on the one hand, of apoenzyme and substrate on the other, and finally

[34] H. Lüers and F. Albrecht, *Fermentforschung* 8, 52 (1924).
[35] R. D. Housewright and R. J. Henry, *J. Bacteriol.* 53, 241 (1947).
[36] B. Cinader, *Biochem. Soc. Symp.* 10, 16 (1953).
[37] P. C. Zamecnik and F. Lipmann, *J. Exp. Med.* 85, 395 (1947).
[38] E. L. Smith, B. V. Jager, R. Lumry, and R. R. Glantz, *J. Biol. Chem.* 199, 789 (1952).
[39] S. Kistner, *Acta Chem. Scand.* 12, 2034 (1958).
[40] S. Kistner, *Acta Chem. Scand.* 13, 1149 (1959).
[41] S. Kistner, *Acta Chem. Scand.* 14, 1441 (1960).
[42] A. J. Samuels, *Biophys. J.* 1, 437 (1961).
[43] R. D. Owen and C. L. Markert, *J. Immunol.* 74, 257 (1955).
[44] M. C. Michaelides, R. Sherman, and E. Helmreich, *J. Biol. Chem.* 239, 4171 (1964).
[45] T. C. Fuller and A. A. Marucci, *J. Immunol.* 106, 110 (1971).
[46] T. E. Mansour, E. Bueding, and A. B. Stavitsky, *Brit. J. Pharmacol.* 9, 182 (1954).
[47] B. Cinader, *Ann. N. Y. Acad. Sci.* 103, 495 (1963).
[48] N. Talal and G. M. Tomkins, *Biochim. Biophys. Acta* 89, 226 (1964).

of apoenzyme and substrate should be compared. Indeed, at least two cases are known in which the difference between simultaneous addition and preincubation can be demonstrated only if enzyme and antibody are added simultaneously with *all* the substrates. The first example of this type was creatine kinase, which requires two substrates and one cofactor, i.e., creatine hydrate, ATP, and Mg^{2+}.[49] Creatine kinase is not protected against antibody-neutralization by simultaneous addition of any one, or any pair, of these molecules, but only by the addition to enzyme, prior to antibody, of all three substrates.[42] Staphylococcal ornithine carbamoyl transferase is not protected against antibody neutralization by either one of its two substrates, alone. It is, however, protected by simultaneous preincubation with both its substrates: L-ornithine and carbamoyl phosphate.[49a]

The difference between the inhibitory capacity of antisera, when preincubated with enzyme, in the absence and in the presence of substrate, appears to be attributable to (i) substrate-induced conformational changes at the catalytic site and antibody directed against determinants in the neighborhood of the catalytic site. Direct evidence for the relation between configurational enzyme changes and combining capacity of different antibodies has been obtained in several systems. Staphylococcal nuclease provides an instructive illustration of such changes and of the functional relation between the effect of these changes on the combining capacity of different functional types of antibodies.[50] The precipitin reaction of nuclease-antinuclease in the presence of deoxythymidine 3′,5′-diphosphate and Ca^{2+} shows two separable peaks. The first and minor peak corresponds to antibodies which react with nuclease identically in the presence or absence of Ca^{2+} or substrate analogs. The second, major peak is due to antibody whose reaction with nuclease is inhibited by Ca^{2+} and certain nucleotides. Furthermore, nuclease, complexed with specific antibodies, is protected from irreversible inactivation by nitration with tetranitromethane.

In dealing with the effect of substrate concentration on the degree of neutralization, another and earlier example of the effect of Ca^{2+} on neutralization will be cited.[36] On the basis of these and similar experiments, the conclusion can be reached that some antibodies are directed against determinants that readily undergo conformational changes and that some, though not all, antibody molecules are able to combine firmly with only one of several configurational forms of a determinant. We shall, in sub-

[49] S. A. Kuby, L. Noda, and H. A. Lardy, *J. Biol. Chem.* **210**, 65 (1954).

[49a] O. Zaharia and E. Soru, *Rev. Roum. Biochim.* **8**, 285 (1971).

[50] S. Fuchs, P. Cuatrecasas, D. A. Ontjes, and C. B. Anfinsen, *J. Biol. Chem.* **244**, 943 (1969).

sequent sections, deal with configurational stabilization and configurational changes that can be induced by yet other types of antibodies. All these phenomena are dependent on antibody specificity and on the flexibility of the relevant antigenic determinant.

c. Effect of Substrate Concentration

To study the effect of concentration of substrate on the combination of enzyme and antibody, it is usually best to estimate the influence of substrate concentration under conditions of simultaneous additions, since it is well known that preincubated complexes of antigens and antibody are only very slowly dissociable.

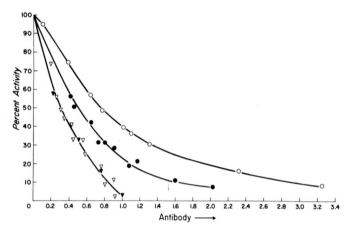

Fig. 5. The effect of $CaCl_2$ concentration on the combination of *Clostridium welchii* lecithinase with *C. welchii* equine antibody under conditions of preincubation (30 minutes, 37°) (—▼—, 0.0004 M $CaCl_2$; —▽—, 0.004 M $CaCl_2$) and of simultaneous addition (— ●—, 0.0004 M $CaCl_2$; —○—, 0.004 M $CaCl_2$). After B. Cinader, *Biochem. Soc. Symp.* **10**, 16 (1953).

No general picture has emerged as to the effect of substrate concentration on the activity of enzyme and antibody complexes. Upon mixing *Clostridium welchii* (*C. perfringens*) lecithinase and substrate, an increase in concentration of the enzyme activator, calcium, was seen to favor the reaction with substrate at the expense of combination between enzyme and antibody (Fig. 5), hence the neutralization curve of lecithinase was shifted toward higher concentrations of antitoxin.[36, 51] The difference between incubation and simultaneous addition might be thought to indicate the competitive nature of inhibition by antibody,[37] as does the effect of Ca^{2+} concentration in the lecithinase system.[36]

[51] B. Cinader, *Bull. Soc. Chim. Biol.* **37**, 761 (1955).

However, in the same system, a noncompetitive relation between antibody and substrate was observed when the substrate concentration was varied.[36] In other studies a marked effect of substrate concentration was observed when antibody was added to enzyme and substrate, or to enzyme and coenzyme.[43, 52-54] It has become apparent that these variations depend on antibody properties and that an antiserum may contain both types of antibody.

Antibodies to Taka-amylase could be separated, by chromatography, into fractions; the inhibitory capacity of one was dependent upon substrate concentration, the others were independent of substrate concentration.[55] In short, antibody inhibition depends on substrate concentration in some cases, and in other instances it does not.

It is important to realize that competitive inhibition cannot be demonstrated when the binding of the inhibitor, in our case antibody, to the enzyme shows much higher affinity than the combination between enzyme and substrate.[56-59] Accordingly, demonstration of competitiveness has much greater evidential value than demonstration of noncompetitive inhibition. At the same time, it must be stressed that competitiveness does not necessarily indicate combination with the catalytic site when a macromolecular inhibitor is involved. The macromolecule may block access to the catalytic site without direct combination with this site. The observation that inhibitory capacity of antibody depends on the molecular weight of substrates supports this view and provides evidence (Section 18.B.2.c) that enzymes can be inhibited by steric hindrance.[60, 61] The apparent paradox of inhibition outside the catalytic space and competitive kinetics will be resolved in a subsequent section.

d. HETEROGENEITY OF ANTIBODY

Antibodies exhibiting different properties are synthesized by different animals and by the same animal in the course of prolonged immunization. The heterogeneity of the responsiveness is the reason for differences ob-

[52] E. Bueding and J. A. MacKinnon, *J. Biol. Chem.* **215**, 507 (1955).

[53] W. F. Henion, T. E. Mansour, and E. Bueding, *Exp. Parasitol.* **4**, 40 (1955).

[54] M. N. Lipsett, R. B. Reisberg, and O. Bodansky, *Arch. Biochem. Biophys.* **84**, 171 (1959).

[55] Y. Matsouka, T. Hamaoka, and Y. Yamamura, *J. Biochem.* (*Tokyo*) **61**, 703 (1966).

[56] W. W. Ackermann and V. R. Potter, *Proc. Soc. Exp. Biol. Med.* **72**, 1 (1949).

[57] A. Goldstein, *J. Gen. Physiol.* **27**, 529 (1944).

[58] L. A. Day, J. M. Sturtevant, and S. J. Singer, *Ann. N. Y. Acad. Sci.* **103**, 611 (1963).

[59] A. H. Sehon, *Ann. N. Y. Acad. Sci.* **103**, 626 (1963).

[60] B. Cinader and K. J. Lafferty, *Ann. N. Y. Acad. Sci.* **103**, 653 (1963).

[61] B. Cinader and K. J. Lafferty, *Immunology* **7**, 342 (1964).

served in the effect of different antisera on the catalytic action of enzymes. Differences are primarily attributable to specificity and extend to firmness of combination and extent of hydrogen bonding (i.e., effective size of the antibody combining area).

A time-dependent increase of inhibitory capacity (antibody excess) was observed with antisera to ribonuclease obtained in the course of prolonged immunization[1] (Fig. 6); differences in inhibitory capacity of

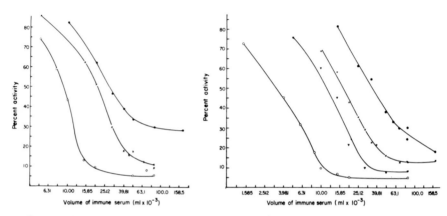

FIG. 6. Changes in the inhibitory capacity of ribonuclease antibody during prolonged immunization. All mixtures contained the same quantity of enzymes and different amounts of antibody. *Left:* Bleeding from rabbit 570: ●——●, serum 5 days after the fifth subcutaneous injection of ribonuclease in adjuvant; ✕——✕, serum 110 days later and 5 days after an intravenous injection in 0.15 M NaCl; ○——○, serum 356 days later and 5 days after the last of five further courses of intravenous injections in 0.15 M NaCl. *Right:* Bleeding from rabbit 619: ●——●, serum 5 days after a course of subcutaneous injections in adjuvant followed by one intravenous injection in 0.15 M NaCl; ✕——✕, serum 33 days later, 5 days after a further intravenous injection; ▽——▽, serum 31 days later, and 5 days after a course of three intravenous injections in 0.15 M NaCl; ○——○, serum 252 days later and 5 days after a course of three intravenous injections. After M. Branster and B. Cinader, *J. Immunol.* **87**, 18 (1961).

univalent Fab fragments I and II were found (Fig. 7) and provided evidence for competition between inhibitory and noninhibitory antibody molecules.[60, 61] The fractionation of ribonuclease antibody (Fig. 3) has provided further evidence for the functional heterogeneity of antibody (Fig. 4) and for the existence of antibodies that distort enzyme specificity and compete with inhibiting antibody.[27] The preceding observations have been confirmed in several systems. The functional heterogeneity of individual bleedings of animals has been demonstrated by chromatographic fractionation,[27, 31] by zonal ultracentrifugation in a sucrose gradient,[31]

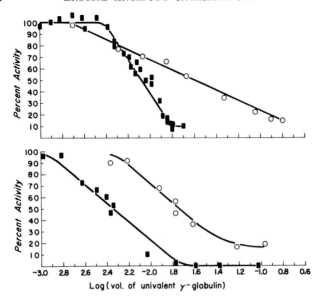

FIG. 7. Relative inhibitory capacities of univalent fragments I and II from papain digests of γ-globulins from two different pools of antisera. Constant amounts of ribonuclease were mixed with different amounts of antibody and incubated for 30 minutes at 37°. The activities of these mixtures were determined manometrically with nucleic acid as substrate at pH 7, and 37°. ■, Fraction I isolated from papain digest; ○, fraction II isolated from papain digest. After B. Cinader and K. J. Lafferty, *Immunology* **7**, 342 (1964).

by isoelectric focusing,[62] by absorption of antisera with limited amounts of the antigen,[29, 50, 63, 64] by absorption with structurally related molecules,[63, 65–67] and by dissociation of antigen–antibody complexes formed with native[68] or with configurationally altered enzyme molecules.[69] In the last-mentioned study, two fractions were obtained from an antiserum against Na^+, K^+-adenosine triphosphatase. One of these appeared to affect a digitalis glycoside receptor site or binding conformation, and the other a catalytic site or site-conformation.

[62] G. Köhler and F. Melchers, *Eur. J. Immunol.* **2**, 453 (1972).
[63] B. G. Carter, B. Cinader, and C. A. Ross, *Ann. N. Y. Acad. Sci.* **94**, 1004 (1961).
[64] N. Zyk and N. Citri, *Biochim. Biophys. Acta* **159**, 317 (1968).
[65] R. Arnon and E. Shapira, *Biochemistry* **6**, 3942 (1967).
[66] R. Arnon and E. Shapira, *Biochemistry* **7**, 4196 (1968).
[67] S. Iida, M. Sasaki, and S. Ota, *J. Biochem.* (*Tokyo*) **73**, 377 (1973).
[68] M. Imanishi, N. Miyagawa, H. Fujio, and T. Amano, *Biken J.* **12**, 85 (1969).
[69] J. L. McCans, L. K. Lane, G. E. Lindenmayer, V. P. Butler, Jr., and A. Schwartz, *Proc. Nat. Acad. Sci. U.S.* **71**, 2449 (1974).

In short, functional heterogeneity of antibodies is a result of heterogeneity of specificity and is a general phenomenon. Similarly, changes of inhibitory capacity in the course of immunization[1] can now be seen as a general phenomenon of the response to enzymes (for instance, chymopapain[70]) and reflect the competition between inhibitory and non-inhibitory antibody.[27, 28, 60, 61, 71] The relative proportion of these two functional types of antibodies appears to change in the course of immunization. This functional change may be attributable (i) to the relative number of determinants that elicit inhibiting and conformationally altering antibodies and/or (ii) to differences in the tolerance barriers against antibody induction by the two types of determinants. Prolonged immunization results in affinity maturation by antigen-mediated selection of receptors[72-75] and in a succession of antibodies directed against different determinants,[76, 77] which result from stimulation of a succession of clones of limited capacity to divide.[78-82] The probability of the formation of inhibitory antibody in prolonged immunization will be favored if the number of determinants, through which enzyme activation can be induced, is relatively very much smaller than the number of determinants through which sterically hindering antibodies can be induced. Fewer receptor-bearing cells will be available for triggering by the numerically inferior determinant type, so that affinity maturation will be relatively slow and the potential pool of precursor cells will be exhausted relatively early. We already know that naturally acquired tolerance controls some aspects of the response to enzymes in that it excludes the catalytic site from immunogenicity.[26, 83, 84] This exclusion occurs because the catalytic site of enzymes is preserved in evolution and is thus usually identical

[70] E. Shapira and R. Arnon, *Immunochemistry* **5**, 501 (1968).
[71] B. Cinader, T. Suzuki, and H. Pelichová, *J. Immunol.* **106**, 1381 (1971).
[72] G. W. Suskind and B. Benacerraf, *Advan. Immunol.* **70**, 1 (1969).
[73] C.-Y. Wu and B. Cinader, *J. Immunol. Methods* **1**, 19 (1971).
[74] C.-Y. Wu and B. Cinader, *Eur. J. Immunol.* **2**, 398 (1972).
[75] L. Brenneman, and S. J. Singer, *Ann. N. Y. Acad. Sci.* **169**, 72 (1970).
[76] J. Fisher, J. Spragg, R. C. Talamo, J. V. Pierce, K. Suzuki, K. F. Austen, and E. Haber, *Biochemistry* **8**, 3750 (1969).
[77] E. Maron, R. Arnon, and B. Bonavida, *Eur. J. Immunol.* **2**, 181 (1971).
[78] K. Eichmann and T. J. Kindt, *J. Exp. Med.* **134**, 532 (1971).
[79] A. Sher and M. Cohn, *Eur. J. Immunol.* **2**, 319 (1972).
[80] K. Eichmann, *J. Exp. Med.* **137**, 603 (1973).
[81] L. L. Pawlak, D. A. Hart, and A. Nisonoff, *J. Exp. Med.* **137**, 1442 (1973).
[82] A. Nisonoff, *in* "La génétique des immunoglobulines et de la réponse immunitaire" *Ann. Immunol.* (*Inst. Pasteur*) *Paris* **125c**, 363 (1974).
[83] B. Cinader, *in* "Regulation of the Antibody Response" (B. Cinader, ed.), p. 3. Thomas, Springfield, Illinois, 1968.
[84] B. Cinader, *Behringwerk-Mitt.* **47**, 16 (1967).

in the tolerance-inducing autologous antigens of the immunized animal and in the donor of the antigen. This barrier is not impenetrable and may yield, in certain circumstances, to immunization with cross-reacting antigens.[85-92]

The determinants through which steric hindrance is induced may tend to be better preserved in evolution than the determinants through which conformational alteration is induced. Were this the case, it would result in the functional changes in inhibitory capacity that have been observed in the course of prolonged immunization.

In this, as in many other experimental situations, it will be important to compare not only antibodies from different individuals of different species, but also antibodies obtained at different stages of immunization, and to analyze not only changes in specificity and function, but also relative rates of affinity maturation. It seems likely that both the above mechanisms will be found to operate.

2. MECHANISM OF MODIFICATION OF ENZYME ACTIVITY BY ANTIBODY

a. INTRODUCTION

Any satisfactory analysis of the mechanism by which antibody inhibits enzyme must be capable of accounting for the following facts: (i) some enzymes are completely inhibited by antibody, some partly, and at least two enzymes are not inhibited at all; (ii) the inhibitory capacity of antibody undergoes changes in the course of immunization; (iii) antibody is a less effective inhibitor when combining with enzyme in the presence rather than in the absence of substrate; (iv) the kinetics of the inhibition of antibody appear often to be noncompetitive, sometimes competitive, and occasionally of intermediate type, and, in at least one instance, uncompetitive[54]; (v) some antibodies have been found to increase, rather than decrease, the activity of an enzyme. Clearly, antibody can have not only an all-or-none inhibitory effect, but can also modify the function of the catalytic site.

[85] B. Cinader and J. M. Dubert, *Brit. J. Exp. Pathol.* **36**, 515 (1955).
[86] B. Cinader and J. H. Pearce, *Brit. J. Exp. Pathol.* **37**, 541 (1956).
[87] K. Rajewsky, *Immunochemistry* **3**, 487 (1966).
[88] J. E. M. St. Rose and B. Cinader, *J. Exp. Med.* **125**, 1031 (1967).
[89] B. Cinader, J. E. M. St. Rose, and M. Yoshimura, *J. Exp. Med.* **125**, 1057 (1967).
[90] J. E. M. St. Rose and B. Cinader, *Eur. J. Immunol.* **3**, 409 (1973).
[91] M. Fujiwara and B. Cinader, *Cell. Immunol.* **12**, 1 (1974).
[92] G. Lakatos, A. Strefling, R. R. Joseph, and D. S. McCann, *Cancer Res.* **34**, 1395 (1974).

b. The Effect of Antibody on the Access of Substrate to the Catalytic Area (Equilibrium Dialysis)

Kinetic studies have led to apparently contradictory, and certainly inconclusive, data on the relation between specificity of binding with antibody and capacity to inhibit catalytic function. The independence of inhibitory capacity with respect to substrate concentration could be due to either of two effects; (i) classical noncompetitive inhibition (in which case all enzyme sites would remain accessible), or (ii) relative irreversibility of antibody binding at the catalytic site in relation to the more reversible binding between enzyme and substrate,[93, 94] in which case enzyme sites on all inhibited molecules would be inaccessible.

The degree of enzyme inhibition by antibody depends on the molecular weight of the substrate (Section 18.B.2.c). This relationship between substrate size and degree of inhibition is relevant here: a fraction of antibody-bound enzyme molecules reacts with a given substrate only if it has a molecular weight below some critical limit. This indicates that at least one fraction of unreactive enzyme molecules is inhibited as a consequence of the distance between catalytic site and site of antibody attachment.

In view of the irreducible residual activity in antibody excess of most enzymes, the question arises whether antibody completely inhibits the activity of individual enzyme molecules or whether all enzyme molecules are reactive, but with changed kinetic properties. This can be tested by comparing the combining capacity of enzyme in the presence and in the absence of antibody. Great care must be taken to do this under strictly comparable conditions, and reference has already been made to difficulties in interpretation of such data. Conclusive data can be obtained by measuring, in a complex of antibody and antigen, the number of sites that remain available for combination with substrate, or with a competitive inhibitor of low molecular weight. This can be done by means of equilibrium dialysis, as described in Vol. II, Chap. 15.B for the study of hapten–antibody equilibrium. The method involves choosing competitive inhibitors that bind firmly, and ascertaining the number of inhibitor molecules that combine with enzyme in the presence of antibody *vs* the number of molecules combining with enzyme in the presence of normal γ-globulin. In order to obtain equilibrium conditions, the enzyme–antibody mixtures should be soluble. Complexes between antigen and divalent antibody are soluble only in extreme antigen excess. To measure soluble complexes in the equivalence region and in antibody excess, univalent

[93] B. Cinader, *Annu. Rev. Microbiol.* **11**, 371 (1957).
[94] A. G. Ogston, *Disc. Faraday Soc.* **20**, 161 (1955).

fragments of antibody, prepared by a method such as Porter's[95] can be used.[61] If the fractional loss of available sites is identical with the fractional loss of enzyme activity, it can be concluded that individual enzyme molecules in the enzyme antibody complex are not "partially inhibited" but consist of two populations of which one is completely inhibited and remains accessible to substrate. Experiments of this type have been car-

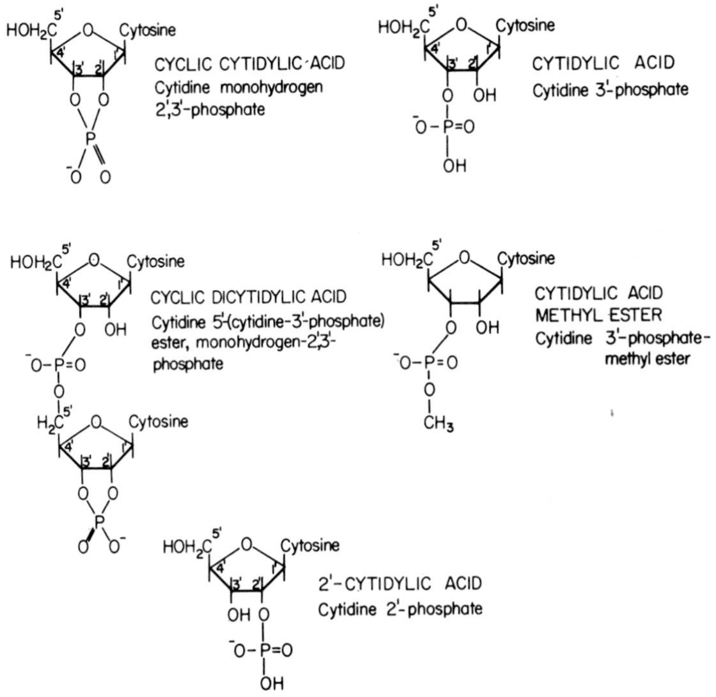

FIG. 8. Structural formulas of cytidylic acid and related compounds.

ried out using ribonuclease and cytidine 2′-phosphate (Fig. 8), and have led to the demonstration of residual accessible catalytic sites in the antibody-excess region.[61]

c. INHIBITION BY STERIC HINDRANCE

i. The Effect of Substrate Size

Steric hindrance by antibody attaching to enzyme will be considered, first, as an "umbrella" term, implying blockade of the catalytic site without combination of the antibody directly with catalytic site. This type

[95] R. R. Porter, Biochem. J. **73**, 119 (1959).

of inhibition is suggested by surveying the activity of various enzymes in the presence of excess antibody, for there is some degree of correlation between the amount of inhibition in antibody excess and the molecular weight of the substrate (Table I). Conclusive evidence for this type of inhibition has been obtained by studies with ribonuclease[1] and has been confirmed with several other enzymes, such as neuraminidase,[2] C′1-esterase,[3,96] and trypsin,[4] papain,[97] bromelain,[98] and acid α-glucosidase,[99] each of which acts on several substrates that differ in molecular weight and each of which is much more effectively inhibited in its action on the large molecular weight substrate.

Ribonuclease, as one example, can bring about esterification of cyclic cytidylic acid, resulting in the synthesis of a dimer or in the formation of an ester with any one of several alcohols added to the reaction mixture (Fig. 8). The reaction can, therefore, result in the formation of a dimer of molecular weight 612 or, if methyl alcohol is present, in the synthesis of the methyl ester of cytidylic acid with a molecular weight of 338.[1] The synthesis of the product of large molecular weight is more effectively inhibited than synthesis of the product of low molecular weight. The relative hydrolytic activity of a mixture of ribonuclease and antibody can be determined on a macromolecule, nucleic acid, or on cytidylic cyclic phosphate (MW 306) used as substrate. The inhibitory effect of antibody on the hydrolytic reaction is greater when the substrate is a macromolecule.[100, 101]

ii. The Role of the Aggregation of Antigen and Antibody (Danysz Phenomenon, Univalent Fragments of Antibody)

Were antibody to possess such a specificity that it would combine at the border of the active center, it could directly prevent access of large substrates to the catalytic area. In this case, *only a fraction of the total antibody* would participate in the inhibition.

Alternatively, divalent antibody could inhibit by virtue of forming a lattice, i.e., an aggregate with multivalent antigen (enzyme). In this case, *any antibody molecule contributing to aggregate formation* would participate in the inhibition.

[96] A. L. Haines and I. H. Lepow, *J. Immunol.* **92**, 479 (1964).

[97] E. Shapira and R. Arnon, *Biochemistry* **6**, 3951 (1967).

[98] M. Sasaki, S. Iida, and T. Murachi, *J. Biochem. (Tokyo)* **73**, 367 (1973).

[99] T. De Barsy, P. Jaquemin, P. Devos, and H.-G. Hers, *Eur. J. Biochem.* **31**, 156 (1972).

[100] R. K. Brown, *Ann. N. Y. Acad. Sci.* **103**, 754 (1963).

[101] R. K. Brown, R. Delaney, L. Levine, and H. Van Vunakis, *J. Biol. Chem.* **234**, 2043 (1959).

By electron microscopy, the visualized structure of aggregates[102, 103] appears quite similar to the patterns proposed by Marrack[104] and Pauling.[105] In moderate antibody excess, there are orderly structures indicative of cross-linking, and cyclic arrangements of antigen are seen frequently. Antibody connects molecules of antigen by a distance which is usually somewhat shorter than the long axis of γ-globulin (240 to 250 Å), so that molecules of diameter greater than this may be unable to penetrate the lattice. The relative importance of such a restriction will depend on the ratio of enzyme (antigen):antibody molecules within the core of the aggregate. This ratio cannot be known from electron microscopic studies. However, in far antibody excess, each individual molecule of antigen is seen to be surrounded by a dense halo of antibody molecules,[102] and cross-linking does not occur. Thus maximal enzyme inhibition occurs when there is no lattice formation. Estimates of the probable contribution of aggregates to enzyme inhibition can be made from study of the Danysz effect, that is from comparison of the different degrees of neutralization encountered when a given amount of a biologically active antigen (originally diphtheria toxin) is added in increments or when it is added all at once to *equine* antibody. The different degrees of neutralization are attributable to the fact that antigen and antibody combine in multiple proportions.[106]

When enzyme (*C. welchii* lecithinase) is added to a fixed amount of antibody (i) in increments and (ii) in a single addition, there is a difference in the enzymatic activity of the two mixtures. Detailed analysis of these results led to the conclusions that a complex of enzyme (E) and antibody (A) of composition (EA_{2n}) can be formed and would then represent the predominant stable compound of high antibody content. Most interestingly, it could be shown that the complex EA_n, formed by E and A at the first addition of E, can combine with still more antibody: accordingly, there is only limited restriction imposed on penetration of antibody into the aggregate following the initial aggregation of E and A. Hence experiments based on the Danysz phenomenon lead to the conclusion that aggregate structure would present little obstacle to the penetration of molecules of the size of γ-globulin.[106]

The contribution of aggregation to steric hindrance can be examined *directly* by comparing the inhibitory capacities of divalent antibody and of Fab fragments.[95] Aggregates will be formed only with the divalent

[102] J. Almeida, B. Cinader, and A. Howatson, *J. Exp. Med.* **118**, 327 (1963).

[103] J. D. Almeida, B. Cinader, and D. Naylor, *Immunochemistry* **2**, 169 (1965).

[104] J. R. Marrack, *Med. Res. Counc. (Gt. Brit.) Spec. Rep. Ser.* **230**, 1 (1938).

[105] L. Pauling, *J. Amer. Chem. Soc.* **62**, 2643 (1940).

[106] B. Cinader, *Brit. J. Exp. Pathol.* **38**, 362 (1957).

antibody. Direct comparisons of this type with enzymes such as car-bamoyl phosphate synthetase,[107] ribonuclease,[60] phosphorylase,[44] and ornithine carbamoyl transferase[49a] have shown little difference between the inhibitory capacities of divalent and univalent antibodies. However, since antibody fragment I and antibody fragment II exhibit different de-grees of inhibitory capacity, and the relative yields of these two fractions may vary, it is inadvisable to rely on a comparison of the inhibitory capacity of isolated univalent fragments and of divalent antibody. Alter-natively, it is possible to convert univalent antibody of known activity into multivalent antibody, by adding a divalent antibody that is directed against univalent fragments.[61] This procedure has shown, in the ribonu-clease–antibody system, that aggregation of the antigen–antibody com-plex does *not* increase the "steric hindrance component" of the inhibitory capacity of antibody,[61] even though it may contribute to the firmness of binding between enzyme and nonavid antibody. Increased firmness of binding may be the mechanism whereby the residual activity of soluble complexes between sheep antibodies and rabbit spleen ribonuclease can be reduced by precipitation with anti-sheep IgG.[108] Arguments for inhibi-tory capacity of aggregates have been based on the observation that the activity of soluble complexes of papain–antipapain does not show the dependence on substrate size that is found with insoluble complexes.[97, 109] This observation, however, may only show that enzymes are not inhibited when they are in complexes consisting of one antibody and two enzyme molecules and, therefore, catalyze transformation of substrates of differ-ent molecular weight at relative rates that are identical with those of free enzyme. Only complexes with two, or more than two, molecules of antibody per enzyme molecule are inhibited (by steric hindrance) and show a dependence of residual activity on the molecular weight of sub-strate. With some substrates, steric hindrance by aggregates does, never-theless, play a part. This occurs with substrates possessing a diameter considerably larger than the long axis of the antibody molecules. An indi-cation of this possibility may be deduced from the previously mentioned analysis of the structure of antigen–antibody complexes,[102] of the Danysz effect,[106] and from the observation, made initially by Goldsworthy,[110] that a greater amount of hemolytic complement could be removed from fresh guinea pig serum if complement was present at the initiation of

[107] M. Marshall and P. P. Cohen, *J. Biol. Chem.* **236**, 718 (1961).

[108] W. Y. Lee and A. H. Sehon, *Immunochemistry* **8**, 743 (1971).

[109] R. Arnon, *in* "Immunological Approaches to Fertility Control" (E. Diczfalusy, ed.) *Karolinska Symp. Res. Methods Reprod. Endocrinol. 7th Symp.* p. 133. Karolinska Institutet, Stockholm, 1974.

[110] N. E. Goldsworthy, *J. Pathol. Bacteriol.* **31**, 220 (1928).

the antigen–antibody interaction than when it was added to preformed complexes.[111-115] Fazekas de St. Groth has provided an example of neutralization in which steric hindrance by the aggregate may directly contribute to inhibition; the inhibition of neuraminidase was very feeble when sialyl lactose (MW 633) served as substrate, was partial when the substrate had a molecular weight of 10^4 daltons and was complete when the molecular weight of the substrate exceeded 10^5 daltons.[2] It is probable that the first of these increments of inhibition is due to steric hindrance dependent on specificity of the antibody, i.e., due to contiguity between the antibody-combining site and the catalytic space and that the second inhibition increment is due to steric hindrance by the aggregate, i.e., it is *not* dependent on the distance of determinants from the catalytic site.

iii. Steric Hindrance and Specificity (Blocking Antibody)

The relative positions of the catalytic site and of the antibody-combining sites on the enzyme molecule determine, in an important way, the effect of antibody on enzyme activity. Three functional types of antibody will be considered here, viz., one type that combines with enzyme but does not affect its catalytic activity, another type that inhibits enzymatic function, and a third type that, though not inhibiting enzymatic function directly, can compete with inhibiting antibody for sites on the enzyme.

The evidence for three "functional" varieties of antibody has been obtained by choosing sera of different inhibiting capacity, and examining the effects of mixtures of antibodies on enzyme activity. For example, rabbit antibodies raised with cell-free penicillinase were compared with those to cell-bound penicillinase. The former combined with and inhibited the cell-free enzyme, the latter combined with but failed to inhibit cell-free enzyme. In mixtures, the two antibodies competed for sites on the enzyme molecules, and the normally inhibiting antibody showed no inhibitory action.[116]

A similar mechanism could be demonstrated, though less directly, in the interaction of ribonuclease with its antibody. Antibody was split and fractionated to yield a univalent fragment I and fragment II, and the two fragments were found to differ in inhibitory capacity, as judged by residual activity, in antibody excess; fraction II left more residual enzymatic activity than fraction I. Mixtures of fraction I and fraction II

[111] R. Feinberg, *J. Immunol.* **81**, 14 (1958).
[112] W. F. Friedewald, *J. Exp. Med.* **78**, 347 (1943).
[113] K. Goodner and F. L. Horsfall, Jr., *J. Exp. Med.* **64**, 201 (1936).
[114] M. Heidelberger, M. Rocha e Silva, and M. Mayer, *J. Exp. Med.* **74**, 359 (1941).
[115] M. Heidelberger and M. Mayer, *J. Exp. Med.* **75**, 285 (1942).
[116] N. Citri and G. Strejan, *Nature (London)* **190**, 1010 (1961).

could be made that inhibited less effectively in antibody excess than did fraction I alone. In other words, a given amount of fraction I inhibited more effectively in the absence than in the presence of fraction II.[61] Thus with penicillinase and with ribonuclease, noninhibiting antibody can compete with inhibiting antibody for the combining sites on the antigen.[60, 61, 116] Different enzyme determinants can be identified that elicit inhibitory or noninhibitory antibodies, respectively. For instance, antibodies specific for the 50-amino acid C-terminal region between residues inhibitory or noninhibitory antibodies, respectively. For instance, antibodies directed against the region which contains two disulfide bridges, located between residues 57 and 107 of hen egg lysozyme.[119-122] On the other hand, antibodies directed against a portion of this lysozyme region between residues 60 and 83, which contains one intrachain disulfide bond do not inhibit catalytic activity.[77, 123] Whether the inhibitory and noninhibitory antibodies against the two overlapping lysozyme regions compete with one another remains a question to be answered in the future. This is clearly a system in which the study of enzyme neutralization could and should be effectively advanced.

d. ACTIVATING ANTIBODY

Purified activating antibody increases ribonuclease activity to a constant maximum level which is reached when one activating antibody molecule saturates one determinant per enzyme molecule. A decrease of this activity level, at greater total antibody concentration, occurs only if small quantities of *inhibiting* antibody are present as an impurity. Fractions of activating antibody, directed against pancreatic bovine ribonuclease, induce activation of hydrolysis of cyclic cytidylic acid and cyclic uridylic acid but not of ribonucleic acid.[27] This difference is not necessarily attributable to steric hindrance and may be due to a change in enzyme specificity or to activation which affects splitting of the cyclic bond but does not affect transphosphorylation. In any case, there is a marked difference in the effect of antibody when cyclic cytidylic and

[117] D. H. Sachs, A. N. Schechter, A. Eastlake, and C. B. Anfinsen, *Biochemistry* **11**, 4268 (1972).

[118] D. H. Sachs, A. N. Schechter, A. Eastlake, and C. B. Anfinsen, *Nature (London)* **251**, 242 (1974).

[119] R. E. Canfield and A. K. Liu, *J. Biol. Chem.* **240**, 1997 (1965).

[120] S. Shinka, M. Imanishi, N. Miyagawa, T. Amano, M. Inouye, and A. Tsugita, *Biken J.* **10**, 89 (1967).

[121] H. Fujio, M. Imanishi, K. Nishioka, and T. Amano, *Biken J.* **11**, 219 (1968).

[122] H. Fujio, N. Sakato, and T. Amano, *Biken J.* **14**, 395 (1971).

[123] R. Arnon, E. Maron, M. Sela, and C. B. Anfinsen, *Proc. Nat. Acad. Sci. U.S.* **68**, 1450 (1971).

cyclic uridylic acid serve as substrates. Clearly, this difference cannot be attributed to steric hindrance, but is due to an antibody-induced change in the substrate specificity spectrum of the enzyme (Fig. 9).

If activating and inhibiting antibodies are present simultaneously, the enzyme activity will depend on the relative number of inhibited and of

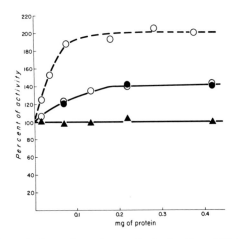

Fig. 9. Activation of ribonuclease by antibody-fractions P1′ (see Fig. 3) using cyclic cytidylic acid, cyclic uridylic acid, and nucleic acid as substrates. Constant quantities of enzyme were mixed with various quantities of each antibody fraction, and the hydrolytic activity of the mixtures was determined manometrically in the Warburg apparatus. From T. Suzuki. H. Pelichová, and B. Cinader, *J. Immunol.* **103**, 1366 (1969).

Symbol	Substrate	Fraction
—○— — ●— —▲—	Cyclic cytidylic acid Cyclic uridylic acid Yeast ribonucleic acid }	P1′ from pooled ribonuclease antisera
--○--	Cyclic cytidylic acid }	P1′ from two individual sera (973,973) from hyperimmunized animals, bled between day 150 and day 300 after beginning of immunization

activated enzyme molecules. At low total antibody concentration (say, one antibody molecule per enzyme molecule), this ratio will depend, primarily, on the relative concentration of activating and inhibiting antibodies. In fact, the extent of activation may be reduced by the admixture of inhibiting antibody. Equivalent quantities of activating (P1) and inhibiting (P10) antibodies (prepared as shown in Fig. 3, and with neutralizing capacities as shown in Fig. 4) were mixed before addition of enzyme; the highest attainable activity of enzyme was reduced from 200% to 142% (Fig. 10).

Maximum activity corresponded to a relatively low quantity of activating antibody. Antibody in fraction P1 induced maximal activation at 200 μg of antibody protein. When P1 was mixed with inhibiting anti-

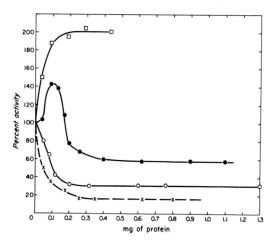

Fig. 10. The effect of the simultaneous presence of activating and inhibiting antibody on ribonuclease activity. Various quantities of antibody were added to constant quantities of bovine pancreatic ribonuclease. After 30 minutes of incubation, the enzymatic activity of these mixtures was measured in the presence of cyclic cytidylic acid. Mixtures of activating and inhibiting antibodies were made in proportions based on units corresponding to the minimal amount of antibody that caused maximal inhibition or activation: □———□, Activating antibody fraction P1 prepared (as shown in Fig. 3) from a pool of antisera from rabbits; ×---×, inhibitory antibody-fraction P10 prepared from a pool of antisera; ●———●, mixture of P1 and P10 (1:1); ○———○, mixture of P1 and P10 (1:9). (See Figs. 3 and 4.) After H. Pelichová, T. Suzuki, and B. Cinader *J. Immunol.* **104,** 195 (1970).

body (P10), only one-fifth of this quantity was required for maximum activation. However, the extent of activation caused by this reduced quantity of P1 was similar, whether or not inhibiting antibody was present. Beyond this limiting concentration of total antibody, the neutralizing capacity of the inhibiting antibody was reduced by the presence of activating antibody. The effect of inhibiting antibody seemed to become dominant at higher total antibody concentration. We would, therefore, expect a decrease of attainable activation with mixtures in which the relative content in inhibiting antibody was increased. This was, in fact, observed: when the relative proportion of the inhibiting fraction, P10, was increased 9-fold, the zone of activation was no longer detected. However, the effect of activating antibody was manifested by a persistent decrease in the inhibitory capacity. Thus, we find that the activating fraction P1 could manifest two properties when inhibiting antibody was present. In antigen excess, activating antibody in the presence of inhibiting antibody could increase enzyme activity above 100%. In antibody excess, it could reduce the inhibitory capacity of inhibiting antibody.

These two types of interaction depended to a different extent on relative concentrations of inhibiting and activating antibody: when the content in activating antibody was relatively low, its effect was more pronounced in the zone of total antibody excess than it was in the zone of antigen excess. It seemed, therefore, as though a factor operated in antibody excess but not in antigen excess. This factor may be competition for determinants of the enzyme: activating antibody molecules may compete with some of the inhibiting antibodies for overlapping determinants. Thus activating antibodies displace some molecules of the inhibiting antibodies but not others, particularly at high antibody concentrations. At low antibody concentrations, this factor would be negligible. At high total antibody concentration, on the other hand, it might reduce the number of inhibited enzyme molecules. To test this hypothesis, we needed criteria by which we could distinguish between activation of individual molecules and reduction in the number of inhibited enzyme molecules.[28] Let us consider the reaction with ribonucleic acid in enzyme–P1 antibody complexes of which the activity toward cyclic cytidylic acid was increased above 100%. In the presence of ribonucleic acid, the activity of these complexes was identical with that of enzyme contained in them. This phenomenon has been encountered not only in examining the activity of fraction P1, but also with fractions such as P5 and P6 (Fig. 4). It follows that the activating effect of antibody *cannot* affect the hydrolysis of ribonucleic acid. When activating antibody is added to inhibiting antibody, it may at first appear paradoxical to find, with ribonucleic acid substrate, an *increase* of residual enzyme activity in antibody excess. To attribute this to activated enzyme molecules would require the absurd assumption that activation of enzymatic hydrolysis of ribonucleic acid can occur only when most enzyme molecules are inhibited or when the same molecule is combined with activating and inhibiting antibody. A process *other than activation* must contribute to the decreased inhibitory power in excess of total antibody. *Competition* between activating and inhibiting antibody for enzyme sites has already been mentioned. As a consequence of such competition, less inhibiting antibody could combine in mixtures and, therefore, less inhibition would be observed in antibody excess. It remains possible that neutralization, particularly in antibody excess, may be affected by antibodies that have no independent influence on enzyme activity, but can compete with inhibiting antibodies as a result of overlapping determinants.

So far, we have assumed that inhibitory and activating antibodies bind enzyme equally firmly and that activation in antigen excess and competition in antibody excess depend primarily on relative concentrations. At times, this may be the only decisive factor. In the enzyme neutralization by intermediary fraction, such as P5 (Fig. 4), the relative binding strength of two types may contribute to the course of the neutralization curve. If inhibiting and noninhibiting antibodies compete for enzyme sites, the resulting enzyme activity in antibody excess (residual activity) will be *independent* of antibody concentration, provided the competing antibodies bind the enzyme *equally firmly*. Under these circumstances, residual activity reflects the relative concentration of the two types of antibodies. Alternatively, neutralization in antibody excess will be *dependent* on antibody concentration if the competing antibodies bind enzyme with *different* firmness. Antibodies that bind relatively firmly, but are present in relatively low concentrations, will "capture" more enzyme sites at a given total antibody concentration. This will lead to a steady increase in enzyme activity after maximal inhibition has been reached. The activity will reach a constant level when the total antibody concentration is proportional to a function of the ratio of binding constants of the inhibiting and the competing noninhibiting antibodies. Thus the increase in enzyme activity with increasing antibody, following maximum inhibition at lower antibody concentrations (Fig. 4, fractions P5 and P6), has been interpreted on the basis of two sets of assumptions: (a) competition for determinants, and (b) unequal firmness of binding of inhibiting and activating antibodies. Competition for sites plays an important role in the zone of antibody excess and may result in reduced inhibition through displacement of inhibiting antibody.

Having examined changes in the spectrum of enzyme specificities and competition that interfere with these changes, we shall now deal with conformational change as a mechanism by which antibody may change the enzyme-specificity spectrum.

e. CONFORMATIONAL CHANGES

Antibody stabilizes the conformation of antigen so that enzymes can be protected by antibody against the denaturing effects of heat or high hydrogen-ion concentration (penicillinase,[64, 124] acetylcholinesterase,[125]

[124] N. Zyk and N. Citri, *Biochim. Biophys. Acta* **159**, 327 (1968).
[125] D. Michaeli, J. D. Pinto, E. Benjamini, and F. P. de Buren, *Immunochemistry* **6**, 101 (1969).

L-amino acid oxidase,[126] β-galactosidase,[127] mutant mouse strain catalase,[128] isozyme A of hexosaminidase.[129] A particularly interesting example
of this type is the stabilization of labile, deficient enzymes by antibodies
which had been elicited with the analogous normal enzymes (e.g., erythrocyte catalase in Swiss-type acatalasemia,[129a] glucose-6-phosphate dehydrogenase in congenital nonspherocytic hemolytic anemia.[129b] Antibodies not only preserve configuration but can also participate in the
restoration of configuration of a heat-denatured enzyme.[130] The most
striking type of restoration of activity has been obtained by the action
of antibody raised against wild-type *E. coli* β-galactosidase on genetically defective mutants of the enzyme. The antibody can induce as much
as a 900-fold increase in activity.[131, 132] Similarly, antibody against
ribonuclease A can induce, in ribonuclease S, the substrate-specificity
spectrum of ribonuclease A.[71] Antibodies elicited by a defective enzyme
do not possess the capacity to correct the defect.[133] It seems reasonable
to conclude that antibodies elicited by wild-type enzyme induce a
wild-type conformation in the mutant enzyme. The question arises
whether the mechanism that produces this type of change might also
produce alterations in the spectrum of substrate specificities of "normal"
enzyme by antibody elicited with normal enzyme.[134] Certainly changes
of this nature can be induced by chemical modification. For example,
treatment of carboxypeptidase with acetic anhydride results in decreased
peptidase activity and *increased* esterase activity.[135]

By physical measurements, it can be shown that antibodies can induce
conformational changes in synthetic polypeptides arising from linear
polymerization of a tripeptide, Tyr-Ala-Glu. These products differ in
chain lengths, the unit being repeated from 1 to 200 times [i.e., $(TAG)_1$
to $(TAG)_{200}$]. The configuration of the compounds was ascertained from

[126] S. E. Zimmerman, R. K. Brown, B. Curti, and V. Massey, *Biochim. Biophys. Acta* **229**, 260 (1971).

[127] F. Melchers and W. Messer, *Biochem. Biophys. Res. Commun.* **40**, 570 (1970).

[128] R. N. Feinstein, B. N. Jaroslow, J. B. Howard, and J. T. Faulhaber, *J. Immunol.* **106**, 1316 (1971).

[129] B. Geiger. Y. Ben-Yoseph, and R. Arnon, *Isr. J. Med. Sci.* **10**, 1172 (1974).

[129a] E. Shapira, Y. Ben-Yoseph, and H. Aebi, *Experientia* **29**, 1402 (1973).

[129b] A. Kahn, P. Boivin, J. Leger, D. Cottreau, and D. Hollard, *Biochim. Biophys. Acta* **343**, 431 (1974).

[130] D. Michaeli, J. D. Pinto, and E. Benjamini, *Immunochemistry* **6**, 371 (1969).

[131] M. B. Rotman and F. Celada, *Proc. Nat. Acad. Sci. U.S.* **60** 660 (1968).

[132] W. Messer and F. Melchers, *in* "The Lactose Operon" (J. R. Backwith and D. Zipser, eds.), p. 305. Cold Spring Harbor Laboratory, Cold Spring Harbor, New York, 1969.

[133] F. Celada, J. Ellis, K. Bodlund, and B. Rotman, *J. Exp. Med.* **134**, 751 (1971).

[134] F. Celada and R. Strom, *Quart. Rev. Biophys.* **5**, 395 (1972).

[135] R. T. Simpson, J. F. Riordan and B. L. Vallee, *Biochemistry* **2**, 616 (1963).

circular dichroism spectra, either directly in the region of the peptide bond transitions (225 to 190 nm), or in the region of the transitions of the tyrosyl residues (300 to 250 nm). At neutral pH, in the presence of salt, the shortest peptides were in a disordered random coil configuration, while the longest one had an ordered helical structure. The values of the ellipticities in the 225 to 190 nm and in the 300 to 250 nm regions were strictly correlated, both being more negative in the helical configuration.[136] Since purified Fab fragments showed relatively little ellipticity in the 300 to 250 nm region, it was possible to investigate changes of circular dichroism of the peptides in the presence of antibody.[57, 137] The ellipticity of $(TAG)_{13}$ underwent a 4- to 7-fold increase toward negative values upon reaction with anti-$(TAG)_{200}$ Fab, substantiating the hypothesis of a conformational change of the peptide toward a more helical form. A different type of evidence for antibody-mediated conformational changes was obtained in the reaction of anti-hapten antibodies with a polymer carrying the hapten in regions not accessible to the solvent. The molecule consisted of a p-azobenzene arsonate group linked to a $(TAG)_{200}$ helical copolymer. The hapten was deeply embedded in the macromolecule, as shown by its inability to induce anti-hapten antibodies and by its high ellipticity at 420 nm, owing to close interaction with the tyrosine chromophores. It could, however, react with anti-hapten antibodies or with the antibody Fab fragment. Upon such reaction, the circular dichroism properties became similar to those of the hapten bound to a random-coil polymer.[138] Local modification around the hapten or a conformational change of the whole polymer had freed the hapten from its environment. Alternatively, there may be an equilibrium between the helical and the random-coiled form of the polypeptide; antibody would combine with the coiled form (in which the hapten is exposed), and the equilibrium would be shifted in favor of the coiled form.

From studies of phosphoglucomutase and of hemoglobin, it has become apparent that the catalytically active site of an enzyme is not a rigid area of the molecule but is flexible and undergoes conformational change as one of the steps of interaction with substrate.[139-143] Substrate-induced

[136] B. Schechter, I. Schechter, J. Ramachandran, A. Conway-Jacobs, and M. Sela, *Eur. J. Biochem.* **20**, 301 (1971).

[137] B. Schechter, A. Conway-Jacobs, and M. Sela, *Eur. J. Biochem.* **20**, 321 (1971).

[138] A. Conway-Jacobs, B. Schechter, and M. Sela, *Biochemistry* **9**, 4870 (1970).

[139] D. E. Koshland, Jr., *Proc. Nat. Acad. Sci. U.S.* **44**, 98 (1958).

[140] D. E. Koshland, Jr., *in* "The Enzymes" (P. D. Boyer, H. Lardy, and E. Myrbäck, eds.), 2nd ed., Vol. 1, pp. 305–346. Academic Press, New York, 1959.

[141] J. A. Thoma and D. E. Koshland, Jr., *J. Amer. Chem. Soc.* **82**, 3329 (1960).

[142] D. E. Koshland Jr., J. A. Yankeelov, Jr., and J. A. Thoma, *Fed. Proc., Fed. Amer. Soc. Exp. Biol.* **21**, 1031 (1962).

[143] D. E. Koshland, Jr., *Ann. N. Y. Acad. Sci.* **103**, 630 (1963).

changes at the catalytic site may not be confined to this site, for they may lead to exposure or to "burial" of other residues of the enzyme molecule's structure. How this may result in the interference of substrate with antibody-mediated neutralization has been discussed in Section 18.B.1.c, dealing with inhibition under conditions of simultaneous addition of enzyme, substrate, and antibody. When enzyme and antibody are incubated prior to substrate addition, antibody may act by modifying a site which, thereafter, affects the configuration of the catalytic space in such manner as to modify the fit required by the substrate, or even so as to completely prevent access of substrate to the site. It is well known that substances other than substrate can affect the properties of a particular site on the protein molecule and that the ensuing changes may affect the configuration of the catalytic site; Monod, Changeux, and Jacob referred to this as the allosteric effect.[144] That antibody might act in a similar way, has been suggested on the basis of indirect evidence,[64-68] and reference has already been made to physical measurements of such changes in synthetic polypeptides. It seems reasonable to assume that it is this type of change that causes antibody-induced alteration of the substrate-specificity spectrum of enzymes as observed with penicillinase,[29, 30] ribonuclease,[26, 28] glutamic dehydrogenase,[145] amylase,[146] Taka-amylase,[155] β-galactosidase,[131] and β-lactamase.[147]

There is direct evidence that antibody, combining outside the catalytic site, can affect the integrity of the catalytic space. In the case of ribonuclease A, this space is known to consist of the N-terminal peptide (particularly histidine in position 12) and of amino acids in positions 41 and 115 to 121.[148-154] Interactions between these parts of the protein chain are involved in enzyme action. The catalytic space of bovine pancreatic ribonuclease can be disrupted by treatment with subtilisin, which splits ribonuclease into the N-terminal S-peptide (residues 1 to 20 or 21) and S-protein (residues 21 or 22 to 124). Upon isolation, neither of these two fragments shows appreciable catalytic activity. However, activity is re-

[144] J. Monod, J. P. Changeux, and F. Jacob, *J. Mol. Biol.* **6**, 306 (1963).
[145] F. G. Lehmann, *Biochim. Biophys. Acta* **235**, 259 (1971).
[146] Y. Okada, T. Ikenaka, T. Yagura, and Y. Yamamura, *J. Biochem. (Tokyo)* **54**, 101 (1963).
[147] N. Gilboa-Garber, C. Weisman, and N. Garber, *Abstr. 41st Meet. Isr. Chem. Soc.* p. 47, 1971.
[148] A. M. Crestfield, W. H. Stein, and S. Moore, *J. Biol. Chem.* **238**, 2413 (1963).
[149] E. A. Barnard and W. D. Stein, *J. Mol. Biol.* **1**, 339 (1959).
[150] W. D. Stein and E. A. Barnard, *J. Mol. Biol.* **1**, 350 (1959).
[151] H. G. Gundlach, W. H. Stein, and S. Moore, *J. Biol. Chem.* **234**, 1754 (1959).
[152] C. H. W. Hirs, *Brookhaven Symp. Biol.* **15**, 154 (1962).
[153] C. B. Anfinsen, *J. Biol. Chem.* **221**, 405 (1956).
[154] J. E. Erman and G. G. Hammes, *J. Amer. Chem. Soc.* **88**, 5607 and 5614 (1966).

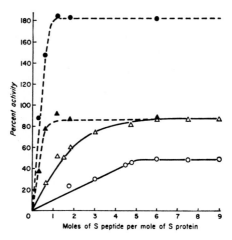

Fig. 11. Effect of antibody on the recombination between components of the catalytic space of ribonuclease A. A first series of mixtures contained constant quantities of S-protein and varying quantities of S-peptide. A second series contained the same reagents and in addition constant quantities of ribonuclease A antiserum fraction P1 (Nos. 971–973, see Fig. 3). To both series of mixtures, constant quantities of ribonuclease A were added and the enzyme activity was determined manometrically. The activity of these mixtures is expressed as the percentage of the activity of ribonuclease A (equivalent on a nitrogen basis to the S-protein in the mixture), in the absence of antibody. From B. Cinader, T. Suzuki, and H. Pelichová, *J. Immunol.* **106**, 1385 (1971).

Mixture	Substrate	Symbol
S-peptide + S-protein	Cyclic cytidylic	○——○
S-peptide + S-protein	Ribonucleic acid	△——△
P1 + S-peptide + S-protein	Cyclic cytidylic acid	●----●
P1 + S-peptide + S-protein	Ribonucleic acid	▲----▲

gained when the two fragments are mixed,[155, 156] although structure and function of native ribonuclease A is not completely restored.[155-159] The molar ratio (S-peptide:S-protein) at which maximum restoration of activity occurs was reduced when S-protein was allowed to combine with ribonuclease A antiserum or with activating-antibody fractions (Fig. 11).

[155] F. M. Richard and R. P. J. Vithayathil, *J. Biol. Chem.* **234**, 1459 (1959).
[156] J. J. Potts, D. M. Young, C. B. Anfinsen, and A. Samdoval, *J. Biol. Chem.* **239**, 3781 (1964).
[157] F. M. Richard and R. P. J. Vithayathil, *Brookhaven Symp. Biol.* **13**, 115 (1960).
[158] E. R. Simons and E. R. Blout, *J. Biol. Chem.* **243**, 218 (1968).
[159] M. S. Dosher and C. H. W. Hirs, *Biochemistry* **6**, 304 (1967).

Antibody also changed the substrate-specificity spectrum of ribonuclease S to one similar to that of ribonuclease A.[71] In short, substrate specificity of the intact catalytic space can be modified and the native configuration of an unstable catalytic space can be reestablished by antibodies that combine at a site distant from the catalytic space. These conclusions gain further support from experiments with genetically defective enzymes and antibodies against the intact (i.e., wild type) enzyme. Most attention has been given to the products of the *E. coli* z gene. In the wild type, the gene product is β-galactosidase (GZ). The activity of wild-type GZ is not affected by antibody, but can be protected from heat denaturation by antibody or by substrate analogs.

A number of genetically distinct mutants have trace activity that can be increased by anti-GZ antibodies.[131, 132] The mutant enzyme activity is very labile at 37°. Antibodies not only cause a net increase in activity (up to 10% of the specific activity of the wild type) but also protect against heat inactivation. The substrate analog TPEG* has similar effects.[160] Antibodies directed against the homologous mutant enzyme do not activate and they compete with activating antibody.[133] Only antibodies directed against wild-type molecules or against certain *other* point mutants protect and activate. Activation can occur only within certain limits: the substrate binding site cannot be "repaired" unless its amino acid sequence is present and is able to bind substrate. If the site is completely defective, it can be replaced only by complementation.

It seems that activation and protection against heat denaturation are two properties that can be distinguished: at least one mutant is not protected from thermal inactivation, but is activated by antibody.[127]

Some mutations of the z gene, resulting in deletions from the N-terminal section of the polypeptide product of the z gene, generate an enzymatically inactive gene product. If the deleted section does not go beyond a certain point, the "barrier," the activity of these molecules (α-acceptors) may be restored by noncovalent interaction with point mutants, or with molecules with deletions in the C-terminal, or even with N-terminal fragments that can be obtained by treatment of GZ with CNBr. Anti-GZ antibodies produce a true activation of α-acceptors in the absence of complementing fragments.[161] The efficiency or velocity of complementation are not affected by either antibody or substrate analog.

C-terminal deletions reducing the size of the GZ monomer to two thirds (ω-acceptor) can be repaired by *in vitro* complementation if the ω frag-

* TPEG, β-phenyl ethyl thiogalactoside.
[160] F. Celada, J. Radojkovic, and R. Strom, *J. Chim. Phys. Phis. Chim. Biol.* **71**, 1007 (1974).
[161] R. S. Accolla, Thesis, University of Rome, 1974.

ment has a molecular weight of at least 40,000. It may be assumed that wild-type conformation of ω is not maintained if the deletion is greater.[162] Immunological cross-reactions between ω and GZ[163] support this view. The acceptor can be reactivated by ω molecules. The substrate analog TPEG[162] and anti-GZ antibody[163] facilitate this complementation. The mechanisms of facilitation by these two agents may be different: the analog acts only when the acceptor is a monomer; antibody acts on both monomer and tetramer.

The catalytic site has a delicate three-dimensional balance, to which many regions of the molecule—some quite distant—contribute. A single amino acid replacement may severely derange this balance or render it unstable. It can be restored in two ways: (a) by introducing a molecule that has high affinity toward different parts of the active cavity and thus maintains the configuration of the cavity; (b) by highly specific antibodies directed toward conformation-dependent determinants of the wild-type molecule.

Residual similarity between the wild-type and the mutant determinant may result in cross-reactivity. The combination of a defective enzyme with antibody against a wild-type determinant may impose a wild-type configuration. Alternatively, the defective enzyme may occur in several configurations that are in equilibrium. Antibody may shift this equilibrium to the predominant presence of a configuration similar to that of the wild-type enzyme. The two postulated pathways $Ab + E^- \rightleftharpoons (Ab.E)^- \rightarrow (Ab.E)^+$ and $E^- \rightleftharpoons E^+ + Ab \rightarrow (Ab.E)^+$ are thermodynamically equivalent. It remains to be seen whether activation is due to an induced change of conformation or to preferential stabilization of one of several configurations.

f. ENZYME NEUTRALIZATION AS A REFLECTION OF SPECIFICITY-HETEROGENEITY AND OF THE FACTORS THAT DETERMINE THIS HETEROGENEITY

In the last decade, knowledge of the neutralization reaction has been elucidated and the mechanisms of activity modification, and variables affecting them have been identified. Neutralization is seen as the interaction between functional properties of sites on the enzyme and combining properties of a very heterogeneous assembly of antibodies. The latter are the resultant of genetic controls of responsiveness and of a "steering

---

[162] A. Ullman and J. Monod, *in* "The Lactose Operon" (J. R. Beckwith and D. Zipser, eds.), p. 265. Cold Spring Harbor Laboratory, Cold Spring Harbor, New York, 1970.

[163] F. Celada, *in* "Immunological Approaches to Fertility Control" (E. Diczfalusy, ed.), *Karolinska Symp. Res. Methods Reprod. Endocrinol. 7th Symp.* p. 150. Karolinska Institutet, Stockholm, 1974.

mechanism,"[164, 165] dependent on naturally acquired tolerance to autologous isofunctional molecules of the immunized animal. Thus, neutralization is approached in terms of the evolution of enzymes on the one hand, and of the regulation of antibody specificity on the other. The factors that determine the antibody-mediated modification of enzyme action will be summarized next as the basis for experimental design in immunoenzymology.

Antibody which is not directed against the catalytic site can inhibit catalytic activity. For instance, antibody directed against the C-terminal fragment of staphylococcal nuclease (residues 94 to 149) inactivates the enzyme with first-order kinetics,[117, 166] yet no amino acid in the fragment is involved in the active site of the enzyme. On the other hand, there are no convincing data of antibody being elicited by the catalytic site of any enzyme. Indeed, this part of the enzyme is preserved in evolution, and hence animals, being tolerant to the majority of catalytic sites, do not produce antibodies that are directed against these sites. For the same reason, the prosthetic group of an enzyme does not function as a determinant; i.e., it does not appear to be capable of eliciting antibody.[167–172] It will affect the antigenic reactivity of an enzyme only when the native conformation of the enzyme depends on the presence of the prosthetic group.[168, 173] Antibody-mediated inhibition of enzyme is therefore not attributable to the combination of antibodies with the catalytic site, but to combination with determinants outside the catalytic site. If these determinants are sufficiently close to the catalytic site, they prevent access of substrate to the catalytic site. The magnitude of the gaps between the blockading antibodies depends on the relative disposition of the many determinants with which antibodies can combine and hence is heterogeneous. More of these gaps bar large substrates than small substrates, and hence the effectiveness of inhibition depends on substrate size. Since the

[164] B. Cinader, *Nature (London)* **188**, 619 (1960).

[165] B. Cinader, *Brit. Med. Bull.* **19**, 219 (1963).

[166] D. H. Sachs, A. N. Schechter, A. Eastlake, and C. B. Anfinsen, *J. Immunol.* **109**, 1300 (1972).

[167] J. L. Hedrick, S. Shaltiel, and E. H. Fischer, *Biochemistry* **5**, 2117 (1966).

[168] S. Shaltiel, *Isr. J. Chem.* **6**, 104 (1968).

[169] I. M. Patrami, K. D. Katsiri, C. G. Dimitropoulos, T. G. Kalogerakos, M. P. Pavlatos, and A. E. Evanglopoulos, *Eur. J. Biochem.* **15**, 293 (1970).

[170] M. Martinez-Charion, J. Baron, W. E. Taylor, E. L. Isaacson, and J. LoSpalluto, *J. Biol. Chem.* **246**, 4143 (1971).

[171] Y. Miyake, K. Yamaji, and T. Yamano, *J. Biochem. (Tokyo)* **65**, 531 (1969).

[172] P. J. Wistrand and S. N. Rao, *Biochim. Biophys. Acta* **154**, 130 (1968).

[173] T. F. O'Brien and J. H. R. Kagi, *Fed. Proc. Fed. Amer. Soc. Exp. Biol.* **27**, 260 (1968).

size of the gap depends on the determinants that have elicited the antibody response, and since this is under genetic control, there are considerable differences in the specificity of the inhibitory antibodies that are found in a given antiserum and considerable differences in inhibitory capacity dependent on dose and duration of immunization. At any rate, the fraction of antibodies which inhibit access of low molecular weight substrate is relatively small. In one case, namely, an antiserum to lysozyme, an inhibitory fraction was obtained by dissociation of antigen–antibody complexes with the lysozyme inhibitor, tri-N-acetyl glucosamine, and was found to comprise 7 to 8% of the total precipitating antibody.[68] Many antibody molecules elicited by an enzyme are directed against determinants that are distant from sites that are relevant to catalysis; most of these antibodies have no effect on catalysis. There is a well-defined delineation between determinants that elicit inhibitory antibodies and those that do not, as exemplified by the already mentioned inhibitory antibodies that can be elicited by the lysozyme fragment between residues 57 and 107, but not by the fragment between residues 60 and 83.[174, 175] Aggregate formation contributes to inhibition by antibodies of low affinity since antigen–antibody combination is less readily dissociable in a complex; it also contributes directly to steric hindrance when the molecular weight of the substrate exceeds 10^5 daltons.

Antibodies of appropriate specificity can change the catalytic site conformation of a defective enzyme to that of the competent enzyme against which the antibody was raised (β-galactosidase, penicillinase, ribonuclease S, action on ribonuclease A of antibody elicited with polyalanine polytyrosine ribonuclease) or can change the substrate specificity spectrum of an enzyme. In the latter case one enzyme molecule per antibody molecule suffices for maximum effect.[28] Antibodies of this type compete with inhibiting antibodies. As a rule, antisera contain predominantly noninhibitory antibodies, which do not interfere with catalysis, and inhibitory antibodies. The much smaller component of competing noninhibitory antibodies manifests itself only in the constant residual activity found in antibody excess. The interaction between inhibitory and competing noninhibitory antibodies depends not only on the relative quantity, but also on the relative affinity of the two types of antibody. The presence of substrate during the combination of antibody with enzyme interferes with antibody combination by steric hindrance and by conformational change of determinants.

In the conversion of proenzyme to enzyme two additional functional indicators of antibody specificity play a role: (i) interference with the

---

[174] N. Sakato, H. Fujio, and T. Amano, *Biken J.* **14**, 405 (1971).
[175] R. Arnon and M. Sela, *Proc. Nat. Acad. Sci. U.S.* **62**, 163 (1969).

initiating step of conversion and (ii) interference with dissociation of the activated enzyme from the proenzyme complex. Antisera against chymotrypsinogen and trypsinogen can interfere with the second of these two steps,[176] and this may well turn out to be attributable to the type of antibody-induced conformational stabilization that has been found in the interaction between two peptides forming the catalytic space of ribonuclease A.[71] The functional effects of antisera depend on the specificity of the antibodies. This, in turn, depends on natural tolerance to autologous antigens and hence on polymorphism and species,[164,177] on the past immunological history of the individual,[1] and on genetic controls for responsiveness.[178-183] All these factors can contribute to a useful analysis, if properly exploited and if the analysis takes account of the often neglected fact that the immune response depends, to a very considerable extent, on the evolutionary distance between antigen donor and antibody producer.[177, 184, 185]

If one wishes to detect determinants that remain stable during the evolution of an order (say mammals), it is best to elicit antisera in animals of a *different* order. If antibodies are wanted against determinants which have been preserved in vertebrate evolution, one can immunize animals which have a complete genetic deficiency of a particular molecule (eniotypy[185]). In short, Landsteiner's "false immunological perspective" can be put to use.[186]

As a rule, it is difficult to determine the effects of genetic controls in the response to multideterminant antigens, but the different functional

[176] J. T. Barrett and M. S. Epperson, *Immunochemistry* 4, 497 (1967).
[177] B. Cinader, S. W. Koh, and D. Naylor, *Int. Arch. Allergy Appl. Immunol.* 35, 150 (1969).
[178] B. Benacerraf, H. G. Bluestein, I. Green, and L. Ellman, in "Progress in Immunology" (B. Amos, ed.), Vol. 1, p. 487. Academic Press, New York, 1971.
[179] "Genetic Control of Immune Responsiveness" (H. O. McDevitt and M. Landy, eds.). Academic Press, New York, 1973.
[180] *Symp. Genetic Control Immune Response, Proc. 2nd Congr. Immunol.* Vol. 2. A.S.P. Biological and Medical Press (North-Holland Division), Amsterdam, 1974.
[181] *Symp. Antigenicity, Proc. 2nd Congr. Immunol.* A.S.P. Biological and Medical Press (North-Holland Division), Amsterdam, 1974.
[182] S. K. Ruscetti, H. W. Kunz, and T. J. Gill, III, *J. Immunol.* 113, 1468 (1974).
[183] V. Würzburg, H. Schutt-Gerowitt, and K. Rajewsky, *Eur. J. Immunol.* 3, 762 (1973).
[184] B. Cinader, "Antibody Specificity as a Factor in Enzyme-Inhibition and in the Classification of Inborn Metabolic Errors," Vol. 2, "Clinical Enzymology" (R. W. Schmidt, ed.), p. 57. Karger, Basel, 1968.
[185] B. Cinader, S. Dubiski, and A. C. Wardlaw, *Nature (London)* 210, 1291 (1966).
[186] K. Landsteiner, "The Specificity of Serological Reactions," rev. ed. Harvard Univ. Press, Cambridge, Massachusetts, 1945.

effects of enzyme antibodies afford a unique opportunity to screen for genetic heterogeneity and, ultimately, to develop strains of animals for further research. For instance, it was possible to identify the rare rabbit which made antibody that activated native ribonuclease when immunized with polytyrosine polyalanine ribonuclease[26] and, in the response to L-asparaginase, 37% of immunized rabbits made activating and 33% made inhibiting antibodies.[186a]

3. IMMUNOENZYMOLOGICAL COMPARISONS

Immunoenzymological comparisons (Table II) are best carried out with antibody directed against either (i) chemically defined determinants or defined subunits or (ii) determinants that can be defined in terms of functional consequences of the enzyme–antibody interaction. For both purposes, antisera can be raised against the intact enzyme and their specificity can be increased by absorption with enzyme fragments or with cross-reacting molecules. Such absorptions should be carried out with molecules that are rendered insoluble so as to guard against persistence of antigen–antibody complexes in the absorbed antisera. The autologous determinants of the immunized animals will limit the range of determinants against which antibodies can be elicited.

The proteins of members of one species differ from the proteins of members of another species by many amino acid changes and by their configurations; proteins of different individuals of any one species differ from one another by considerably fewer amino acid substitutions. For example, although the proteins of different mice differ from one another in varying degrees, they all differ greatly from those of chickens. However, the proteins of mice differ in general from those of chickens more than they differ from those of animals of a species more closely related to mice (that is, of the same mammalian order); for example, they resemble the proteins of rats more closely than those of chickens. Therefore, for producing antiserum, at least three possibilities should be considered. In the case of a mouse, these could be as follows: (1) a member of the same species whose proteins differ in only some respects from those of the donor of the antigen (another mouse); (ii) a member of a closely related species (a rat); (iii) a member of a distantly related species (a rabbit).

Figure 12 illustrates some of the factors involved in making antibody against one individual in another member of the same species, differing from the donor in allotype. We shall consider this situation in mice.

The antigen molecule illustrated on the left (Fig. 12) represents the

[186a] E. Soru and O. Zaharia, *Immunochemistry* **11**, 791 (1974).

TABLE II
SOME IMMUNOCHEMICAL STUDIES ON STRUCTURALLY RELATED PROTEINS OF WHICH
AT LEAST ONE HAS ENZYMATIC ACTIVITY

Relation between molecules	Enzyme	Source	Reference[a]
Multiple forms of enzymes	Alcohol dehydrogenase	Horse liver	1, 2
	Amylase	*Bacillus licheniformis*	3
		Mammalian	4–8
	β-Glucuronidase	Rabbit liver	9
	Carbonic anhydrase	Erythrocytes	10–13
	DNA polymerase (6 S, 8 S)	Calf thymus	14
	Esterases	Human	15, 16
	Fructose diphosphate aldolase	Rabbit	17
	Glutamic dehydrogenase	Bovine liver	18, 19
	Glycogen phosphorylase *b*	Rabbit muscle	20
	Lactate dehydrogenase	Vertebrate	21–29
	Mitochondrial monoamine oxidase	Bovine liver	30
	Peroxidases	Human	31
	Phosphorylase	Canine	32
	Ribonuclease	Bovine	33, 34
Mutationally altered enzymes with aberrant enzyme activity	Alkaline phosphatase	*Escherichia coli*	35
	β-Galactosidase	*E. coli*	36–44
	Penicillinase	*Bacillus cereus*	45–50
	Tryptophan synthetase	*E. coli*	51–54
		Neurospora crassa	55
Proenzyme/ enzyme	Carboxypeptidase A	Bovine	56–59
	Carboxypeptidase B	Porcine	60
	Chymotrypsin	Bovine	61–66
	Cocoonase	Silk moth	67–69
	Pepsin	Porcine	70–76
		Chick	77
		Dogfish	78
	Plasmin	Human	79
	Thrombin	Human	80, 81
	Trypsin	Bovine	63, 82
Components of allosteric enzymes	Alkaline phosphatase	*E. coli*	83
		B. licheniformis	84
	Aspartate transcarbamylase	*E. coli*	85, 86
	Fructose diphosphate aldolase	Rabbit	17, 87

[a] Key to references:
[1] R. Pietrusko and H. J. Ringold, *Biochem. Biophys. Res. Commun.* **33,** 497 (1969).
[2] R. Pietruszko, H. J. Ringold, N. O. Kaplan and J. Everse, *Biochem. Biophys. Res. Commun.* **33,** 503 (1969).

[3] N. Saito, *Arch. Biochem. Biophys.* **159**, 409 (1973).

[4] R. L. McGeachin and J. M. Reynolds, *J. Biol. Chem.* **234**, 1456 (1959).

[5] R. L. McGeachin and J. M. Reynolds, *Biochim. Biophys. Acta* **39**, 531 (1960).

[6] R. L. McGeachin and J. M. Reynolds, *Ann. N. Y. Acad. Sci.* **94**, 996 (1961).

[7] R. L. McGeachin, J. M. Reynolds, and J. I. Huddleston, Jr., *Arch. Biochem. Biophys.* **93**, 387 (1961).

[8] R. L. McGeachin, *Ann. N. Y. Acad. Sci.* **103**, 1009 (1963).

[9] R. T. Dean, *Biochem. J.* **138**, 407 (1974).

[10] P. O. Nyman, *Biochim. Biophys. Acta* **52**, 1 (1961).

[11] P. J. Wistrand and S. N. Rao, *Biochim. Biophys. Acta* **154**, 130 (1968).

[12] S. Funakoshi and H. F. Deutsch, *J. Biol. Chem.* **245**, 2852 (1970).

[13] Y. Ben-Yoseph, E. Shapira, and A. Russell, *Isr. J. Med. Sci.* **7**, 1050 (1971).

[14] L. M. S. Chang and F. J. Bollum, *Science* **175**, 1116 (1972).

[15] A. Micheli and P. Grabar, *Ann. Inst. Pasteur Paris* **100**, 569 (1961).

[16] J. Uriel, *Ann. N. Y. Acad. Sci.* **103**, 956 (1963).

[17] E. E. Penhoet and W. J. Rutter, *J. Biol. Chem.* **246**, 318 (1971).

[18] N. Talal, G. M. Tomkins, J. F. Mushinski, and K. L. Yielding, *J. Mol. Biol.* **8**, 46 (1964).

[19] N. Talal and G. M. Tomkins, *Biochim. Biophys. Acta* **89**, 226 (1964).

[20] L. H. Schlisefeld, C. H. Davis, and E. G. Krebs, *Biochemistry* **9**, 4959 (1970).

[21] C. L. Markert and E. Appella, *Ann. N. Y. Acad. Sci.* **103**, 915 (1963).

[22] J. S. Nisselbaum and O. Bodansky, *Ann. N. Y. Acad. Sci.* **103**, 930 (1963).

[23] R. D. Cahn, N. O. Kaplan, L. Levine, and E. Zwilling, *Science* **136**, 962 (1962).

[24] N. O. Kaplan and S. White, *Ann. N. Y. Acad. Sci.* **103**, 835 (1963).

[25] G. W. Nace, *Ann. N. Y. Acad. Sci.* **103**, 980 (1963).

[26] K. Rajewski, S. Avrameas, P. Grabar, G. Pfleiderer, and E. D. Wachsmuth, *Biochim. Biophys. Acta* **92**, 248 (1964).

[27] K. Rajewski, *Immunochemistry* **3**, 487 (1966).

[28] G. F. Sensabaugh and N. O. Kaplan, cited by A. Arnon and B. Cinader, *in* "Progress in Immunology" (B. Amos, ed.), p. 1199. Academic Press, New York, 1971.

[29] E. Goldberg, *Proc. Nat. Acad. Sci. U.S.* **68**, 349 (1971).

[30] B. K. Hartman, K. T. Yasunobu, and S. Udenfriend, *Arch. Biochem. Biophys. Acta* **107**, 115 (1971).

[31] N. Rose, F. Peetoom, S. Ruddy, A. Micheli, and P. Grabar, *Ann. Inst. Pasteur Paris* **98**, 70 (1960).

[32] W. F. Henion and E. W. Sutherland, *J. Biol. Chem.* **224**, 477 (1957).

[33] B. G. Carter, B. Cinader, and C. A. Ross, *Ann. N. Y. Acad. Sci.* **94**, 1004 (1961).

[34] R. K. Brown, *Ann. N. Y. Acad. Sci.* **103**, 754 (1963).

[35] G. T. Cocks and A. C. Wilson, *Science* **164**, 188 (1969).

[36] M. Cohn and A. M. Torriani, *J. Immunol.* **69**, 471 (1952).

[37] D. Perrin, A. Bussard, and J. Monod, *C. R. Soc. Biol.* **249**, 778 (1959).

[38] J. R. S. Fincham, *Proc. Int. Congr. Genet. 10th Montreal, 1958*, Vol. 1, p. 355 (1959).

[39] D. Perrin, *Ann. N. Y. Acad. Sci.* **103**, 1058 (1963).

[40] A. V. Fowler and I. Zabin, *J. Mol. Biol.* **33**, 35 (1968).

[41] M. B. Rotman and F. Celada, *Proc. Nat. Acad. Sci. U.S.* **60**, 660 (1968).

[42] F. Celada, J. Ellis, K. Bodlund, and B. Rotman, *J. Exp. Med.* **134**, 751 (1971).

[43] W. Messer and F. Melchers, *in* "The Lactose Operon" (J. R. Beckwith and D. Zipser, eds.), p. 305. Cold Spring Harbor Laboratory, Cold Spring Harbor, New York, 1969.

[44] F. Melchers and W. Messer, *Biochim. Biophys. Res. Commun.* **40**, 570 (1970).

[45] N. Citri, *Ann. N. Y. Acad. Sci.* **103**, 1006 (1963).

[46] N. Citri and G. Strejan, *Nature (London)* **190**, 1010 (1961).

[47] M. R. Pollock, *J. Gen. Microbiol.* **14**, 90 (1956a).

[48] M. R. Pollock, *J. Gen. Microbiol.* **15**, 154 (1956b).

[49] N. Citri, *Bull. Res. Counc. Isr. Sect. A* **9**, 28 (1960).

[50] M. R. Pollock, J. Fleming, and S. Petrie, *in* "Antibodies to Biologically Active Molecules" (B. Cinader, ed.), p. 139. Pergamon, Oxford, 1967.

[51] C. Yanofsky, *Ann. N. Y. Acad. Sci.* **103**, 1067 (1963).

[52] C. Yanofsky, and J. Stadler, *Proc. Nat. Acad. Sci. U.S.* **44**, 245 (1958).

[53] P. Lerner and C. Yanofsky, *J. Bacteriol.* **74**, 494 (1957).

[54] T. M. Murphy and S. E. Mills, *Arch. Biochem. Biophys.* **127**, 7 (1968).

[55] S. R. Suskind, M. L. Wickham, and M. Carsiotis, *Ann. N. Y. Acad. Sci.* **103**, 1106 (1963).

[56] J. T. Barrett, *Immunology* **8**, 129 (1965).

[57] H. I. Lehrer and H. Van Vunakis, *Immunochemistry* **2**, 255 (1965).

[58] H. N. Beaty, *Biochim. Biophys. Acta* **124**, 362 (1966).

[59] K. Amiraian and T. H. Plummer, Jr., *J. Immunol.* **107**, 547 (1971).

[60] J. T. Barrett, *Int. Arch. Allergy Appl. Immunol.* **26**, 158 (1965b).

[61] E. E. Rickli and D. H. Campbell, *Fed. Proc., Fed. Amer. Soc. Exp. Biol.* **22**, 555 (1963).

[62] J. T. Barrett and L. D. Thompson, *Immunology* **8**, 136 (1965).

[63] J. T. Barrett and M. S. Epperson, *Immunochemistry* **4**, 497 (1967).

[64] E. Bucci and D. E. Bowman, *Immunochemistry* **7**, 289 (1970).

[65] H. G. Gundlach, *Hoppe-Seyler's Z. Physiol. Chem.* **351**, 696 (1970).

[66] R. S. Temler and J.-P. Felber, *Biochim. Biophys. Acta* **236**, 78 (1971).

[67] E. Berger and F. C. Kafatos, *Immunochemistry* **8**, 391 (1971).

[68] E. Berger and F. C. Kafatos, *Develop. Biol.* **25**, 377 (1971).

[69] E. Berger, F. C. Kafatos, R. L. Felsted, and J. H. Law, *J. Biol. Chem.* **246**, 4131 (1971).

[70] J. H. Northrop, *J. Gen. Physiol.* **13**, 739 (1930).

[71] C. V. Seastone and R. M. Herriot, *J. Gen. Physiol.* **20**, 797 (1937).

[72] O. V. Lobochevskaya, *Ukr. Biokhim. Zh.* **28**, 385 (1956).

[73] H. Van Vunakis, H. I. Lehrer, W. S. Allison, and L. Levine, *J. Gen. Physiol.* **46**, 589 (1963).

[74] R. Arnon and G. E. Perlmann, *J. Biol. Chem.* **238**, 963 (1963).

[75] J. F. Gerstein, L. Levine, and H. Van Vunakis, *Immunochemistry* **1**, 3 (1964).

[76] M. Bustin and A. Conway-Jacobs, *J. Biol. Chem.* **246**, 615 (1971).

[77] S. T. Donta and H. Van Vunakis, *Biochemistry* **9**, 2798 (1970).

[78] T. G. Merrett, L. Levine, and H. Van Vunakis, *Immunochemistry* **8**, 201 (1971).

[79] K.C. Robbins and L. Summaria, *Immunochemistry* **3**, 29 (1966).

[80] S. S. Shapiro, *Science* **162**, 127 (1968).

[81] S. S. Shapiro and R. Arnon, in preparation.

[82] R. Arnon and H. Neurath, *Immunochemistry* **7**, 241 (1970).

[83] M. J. Schlesinger, *J. Biol. Chem.* **242**, 1599 (1967).

[84] F. M. Hulett-Cowling and L. L. Campbell, *Biochemistry* **10**, 1364 (1971).

[85] M. R. Bethell, R. von Fellenberg, M. E. Jones, and L. Levine, *Biochemistry* **7**, 4315 (1968).

[86] R. von Fellenberg, M. R. Bethell, M. E. Jones, and L. Levine, *Biochemistry* **7**, 4322 (1968).

[87] E. E. Penhoet, M. Kochman, and W. J. Rutter, *Biochemistry* **8**, 4396 (1969).

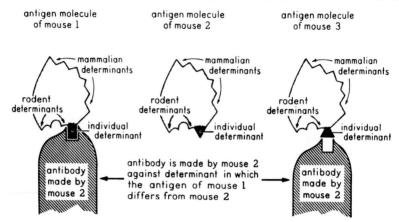

FIG. 12. Antibody formation when donor of antigen and donor of antibody show allotypic differences. From B. Cinader, S. Dubiski, and A. C. Wardlaw, "Studies of Rheumatoid Disease" (*Proc. 3rd Can. Conf. Res. Rheum. Dis.*). Univ. of Toronto Press, Toronto, 1966.

antigen of one kind of inbred mouse (mouse 1). It is injected into a second type of inbred mouse (mouse 2), whose corresponding antigen molecule is shown in the middle. It is seen that all but one of the determinants are identical in both mice; hence both mice are tolerant to these particular determinants, which consequently do not elicit antibody formation. Mouse 2, therefore, makes antibody only against the one determinant (shown in black) in which the antigen of mouse 1 and that of mouse 2 differ from one another. When this antibody is mixed with the corresponding antigen of mouse 3 (shown on the right), it does not react with the one determinant that is different in mouse 3 because this determinant is different from the determinant in mouse 1 to which antibody was made. The antibody that is made in mouse 2 is, therefore, extremely specific for one individual strain of inbred mice (mouse 1), but not for other members of the species.

The situation obtaining when a member of a distantly related species is used for making antibody is shown in Fig. 13.

The antigen of the donor rodent (mouse 1) is shown on the left (Fig. 13), while the corresponding antigen molecule of the rabbit into which the antigen of the mouse 1 is injected is depicted in the middle. The antigens of the rabbit show extensive differences from those of the rodent and hence the rabbit is tolerant to only a few determinants (called "mammalian determinants" in Fig. 13), and consequently antibodies are synthesized against many of the determinants of the rodent antigen. When this antiserum is mixed with the antigens of a second mouse (shown

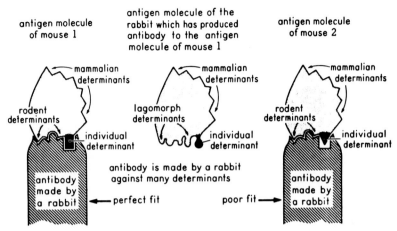

Fig. 13. Antibody formation when a member of a distantly related species is used for making antibody. From B. Cinader, S. Dubiski, and A. C. Wardlaw. "Studies of Rheumatoid Disease" (*Proc. 3rd Can. Conf. Res. Rheum. Dis.*). Univ. of Toronto Press, Toronto, 1966.

on the right), the antibody reacts strongly with all these determinants except the one shown in black. In this situation, virtually all the antibody made against one type of rodent can react with another type of rodent.

Thus, "faulty immunological perspective" depends on the structural relationship between the autologous macromolecules of the donor of antibody and the donor of antigen. If the antigen donor and the antibody donor possess very similar determinants, antibody is made only to the few determinants that differ and that are to be found only in animals closely related to the donor of antigen. The antibody therefore discriminates between the antigen donor and its closest relative but shows little cross-reactivity with antigens of distantly related species. Conversely, when the macromolecules of the antigen donor and the antibody donor differ considerably from one another, antibody is made to very many determinants. This multispecific antibody will react to a very similar extent with the antigens of the donor, with those of animals closely related to the donor, and even with antigens of distantly related species.

It is possible to change the "perspective" of the immunized animal by prior induction of tolerance. For instance, hen and turkey egg-white lysozyme differ from one another by seven amino acid replacements. Rabbit antisera are directed against the many common determinants of the lysozymes and do not detect their differences.[187] Antibodies specific only

[187] B. Scibienski, A. Miller, B. Bonavida, and E. Sercarz, *Fed. Proc., Fed. Amer. Soc. Exp. Biol.* **28**, 767 (1969).

for the turkey enzyme could be elicited in rabbits previously made tolerant to hen's lysozyme.[188]

a. IMMUNOCHEMICAL STUDY OF MULTIPLE MOLECULAR FORMS OF ENZYMES

Enzymes, possessing broadly the same substrate specificity, can be present in multiple forms in the same organism (Table II).[188a, 188b] The enzymatic properties of proteins that migrate differently in an electrical field have been studied by staining methods, based on the conversion of the substrate product into a colored compound (Vol. III, Chap. 14.E.1.d).[188c] The same method has been applied to antigen–antibody precipitin zones observed in immunoelectrophoretic studies (Vol. III, Chap. 14.E.1).[5-11, 189-191]

Heart and muscle dehydrogenases (LDH) of the chicken show considerable differences. In fact, dehydrogenases of an animal's heart and muscle resemble one another less than do the heart enzymes of two different vertebrates.[192-195] The lactic dehydrogenases of most species can be separated into five components by starch gel electrophoresis.[195a] Both the heart and muscle enzymes can be dissociated into four subunits of equal molecular weight.[192, 196] Thus both heart and muscle enzymes are tetramers, BBBB (LDH-I) and AAAA (LDH-V), respectively under the control of two different genes.[196a] Recombination of the primary gene products yield three further species, BBBA, BBAA, and BAAA. Thus, formation of "hybrid molecules" increases the number of molecular species beyond the number to be expected from the genes participating in the formation

[188] B. Bonavida, Dissertation Abstracts, Part B. 3369, University Microfilms, 1968.
[188a] C. L. Markert, and F. Møller, Proc. Nat. Acad. Sci. U.S. 45, 753 (1959).
[188b] C. L. Markert, Ann. N. Y. Acad. Sci. 151, 14 (1968).
[188c] R. L. Hunter and C. L. Markert, Science 125, 1294 (1957).
[189] A. Micheli and P. Grabar, Ann. Inst. Pasteur Paris 100, 569 (1961).
[190] A. Micheli, F. Peetoom, N. Rose, S. Ruddy, and P. Grabar, Ann. Inst. Pasteur Paris 98, 694 (1960).
[191] N. Rose, F. Peetoom, S. Ruddy, A. Micheli, and P. Grabar, Ann. Inst. Pasteur Paris 98, 70 (1960).
[192] R. D. Cahn, N. O. Kaplan, L. Levine, and E. Zwilling, Science 136, 962 (1962).
[193] N. O. Kaplan, M. M. Ciotti, M. Hamolsky, and R. E. Bieber, Science 131, 392 (1960).
[194] N. O. Kaplan and M. M. Ciotti, Ann. N. Y. Acad. Sci. 94, 701 (1961).
[195] N. O. Kaplan and S. White, Ann. N. Y. Acad. Sci. 103, 835 (1963).
[195a] C. L. Markert, in "Cytodifferentiation and Macromolecular Synthesis" (M. Locke, ed.), pp. 65–84. Academic Press, New York, 1963.
[196] E. Appella and C. L. Markert, Biochem. Biophys. Res. Commun. 6, 171 (1963).
[196a] C. Shaw and E. Barto, Proc. Nat. Acad. Sci. U.S. 50, 211 (1963).

of an enzyme.[192, 195, 197] Hybridization can lead to the appearance of the five molecular species that have been observed experimentally. In addition to the five above-mentioned multiple forms of dehydrogenase, there is a unique form, LDH (LDH-X), in sperm-producing testis of mammals and birds. It is also a tetramer but composed of different subunits (C) which differ from B and A and are under separate gene control.[198]

Isozymic forms of *some* enzymes have been reported to be antigenically distinct. This was the case for LDH,[192, 199] glutamic dehydrogenase,[48, 200] carbonic anhydrase,[201, 202] and myosin which possesses adenosine triphosphatase activity.[203, 204] Isozymic forms of other enzymes have been reported to be antigenically similar. This was the case for horse liver alcohol dehydrogenase,[205, 206] mitochondrial monoamine oxidase,[207] and the muscle type of rabbit glycogen phosphorylase[208] (Table II). It must be remembered that cross-reactivity is a relative property that depends on the autologous molecules to which the immunized animal is naturally tolerant and, thus, on the extent to which various determinants of the antigen can be recognized as foreign. Failure to "recognize" differences may result from similar differences in the autologous isofunctional enzymes of the immunized species and should, therefore, not be regarded as an absolute measure of structural relationship between molecules. In fact, LDH-I and LDH-V could be shown to have common determinant following acetylation of both subunits,[209] and cross-reactions were found to occur between chick heart LDH-I and haddock muscle LDH-V.[210]

The occurrence of multiple molecular forms need not invariably be due to multiple gene control, nor indeed to differences in the amino acid com-

---

[197] C. L. Markert and E. Appella, *Ann. N. Y. Acad. Sci.,* **103**, 915 (1963).
[198] A. Blanco and W. H. Zinkham, *Science* **139**, 601 (1963).
[199] D. T. Lindsay, *J. Exp. Zool.* **152**, 75 (1963).
[200] N. Talal, G. M. Tomkins, J. F. Mushinski, and K. L. Yielding, *J. Mol. Biol.* **8**, 46 (1964).
[201] S. Funakoshi and H. F. Deutsch, *J. Biol. Chem.* **245**, 2852 (1970).
[202] Y. Ben-Yoseph, E. Shapira, and A. Russel, *Isr. J. Med. Sci.* **7**, 1050 (1971).
[203] U. Groschel-Stewart and D. Doniach, *Immunology* **17**, 991 (1969).
[204] U. Stewart, *in* "Progress in Immunology" (B. Amos, ed.), p. 1199. Academic Press, New York, 1971.
[205] R. Pietruszko and H. J. Ringold, *Biochem. Biophys. Res. Commun.* **33**, 497 (1969).
[206] R. Pietruszko, H. J. Ringold, N. O. Kaplan, and J. Everse, *Biochem. Biophys. Res. Commun.* **33**, 503 (1969).
[207] B. K. Hartman, K. T. Yasunobu, and S. Udenfriend, *Arch. Biochem. Biophys.* **147**, 797 (1971).
[208] L. H. Schlisefeld, C. H. Davis, and E. G. Krebs, *Biochemistry* **9**, 4959 (1970).
[209] K. Rajewsky, and B. Muller, *Immunochemistry* **4**, 151 (1967).
[210] G. F. Sensabaugh and N. O. Kaplan, *in* "Progress in Immunology" (B. Amos ed.). p. 1199. Academic Press, New York, 1971.

positions of the different molecular species. Enzymes that are found to exist in multiple molecular forms by electrophoretic mobility may reflect the attachment of small molecules, such as sugars or phosphate groups,[211, 212] to a constituent peptide chain that is controlled by the structural gene. This situation seems to exist in the case of alkaline phosphatase of *Escherichia coli* mutants, in which the synthesis of four to five forms of the enzyme is controlled by a single gene. This conclusion is based on the fact that a single mutation leads to disappearance of all the molecular forms of the enzyme.

Whatever the causes may be for the production of multiple molecular forms, the recognition of differences can be assisted greatly by enzyme–antibody reactions. Sometimes multiple molecular forms of one enzyme, or isofunctional enzymes derived from different organs, differ sufficiently to be detected by interaction with corresponding and cross-reacting antibodies[213-221] (Table II). As a rule, however, it is quite difficult to distinguish such enzyme molecules, particularly when they are structurally closely related. It is not very likely that universal methods of high resolving power will be found, so that a number of special methods need to be considered, of which one or the other may turn out to be the best in a given case, or most suitable for a given objective. One approach depends upon selection of antibodies existing within a population of heterogeneous antibodies.

A particularly interesting relationship between very similar molecules has been observed in the synthesis of β-galactosidase (GZ) by *E. coli*.[222-225] Cohn, Monod, and Torriani found an antigen (PZ) in nonin-

[211] M. L. Bach, E. R. Signer, C. Levinthal, and I. W. Sizer, *Fed. Proc., Fed. Amer. Soc. Exp. Biol.* **20**, 255 (1961).

[212] C. Levinthal, E. R. Signer, and K. Fetherolf, *Proc. Nat. Acad. Sci. U.S.* **48**, 1230 (1962).

[213] W. F. Henion and E. W. Sutherland, *J. Biol. Chem.* **224**, 477 (1957).

[214] R. L. McGeachin and J. M. Reynolds, *J. Biol. Chem.* **234**, 1456 (1959).

[215] R. L. McGeachin and J. M. Reynolds, *Biochim. Biophys. Acta* **39**, 531 (1960).

[216] R. L. McGeachin and J. M. Reynolds, *Ann. N. Y. Acad. Sci.* **94**, 996 (1961).

[217] R. L. McGeachin, J. M. Reynolds, and J. I. Huddleston, Jr., *Arch. Biochem. Biophys.* **93**, 387 (1961).

[218] J. S. Nisselbaum and O. Bodansky, *J. Biol. Chem.* **234**, 3276 (1959).

[219] J. S. Nisselbaum and O. Bodansky, *J. Biol. Chem.* **236**, 401 (1961).

[220] M. Schlamowitz, *J. Biol. Chem.* **206**, 369 (1954).

[221] M. Schlamowitz and O. Bodansky, *J. Biol. Chem.* **234**, 1433 (1959).

[222] M. Cohn and J. Monod, *Biochim. Biophys. Acta* **7**, 153 (1951).

[223] M. Cohn and A. M. Torriani, *J. Immunol.* **69**, 471 (1952).

[224] M. Cohn and A. M. Torriani, *Biochim. Biophys. Acta* **10**, 280 (1953).

[225] J. Monod and M. Cohn, *Prof. Int. Congr. Microbiol., 6th, Microbiol. Metabolism*, p. 42, 1953.

duced *E. coli* that possessed negligible β-galactosidase activity, but reacted with antiserum to the enzyme. GZ was precipitated preferentially by GZ antisera, and PZ was precipitated only after all the GZ was removed.

Differences in the exocellular penicillinases of two strains of *Bacillus cereus* could be detected by using a partially absorbed antibody as enzyme inhibitor.[226] Antibody to the enzyme from strain 569 gave a 40% higher neutralization titer against the homologous enzyme than the heterologous enzyme. When a considerable part of the antibody was removed, by either enzyme, the difference in the neutralization titers became still more marked. Other examples of this general type may be found in the references cited in Table II.

Under certain circumstances, it is possible to show differences between multiple molecular forms of an enzyme providing that the forms differ in solubility of the antigen–antibody complex. This has been demonstrated with ribonuclease A and B, which differ from one another by a single carboxyl group, or conversely, by a single amide group.[227] Ribonuclease A and ribonuclease B were found to precipitate similar amounts of antibody, but if the two antigens were allowed to interact with antisera, from which part of the antibody had been previously removed by the addition of ribonuclease A, the residual antibody gave a much larger precipitate with ribonuclease A than it did with ribonuclease B.[63]

The types of problems encountered can be illustrated by further details regarding the reaction of antibodies with these two forms of ribonuclease. A ribonuclease antiserum was found to contain 16% of combining but nonprecipitating antibody, which explained the marked discrepancy between the calculated and the experimentally observed antibody content of residual antibody. Yet the residual antibody neutralized both ribonucleases A and B to the same extent. Apparently the differences between ribonucleases A and B observed in quantitative precipitin tests reflect differences in the hydrophobic properties of the two forms of enzyme, and heterogeneity of antibodies. A portion of the antibody molecules would form insoluble complexes with both antigens, another portion would form soluble complexes, and a third fraction of antibody, with intermediate properties, would give soluble or insoluble complexes depending upon the contribution made by the particular antigen to the solubility of the complex.[63]

One sees clearly, then, how different factors in the heterogeneity of antibody can be used to discriminate between structurally similar antigens.

[226] M. R. Pollock, *J. Gen. Microbiol.* **14**, 90 (1956).
[227] C. Tanford and J. D. Hauenstein, *Biochim. Biophys. Acta* **19**, 535 (1956).

The complement consumption method* has been successfully applied to the discrimination of multiple molecular forms of enzymes. Antigen and antibody are mixed and the capacity of the antigen–antibody complexes to fix complement is measured by means of a quantitative microcomplement fixation test,[228] based on the technique developed by Mayer and his co-workers (Chap. 17.B.3.a.iii)., By using complement consumption tests, it was shown that two isolated forms among the five multiple molecular forms of dehydrogenase cannot cross-react at all, and that the antibodies directed to the two molecular forms which do not cross-react with one another[192, 195] gave cross-reactions of variable extent with the remaining three molecular forms of dehydrogenase. Although this result could presumably also have been obtained with quantitative precipitin tests, the amount of precipitable nitrogen might well have been far too small, and the increased sensitivity of the test obtained upon conversion into a complement assay clearly has advantages when a high level of sensitivity is required.

Much recent work of immunoenzymological comparison[229] was devoted to enzyme structure, the relation between components of allosteric enzymes, between proenzymes and enzymes and between isozymes (Table II). Attention has also been given to questions of enzyme evolution[187, 188, 230–243] and to immunological studies of conformation.[244]

---

* The limitations and advantages of this technique have been discussed in detail [see A. G. Osler, *Bacteriol. Rev.* **22**, 256 (1958)]. It is suitable for the study of cross-reacting antigens, particularly when only very small quantities of antigen and antibody are available. The method is less suitable if antibody fractions or antibodies, obtained from one and the same animal in the course of immunization, are to be compared, since the extent of complement fixation by different classes and subclasses of antibodies varies considerably. Tests based on radioimmunoassay techniques [see Radioimmunoassay and saturation analysis, *Brit. Med. Bull.*, **30**, 1–99 (1974)] or on phage inactivation (Chap. 18, Section C) may be considered as useful alternatives.

[228] E. Wasserman and L. Levine, *J. Immunol.* **87**, 290 (1961).
[229] R. Arnon, *in* "The Antigens" (M. Sela, ed.), Vol. 1, p. 88. Academic Press, New York, 1973.
[230] A. Nisonoff, M. Reichlin, and E. Margoliash, *J. Biol. Chem.* **245**, 940 (1970).
[231] H. Fujio, Y. Saiki, M. Imanishi, S. Shinka, and T. Amano, *Biken J.* **5**, 201 (1962).
[232] N. Arnheim, Jr. and A. C. Wilson, *J. Biol. Chem.* **242**, 3951 (1967).
[233] E. Maron, R. Arnon, M. Sela, J.-P. Perin, and P. Jollès, *Biochim. Biophys. Acta* **214**, 222 (1970).
[234] E. M. Prager and A. C. Wilson, *J. Biol. Chem.* **246**, 5978 (1971).
[235] E. M. Prager and A. C. Wilson, *J. Biol. Chem.* **246**, 7010 (1971).
[236] A. Miller, B. Bonavida, S. A. Stratton, and E. Sercarz, *Biochim. Biophys. Acta* **243**, 520 (1971).
[237] K. Bauer, *Humangenetik* **8**, 27 (1969).

b. STUDIES OF ENZYME EVOLUTION

The major impetus to studies on evolutionary development has come and will continue to come from amino acid sequence studies.[245] The potential contribution of immunochemistry to advances in this field will be illustrated by studies of cytochrome c and of sets of molecules which, though not isofunctional, may have common ancestry. It is clear that common determinants do not necessarily indicate a close relationship between donor species; the same determinant could have arisen several times and independently. An intriguing example of this kind has emerged from studies of cytochrome c evolution in which antibodies have been used to identify antigenic determinants possessed in common by cytochromes of different species. The test is based on displacement of ^{125}I-labeled human cytochrome c from an antigen–antibody complex between human cytochrome c and an antibody elicited by cytochrome c of another species.[239] A determinant containing isoleucine was found in human, *Macaca mulatta,* and kangaroo proteins. This kind of determinant might deserve functional study to establish the physiological circumstances in which a mutation of this type is preserved in speciation and circumstances in which it is not preserved. The shared kangaroo-primate determinant probably indicates the occurrence of two independent mutational events. On the other hand, the determinant common to bovine lactalbumin and hen egg white α-lactalbumin[243] (Section 18.B.3.c) and common to plasminogen and fibrinogen,[237, 238] respectively, might each indicate preservation of a limited structural region which was encoded in common ancestral genes.

c. DIAGNOSIS AND THERAPY (GENETIC DEFECTS AND
TUMOR-VIRUS ENZYMES)

Challenging opportunities for application of immunoenzymology occur in the study of inborn errors of metabolism. Distinctions between de-

---

[238] K. Bauer, *Klin. Wochenschr.* **48**, 443 (1970).

[239] A. Szeinberg, E. Zoreff, and R. Golan. *Biochim. Biophys. Acta* **188**, 287 (1969).

[240] V. R. Linke, R. Zwilling, D. Herbold, and G. Pfleiderer, *Hoppe Seyler's Z. Physiol Chem.* **350**, 877 (1969).

[241] D. Herbold, R. Zwilling, and G. Pfleiderer, *Hoppe Seyler's Z. Physiol. Chem.* **352**, 583 1971).

[242] S. A. Aaronson, W. P. Parks, E. M. Scolnik, and G. T. Todaro, *Proc. Nat. Acad. Sci. U.S.* **68**, 920 (1971).

[243] E. Maron, C. Webb, D. Teitelbaum, and R. Arnon, *Eur. J. Immunol.* **2**, 294 (1972).

[244] F. Celada and R. Strom, *Quart. Rev. Biophys.* **5**, 31 (1972).

[245] N. Arnheim, *in* "The Antigens" (M. Sela, ed.), Vol. 1, p. 377. Academic Press, New York, 1973.

ficiencies that are caused by total absence of a competent molecule (eniotypy) and those due to mutations that result in incompetent molecules (allotypy) can be made by immunological techniques.[184] The question of the immunological consequences of eniotypy with respect to enzymes or enzyme-modifying macromolecules can be approached by similar methods: analysis of the murine deficiency of C5 has led to the finding that animals showing absolute deficiency (eniotypy) of this complement component would, when immunized with C5, produce unusually widely cross-reacting antibodies.[246] This was attributable to the absence of tolerance to any part of the macromolecule and constituted one of the criteria for distinguishing eniotypy from allotypy. Inborn abnormalities of a given molecule may be eniotypic or allotypic and may result in similar pathological consequences. This is the case in patients with hereditary angioneurotic edema (Chap. 17.E.2.a). Such individuals lack a functional protein, $C\bar{1}$ esterase inhibitor ($C\bar{1}INH$), which protects the synthetic amino acid ester substrate N-acetyl-L-tyrosine ethyl ester from the esterolytic action of $C\bar{1}s$.[247] In most patients, neither this molecule nor a cross-reacting inactive analog can be found. In certain persons with hereditary angioedema, the sera of affected individuals contain normal quantities of an antigenically intact but nonfunctional inhibitor protein.[248] Kindreds with this form breed true, and the autosomal dominant mode of inheritance is the same as in the more common form of the disease, in which there is no analog of the competent molecule. Electrophoretic analyses of $C\bar{1}INH$ protein from five related individuals with "genetic variant" hereditary angioedema have revealed several unique mobilities that are constant for all affected members of a given kindred.[249] This allotypic form of angioedema represents a structural mutation. Many other examples, in which eniotypy and allotypy result in a similar disease, have been found in the clotting system.[249a]

At the present stage of our knowledge, the basic enzyme lesions of metabolic inborn errors are often unidentified, and research is thus preoccupied with identification of the defective molecules. It is clear that success in such analysis will result in the availability of diagnostic tools and, ultimately, in rational replacement therapy. The present experimental approach to this analysis may be illustrated by reference to ex-

[246] B. Cinader, S. Dubiski, and A. C. Wardlaw, in "Studies of Rheumatoid Diseases," p. 202. Univ. of Toronto Press, Toronto, 1966.

[247] V. H. Donaldson and R. R. Evans, Amer. J. Med. 35, 37 (1973).

[248] F. S. Rosen, P. Charache, J. Pensky, and V. Donaldson, Science 148, 957 (1965).

[249] C. A. Alper, F. S. Rosen, J. Pensky, M. R. Klemperer, and V. H. Donaldson, J. Clin. Invest. 49, 3a (1970).

[249a] O. Ratnoff, in "Progress in Haemostasis" (T. H. Spaet, ed.), p. 39. Grune & Stratton, New York, 1972.

ploration of the hypothesis that some inborn errors, affecting glycosidases, may be attributable to a defect in the synthesis of "specifier" molecules which alter the spectrum of substrate specificities of enzymes,[250] i.e., molecules that function like the substrate-specificity modifying antibodies described in Section 18.B.2.d.

Perhaps the best understood example of operation of a specifier protein is the case of lactose synthetase. Mammary tissue contains a galactosyl transferase that will catalyze the transfer of galactose from UDP-galactose to N-acetyl-D-glucosamine to form N-acetyllactosamine.[251] In the presence of lactalbumin the specificity of this enzyme is altered to become lactose synthetase. This modified enzyme catalyzes the transfer of galactose from the same nucleotide sugar but to the acceptor glucose, forming lactose (Section 18.B.3.a).

A number of inborn errors, particularly of glycolipid metabolism, are known to be due to deficiencies of the activity of certain glycosidases. Glycosidases occur often in multiple forms; genetically determined deficiencies of these mutiple forms, both complete and partial, have been described. Enzymes of any one type may have a common polypeptide unit conferring the fundamental catalytic activity toward a particular nonreducing terminal sugar; this may be associated with other subunits, which function as "specifier" proteins and modify the catalytic activity so as to render it more specific toward its natural substrate.[250] This concept may be illustrated by the specific enzymatic lesions involved in the etiology of Tay–Sachs disease and Sandhoff's disease. In both diseases a particular glycolipid (the ganglioside GM_2, containing a terminal β-N-acetylgalactosamine residue) accumulates in certain tissues. The enzymatic defect in both diseases involves a deficiency of N-acetyl-β-hexosaminidase (hexosaminidase) activity. Two main forms of this enzyme, A and B, have been demonstrated; Tay–Sachs disease is characterized by a marked deficiency of the former and overproduction of the latter, whereas in Sandhoff's disease both forms are markedly deficient. There is immunologic evidence to suggest that both hexosaminidase A and B may contain the same fundamental catalytic subunit, but that hexosaminidase A may contain, in addition, a "specifier" subunit,[252–254] possibly a sialic-acid containing polypeptide. In Sandhoff's disease, the basic de-

[250] D. Robinson, in "Enzymes" (J. Frei, W. E. Knox, and O. Greengard, eds.), p. 114. Karger, Basel, 1974.
[251] K. Brew, T. C. Vanaman, and R. L. Hill, Proc. Nat. Acad. Sci. U.S. 59, 491 (1968).
[252] M. Carroll and D. Robinson, Biochem. J. 131, 91 (1973).
[253] M. Carroll and D. Robinson, Lancet 1, 322 (1972).
[254] S. K. Srivastava and E. Beutler, Biochem. Biophys. Res. Commun. 47, 753 (1972).

fect is presumed to be a mutation of the catalytic subunit, thus resulting in loss of both A and B activities. A defect of synthesis of the putative sialic acid-containing specifier subunit would result in a loss of A activity, and would permit hexosaminidase B to be formed in elevated amounts, the situation that occurs in Tay–Sachs disease. Immunological evidence for these concepts comes from: (i) the demonstration of the antigenic cross-reactivities between hexosaminidase A and B[252, 254] (ii) the recent demonstration of a specific non-cross-reacting antibody against hexosaminidase A[255]; (iii) the demonstration that immunoelectrophoresis of liver tissue extract from a patient with Sandhoff's disease gave two precipitin zones when reacted against a hexosaminidase B antiserum. This finding might be attributable to the presence of abortive enzyme proteins, corresponding to the A and B activities; furthermore, no such cross-reacting material could be found in the position of hexosaminidase A in liver extracts from Tay–Sachs patients; and (iv) the tentative identification of a low molecular weight protein in fractions of liver from patients with Tay–Sachs or Sandhoff's liver which had some of the expected features of the proposed subunit.[256]

A brief consideration of the pathogenesis of Fabry's disease, another inborn error of glycolipid metabolism (due to a deficiency of activity of an α-galactosidase) is relevant here. As in the case of hexosaminidase, two types of α-galactosidase (A and B) are demonstrable in many tissues.[257] Fabry's disease is due to a deficiency of the activity of the A form. Immunological distinction between the two forms of α-galactosidase led to the conclusion[258] that any resemblance between the precise mechanisms involved in Tay-Sachs and Fabry's disease is superficial, and that a common pathogenesis is unlikely. Before this conclusion is accepted, the specificity of the antibody employed in this study should be considered. The liver α-galactosidase of a number of species has been shown to have a molecular weight of 90,000,[259] whereas the human placental form, which was used for immunization,[258] has a molecular weight of 150,000. It is thus possible that the antiserum raised to the latter enzyme was, in fact, directed against a "specifer" subunit present in the larger aggregated form. Furthermore, findings made during the successful replacement therapy in a Fabry patient may also be interpreted in terms of a subunit hypothesis.[260] The infusion of normal plasma into

[255] S. K. Srivastava and E. Beutler, *Nature (London)* **241**, 463 (1973).
[256] D. Robinson, M. Carroll, and J. L. Stirling, *Nature (London)* **243**, 415 (1973).
[257] E. Beutler and W. Kuhl, *Amer. J. Hum. Genet.* **24**, 234 (1972).
[258] E. Beutler and W. Kuhl, *Nature (London) New Biol.* **239**, 207 (1972).
[259] M. W. Ho, E. Beutler, L. Tennant, and J. S. O'Brien, *Amer. J. Hum. Genet.* **24**, 256 (1972).
[260] C. A. Mapes, R. L. Anderson, C. C. Sweeley, R. J. Desnick, and W. Krivit, *Science* **169**, 987 (1970).

the patient resulted in the appearance of a serum α-galactosidase activity, 22 to 35 times that present initially. A similar increase could not be achieved by simple *in vitro* mixing of the patient's and control sera.[261] An enzyme subunit present in the organs of the Fabry patient may have been potentiated and released by combination with a specifier subunit contained in normal serum. A mechanism of this latter type has been demonstrated in Gaucher's disease, another inborn error of glycolipid metabolism due to a β-glucosidase deficiency. A low molecular weight glycoprotein from the spleen of Gaucher patients associates on incubation with a membrane fragment from normal spleen to produce *"de novo"* glucocerebrosidase activity.[262] A subunit hypothesis may also be invoked in postulating an etiologic basis for hereditary lactase deficiency. A hereditary lack of this enzyme was associated in a number of cases with loss of a low molecular weight heterogalactosidase.[263] This latter enzyme had no action on lactose, yet was absent, along with a specific high molecular weight lactase, while a broadly specific enzyme of intermediate size was present, but ineffective as a digestive enzyme. It is apparent that many problems in this area can be resolved by the application of immunoenzymological techniques, particularly with antibodies of specificity for defined determinants (Section 18.B.3).

It seems likely that enzyme–antibody studies will augment our understanding of other disease processes and may provide a basis for the development of procedures for successful immunotherapy and for diagnosis. Such potential is of particular interest in the case of the RNA-dependent DNA polymerase enzyme (reverse transcriptase) of RNA tumor viruses, both B-type and C-type,[264, 265] and other RNA viruses.[265] Antibody to highly purified enzymes have now been prepared which show marked specificity, although some cross-reactivity is observed between enzymes isolated from closely related virus species.[266-268] Thus antiserum to reverse transcriptase of one strain of avian RNA tumor virus inhibits the activity of the analogous enzyme present in other avian C-type RNA viruses,

[261] H. E. Sutton and G. S. Omenn, *Amer. J. Hum. Genet.* **24**, 343 (1972).
[262] M. W. Ho and J. S. O'Brien, *Proc. Nat. Acad. Sci. U.S.* **68**, 2810 (1971).
[263] G. M. Gray, N. A. Santiago, E. H. Colver, and M. Genel, *J. Clin. Invest.* **48**, 729 (1969).
[264] H. Temin and D. Baltimore, *Advan. Virus Res.* **17**, 129 (1972).
[265] G. J. Todaro, *in* "The Nature of Leukaemia" (P. C. Vincent and V. C. N. Blight, eds.), pp. 79–88. Government Printer, Sydney, Australia, 1972.
[266] W. P. Parks, E. M. Scolnick, J. Ross, G. J. Todaro, and S. A. Aaronson, *J. Virol.* **9**, 110 (1972).
[267] R. C. Nowinski, K. F. Watson, A. Yaniv, and S. Spiegelman, *J. Virol.* **10**, 959 (1972).
[268] H. Bauer, *Advan. Cancer Res.* **20**, 275 (1974).

but has no effect on C-type RNA viruses of mammals. Among the mammalian viruses there is immunological cross-reactivity between the reverse transcriptases of murine, rat, hamster, and feline origin. The enzymes of C-type viruses of primates are similarly related to each other, but not to enzymes of avian or other mammalian viruses.[265-268] The reverse transcriptase of the B-type RNA viruses are immunologically distinct from the enzymes of C-type viruses[264, 269] and also show species specificity.[270]

Hard upon the discovery of viral reverse transcriptase came reports of the presence of enzymes with similar activity in apparently normal tissues. The significance of these enzymes is not yet entirely clear. Of importance in the present context is the observation that antibody to reverse transcriptase from some C-type RNA viruses shows limited cross-reactivity with cellular enzyme.[271-273]

At the present time, antibody to reverse transcriptase has no obvious application as a tool in immunotherapy of diseases induced by viruses carrying this enzyme. This enzyme is present in the core of virions, where it is inaccessible to specific antibody. Tissue cells, in which the enzyme would be accessible, are themselves not permeable to the appropriate antibody.

Yet, as a diagnostic tool, the use of antibody to reverse transcriptase is very appealing, particularly for diseases of human beings. Animals carrying RNA-virus-induced tumors have serum antibody against specific reverse transcriptase.[242] This observation carries with it the potentiality for serum antibody screening—for previous or present infection—by specific reverse transcriptase-carrying viruses.

Numerous reports of the presence of human B- and C-type RNA viruses which may be oncogenic have been made.[271, 274, 275] Reverse transcriptase, with properties similar to the enzymes of the oncogenic and nononcogenic RNA tumor viruses, have been detected in the serum of patients with leukemic and a variety of other neoplastic diseases.[275, 276] Studies with partially purified enzyme and antibody to pri-

[269] A. S. Dion, A. B. Vaidya, G. A. Fout, and D. H. Moore, *J. Virology* **14**, 40 (1974).

[270] A. Yaniv, T. Ohno, D. Kacian, D. Colcher, S. Witkin, J. Schlom, and S. Spiegelman, *Virology* **59**, 335 (1974).

[271] R. C. Gallo, *Blood* **39**, 117 (1972).

[272] D. M. Livingston, L. E. Serxner, D. J. Howk, J. Hudson, and G. J. Todaro, *Proc. Nat. Acad. Sci. U.S.* **71**, 57 (1974).

[273] S. Mizutani and H. M. Temin, *J. Virol.* **13**, 1020 (1974).

[274] K. H. Hollmann, *Biomedicine* **18**, 103 (1973).

[275] T. W. Mak, M. T. Aye, H. A. Messner, R. Sheinin, J. E. Till, and E. A. McCulloch, *Brit. J. Cancer* **29**, 433 (1974).

[276] T. W. Reid and D. M. Albert, *Biochem. Biophys. Res. Commun.* **46**, 383 (1972).

mate and nonprimate purified reverse transcriptases suggest that enzyme of human origin may be immunologically related to reverse transcriptase isolated from C-type virus of primates, but not of subprimate origin.[277]

Definitive assessment of antigenic relatedness must await purification of the reverse transcriptase(s) of human origin. Antibody raised in non-human hosts to such purified enzyme can be used to characterize the species of origin of the enzyme. More important is the potential use of such antibody in the assessment of the association of specific enzymes with specific disease states, both at the qualitative and quantitative level. Such studies could provide the basis for the development of immunotechnology, with which to answer questions concerning the relatedness of reverse transcriptase(s) with specific disease states and the diagnostic value of this enzyme.

Once the reverse transcriptase(s) of human origin have been well characterized, it should open the way for the screening of patient sera and tissues for specific antibody. Such studies should permit assessment of the diagnostic potential of human serum antibody to reverse transcriptase in the study of various disease states.

It may be possible to suppress tumors with antibodies directed against membrane-bound enzymes that are antigenically distinct from isofunctional enzymes of normal tissues. In fact, there is a report of prolonged remission of lymphatic leukemia, induced in DBA/2 mice which had been immunized with porcine lactate dehydrogenase[92] so that a cross-reacting antibody appeared to be implicated in tumor destruction.

---

[277] R. E. Gallagher, G. J. Todaro, R. G. Smith, D. M. Livingston, and R. C. Gallo, *Proc. Nat. Acad. Sci. U.S.* **71**, 1309 (1974).

C. Virus Neutralization

1. THE IMMUNOLOGICAL REACTIONS OF BACTERIOPHAGES*

Immunological procedures have proved to be a useful tool in the study of the biology and chemistry of the bacterial viruses or phages. These methods are used for the identification and classification of various phages, for the study of formation of phage antigens in infected bacterial

---

* Section 18.C.1 was contributed by M. A. Jesaitis and N. D. Zinder.

cells, and for the investigation of structural constituents of the viruses.[1-4] In addition, because of the extreme sensitivity of the neutralization reaction, phages have been used as antigens in the studies of antibody synthesis by single cells and of the early stages of the immune response in animals.[5, 6]

a. Preparation and Properties of Antiphage Sera

Rabbits are usually chosen for the preparation of antiviral sera. Since phages are potent antigens, the amount of virus necessary for immunization is relatively small. As a rule, a group of three rabbits, weighing about 5–6 pounds each, are injected intravenously with increasing amounts of phage suspensions, containing between 10^9 and 10^{11} particles (0.5 to 50 μg) per dose.* The injections are given every second or third day for a period of 4 weeks. At 5 to 7 days after the last injection, the animals are test bled from the marginal ear vein, and the potency of the antisera is determined. If they are found to be satisfactory, the rabbits are bled by cardiac puncture. Otherwise, a second course of injections is administered and the tests are repeated. When it is desired to prepare antibodies to a minor phage component, such as the internal protein, or to a weakly antigenic material such as the nucleic acids of T-even phages, the animals are immunized intravenously with a large quantity (10^{14} particles or more) of ruptured alum-precipitated virus.[7, 8] The subcutaneous route of immunization and Freund's adjuvant also have been used for preparation of antiviral sera[3, 9, 10] and of antisera to viral nucleic acids.[10a] Since viral vaccines are often contaminated with the

---

[1] F. M. Burnet, E. V. Keogh, and D. Lush, *Aust. J. Exp. Biol. Med. Sci.* **15**, 227 (1937).

[2] S. E. Luria, "General Virology," pp. 116–127. Wiley, New York, 1953.

[3] M. H. Adams, "Bacteriophages," pp. 97–119, 421–431, and 461–466. Wiley (Interscience), New York, 1959.

[4] G. S. Stent, "Molecular Biology of Bacterial Viruses," pp. 57–63. Freeman, San Francisco, California, 1963.

[5] G. Attardi, M. Cohn, K. Horibata, and E. S. Lennox, *J. Immunol.* **92**, 335 (1964); **93**, 94 (1964).

[6] J. W. Uhr, *Science* **145**, 457 (1964).

* The particle numbers given in this discussion refer to the large phages, such as the T-even viruses. When other phages are used, different quantities may be optimal.

[7] L. Levine, J. L. Barlow, and H. Van Vunakis, *Virology* **6**, 702 (1958).

[8] L. Levine, W. T. Murakami, H. Van Vunakis, and L. Grossman, *Proc. Nat. Acad. Sci. U.S.* **46**, 1038 (1960).

[9] F. Lanni, and Y. T. Lanni, *Cold Spring Harbor Symp. Quant. Biol.* **18**, 159 (1953).

[10] G. M. Edelman, D. E. Olins, J. A. Gally, and N. D. Zinder, *Proc. Nat. Acad. Sci. U.S.* **50**, 753 (1963).

[10a] O. J. Plescia, W. Braun, and N. C. Palczuk, *Proc. Nat. Acad. Sci. U.S.* **52**, 279 (1964).

antigens of the microorganisms used for propagation of phages, the anti-viral sera may contain antibacterial antibodies. If such sera are to be used for complement fixation or agglutination tests, this antibody has to be removed by absorption of the antisera with bacterial cells.

The sera of animals immunized with bacteriophage contain antibodies to all surface constituents of the virus. In the case of the T-even phages, these are the antibodies to phage membranes and to the phage tail fibers and sheaths.[9, 11] If ruptured phages are used as antigens, the antisera may contain also the antibodies to internal proteins and nucleic acids.[7, 8] Some small phages, such as f2 and ϕX174, are structurally simpler than complex large phages, and therefore they evoke fewer kinds of antibody.[12-14] The antibodies elicited by a virus are not necessarily homogeneous with respect to their specificity. Some react only with the constituents of the virus used for immunization, whereas others combine also with those of serologically related phages.[3] A major portion of the cross-reacting antibodies can, however, be removed by absorbing the antiserum with such heterologous virus.[11, 15, 16, 16a]

b. NEUTRALIZATION REACTION

When an antiphage serum is mixed with a viral suspension, each of the antibodies combines with appropriate viral constituent. As a result, the phage may be neutralized, agglutinated, and acquire the ability to fix complement. Each of these reactions can be used for identification and quantitation of phages or of their constituents, as well as for the detection of virus-specific antibodies in the antiserum.

The most frequently employed serological reaction with viruses is their neutralization.[1, 17] This reaction is followed by measuring the decrease of the number of infectious particles in the phage–antiserum mixture. The virus is neutralized, or inactivated, when antibodies combine with those viral constituents that are essential for infection of bacteria. In the case of T-even phages these constituents are the tail fibers and sheaths. Consequently, the neutralizing antibodies for such viruses are those that are directed against the two tail components.[9, 11] The number of infectious particles also can decrease as a result of the aggregation of virus by antibody. However, as long as the viral concentration is less than 10^7 particles per milliliter, this process is very slow; therefore, phage suspensions con-

---

[11] N. C. Franklin, *Virology* **14**, 417 (1961).
[12] B. U. Bowmann and R. A. Patnode, *J. Immunol.* **92**, 507 (1964).
[13] U. Rolfe and R. L. Sinsheimer, *J. Immunol.* **93**, 18 (1964).
[14] H. F. Lodish, K. Horiuchi, and N. D. Zinder, *Virology* **27**, 139 (1965).
[15] G. Streisinger, *Virology* **2**, 377 (1956).
[16] A. R. Fodor and M. H. Adams, *J. Immunol.* **74**, 228 (1955).
[16a] M. A. Jesaitis, *J. Exp. Med.* **121**, 133 (1965).
[17] S. Fazekas de St. Groth, *Advan. Virus Res.* **9**, 1 (1962).

taining between 10^3 and 10^6 particles per milliliter are used in the neutralization tests.[9, 16]

i. Theoretical

When antibody is present in the phage–antiserum mixture in excess, the neutralization reaction follows approximately first-order kinetics, and may therefore be described by the relation

$$\frac{dp}{dt} = \frac{KP}{D} \qquad (1)$$

which after integration can be written as

$$K = \frac{2.3D}{t} \log \frac{P_0}{P_t} \qquad (2)$$

In these equations, K is the fractional rate of neutralization, or neutralization constant; D is the reciprocal of the final dilution of antiserum; t is time, in minutes, elapsed after mixing the virus with the antiserum; and P_0 and P_t are the initial and final phage titers, respectively. The value of K for a given phage depends upon characteristics of the particular antiserum and varies from one lot to another. It is also dependent on the temperature and ionic strength of the medium.[1, 18-22]

It is apparent from Eq. (2) that the plot of $\log P_t/P_0$ against t should be a straight line, and that the slope of this line should give the negative value of K at the dilution of antiserum employed in the test. In many instances, however, the reaction follows the first-order kinetics only until some 90 to 99% of virus is inactivated. These apparently serum-resistant phages are not genetic variants, for their progeny are inactivated at the same rate as the viral population from which they were derived.[23, 24]

ii. Procedure

(a) *Phage Stock Assay.*[3] The phage stock is diluted serially by 10 in nutrient broth, and 0.1-ml portions of each dilution are added to tubes containing 3 ml of 0.5% nutrient agar inoculated with approximately 5×10^8 cells of sensitive bacterial strain and kept at 45 to 50°. The con-

[18] A. D. Hershey, *J. Immunol.* **41**, 209 (1941).

[19] A. D. Hershey, G. Kalmanson, and J. Bronfenbrenner, *J. Immunol.* **46**, 267 (1943).

[20] A. D. Hershey, G. Kalmanson, and J. Bronfenbrenner, *J. Immunol.* **46**, 281 (1943).

[21] N. K. Jerne, *Nature (London)* **169**, 117 (1952).

[22] N. K. Jerne and L. Snovsted, *Ann. Inst. Pasteur Paris* **84**, 73 (1953).

[23] C. H. Andrewes and W. J. Elford, *Brit. J. Exp. Pathol.* **14**, 367 (1933).

[24] M. Delbrueck, *J. Bacteriol.* **50**, 137 (1945).

tent of the tubes is poured on petri plates containing 1.5% nutrient agar and allowed to solidify at room temperature. The plates are then incubated at 37° for 6 to 18 hours, and viral plaques that appear on the bacterial lawn are counted. The count multiplied successively by the reciprocals of the dilution and of the plated volume (in milliliters) of the sample gives the phage titer of the stock solution.

(b) *Determination of Neutralization Constant.* Serum is diluted serially by factors of 10 or of 3 in broth. Portions of each dilution are mixed with an equal volume (usually 1 ml) of phage suspension diluted from stock to contain about 2×10^5 particles per milliliter. A mixture of phage and nutrient broth serves as a control. The tubes are incubated in water bath at 37° for 30 minutes and then are transferred to an ice bath. Samples (0.1 ml) are taken from each tube and diluted a hundred-fold in 10 ml of ice-cold broth. Aliquots of these dilutions are plated with indicator bacteria as in the phage assay. The plaques are counted, then the percentage of inactivated phage at various dilutions of antiserum is calculated, and thus, the antiserum dilution that will inactive about 50% of the added phage is determined. From these data the neutralization constant of the serum can be approximately calculated using Eq. (2).

When it is necessary to know the exact value of the neutralization constant, the percentage of inactivated particles in the phage antiserum mixture is determined at various time intervals. In this instance, an aliquot of antiserum dilution capable of inactivating some 90% of phage in 30 minutes is added to an equal volume of phage suspension and the mixture is incubated at 37°. Aliquots of the mixture are removed after 1, 5, 10, 20, 30, 45, and 60 minutes and diluted in ice cold broth; aliquots of the dilutions are mixed with bacteria and plated as described above. A control containing equal volumes of phage and broth is also incubated, and samples of this mixture are plated at the beginning and the end of the experiment. After the plaques have been counted, the fraction (P_t/P_o) of surviving phage at various time intervals is determined and the data are plotted as illustrated in Fig. 1. When the experimental points form a straight line, Eq. (2) is followed and the neutralization constant can be calculated at any time point. Depending on the nature of the phage used as immunogen and the duration of immunization, the neutralization constants of antisera (K values) may vary between 10 and more than 10,000 per minute.

iii. Applications of the Neutralization Reaction

Since phages of various species differ in their serological specificity, the neutralization reaction is used for identification and classification of bacterial viruses. This is achieved by exposing the unknown virus to the

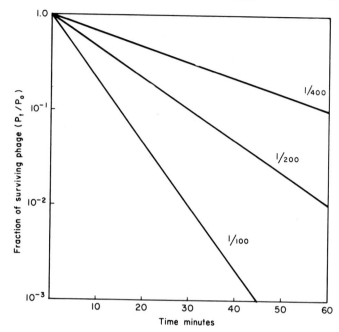

FIG. 1. Neutralization of bacteriophage by antiserum. Shown are idealized curves of the inactivation of phage by various dilutions of antiserum. See text [Section 18.C.1.b.ii(b)] for explanation.

action of a number of known antisera.[25] If the phage tested is neutralized by a certain antiviral serum, it is very likely that it is a member of the same viral species as the phage used for immunization. A negative reaction indicates that the two viruses belong most likely to different species.[3]

By studying the neutralization reaction it is also possible to determine the degree of homogeneity of a viral preparation. Thus, when 95% or more of viral particles are found to be neutralized by an antiserum at a constant rate, the preparation can be considered to contain but one type of virus. If the rate changes earlier, the viral population may be assumed to be nonhomogeneous.

The neutralization reaction can be used to detect viral tail antigens in bacterial cells or in their extracts. This is achieved by immunizing animals with the material under investigation and testing their antisera for the presence of a neutralizing antibody.[26, 27] Since viral tail fibers

[25] F. M. Burnet, *J. Pathol. Bacteriol.* **36**, 307 (1933).
[26] G. T. Barry, *J. Exp. Med.* **100**, 163 (1954).
[27] E. M. Miller and W. F. Goebel, *J. Exp. Med.* **100**, 525 (1954).

and sheaths are serologically different and since they both participate in the neutralization, this technique has been used to determine the specificity of each of the two tail components in hybrids obtained upon crossing the T-even phages.[11, 16a]

Finally, the neutralization reaction has found its way into studies on the formation of antibodies in tissue cultures and on the production of antibody in mammals. The absence of a serological relationship between viral and animal antigens, as well as the possibility of detecting very small quantities of antiviral antibodies by means of the neutralization test were the reasons for selecting this method.[5, 6]

c. DETERMINATION OF SERUM-BLOCKING POWER

The neutralization reaction also can be used for a direct quantitation of viral antigens that react with a neutralizing antibody. This is achieved by measuring the serum-blocking power (SBP) of an unknown material and by comparing it with that of a known phage. The SBP is defined as the ability of a material to decrease the neutralizing activity of an antiphage serum.[28, 29]

i. Procedure for T2[29]

The determination of SBP of a lysate of T2-infected bacteria is carried out as follows: First, the SBP of a standard virus preparation is determined. For this purpose anti-T2 serum is diluted in nutrient broth so as to inactivate phage with $K = 0.04$ min^{-1}. A purified suspension of T2 phage is diluted in the same medium to contain 1.4×10^{10} P/ml and then serially by 2. Portions (0.7 ml) of each of the viral dilutions are added to tubes containing 0.9 ml of diluted antiserum, and the mixtures are incubated for 8 hours at 48°. Then 0.2-ml portions of a suspension of test phage, T2 *rh*, containing 2×10^7 particles per milliliter, are added to each tube and to controls containing broth–antiserum mixture and broth alone. After 2 hours of incubation, the contents of each tube are diluted a hundredfold and aliquots of these dilutions are plated with *Escherichia coli* B/2. After the plaques have been counted, the percentage of surviving phage in each tube is determined. From these data the quantity of standard T2 phage necessary to decrease the neutralizing capacity of the antiserum by 50% is calculated. The experiment is then repeated using serial dilutions of bacterial lysate instead of known phage; from the data obtained, the quantity of the lysate necessary to decrease the neutralizing capacity of the antiserum by 50% is calculated. By compar-

[28] R. I. DeMars, S. E. Luria, H. Fisher, and C. Levinthal, *Ann. Inst. Pasteur Paris* **84**, 113 (1953).
[29] R. I. DeMars, *Virology* **1**, 83 (1955).

ing the results of the two experiments, the serum-blocking power of bacterial lysate can be expressed in terms of SBP of a certain number of phage particles.

The use of T2 phage as absorbing antigen, T2*h* as tester virus, and *E. coli* B/2 as a plating microorganism, permits scoring the test phage in the presence of various amounts of nonneutralized T2, because T2 will not infect *E. coli* B/2. This technique for differentiation between the absorbing and the tester phages is applicable in all instances when a virus and its host-range mutants are available. In those instances, however, when such mutants cannot be had, the serum-blocking power of a given virus can be determined by using, as the absorbing antigen, a virus which has been inactivated with ultraviolet light and the infectious virus as the tester phage.

ii. Applications of SBP Determinations

The measurement of the serum-blocking power is a convenient method for determination of the phage antigens reacting with neutralizing antibody, regardless of whether they are free or incorporated in infectious particles. By this method it has been shown that the lysates of phage-infected bacteria, grown in the presence of proflavin, which prevents formation of infectious virus, contain essentially the same quantity of the antigen in question as do the normal lysates.[28, 29] This assay has also been employed in studies of production of tail components by phage mutants incapable of forming infectious particles in certain bacteria.[14, 30, 31]

d. AGGLUTINATION AND PRECIPITATION REACTIONS

When a phage reacts with a specific antiserum at a concentration higher than 10^7 particles/ml, the virus is not only neutralized, but also agglutinated.[8, 14] The agglutination of viral particles can be caused both by the antibodies to the phage tail constituents and by those directed against viral head membranes. Electron microscopy has revealed that the former antibodies aggregate the viruses by binding their tails whereas the latter agglutinate the phages by coalescing their heads.[9]

If concentration of the virus is less than 10^{10} particles per milliliter, the amount of virus–antibody complexes is too small to be detected visually.[32, 33] In such instances, the agglutination tests can be performed

[30] R. H. Epstein, A. Bolle, C. M. Steinberg, E. Kellenberger, E. Boy de la Tour, R. Chevalley, R. S. Edgar, M. Susman, G. H. Denhardt, and A. Lielausis, *Cold Spring Harbor Symp. Quant. Biol.* **28**, 375 (1963).

[31] R. S. Edgar and I. Lielausis, *Genetics* **52**, 1187 (1965).

[32] F. M. Burnet, *Brit. J. Exp. Pathol.* **14**, 302 (1933).

[33] M. H. Merrill, *J. Immunol.* **30**, 169 (1936).

using the phage-coated microorganisms as an antigen.[34] When the concentration of a virus is 10^{10} particles per milliliter or higher, the amount of phage–antibody aggregates become large enough to be seen, and, therefore, the agglutination and precipitation of phages can be studied in the same manner as that of other particulate antigens.[1, 19, 32]

i. Determination of Agglutinating Capacity

The capacity of an antiserum to agglutinate phage is determined as follows.[19] The phage stock is diluted in broth to contain approximately 10^{11} particles per milliliter, and 0.5-ml portions are distributed into a series of agglutination tubes. The antiserum is diluted serially by 2 in the same medium, and 0.5-ml portions of each dilution are added to tubes containing phage. The phage and antiserum controls are also included. All tubes are placed at 4° for 2–3 days and then examined for agglutination. The highest dilution of antiserum causing a still perceptible flocculation of the virus is considered to be an end point. The reciprocal of this dilution is termed the agglutination titer of the antiserum for given phage.

An antiserum can be titered more rapidly by measuring the changes in turbidity of the phage–antiserum mixture in photoelectric turbidimeter.[16a, 35] The agglutination titers determined in this manner are about 8 times higher than those determined visually. (See also Vol. II, Section 10.B, and Vol. III, Sections 13.D and E.)

ii. Determination of Antibody Concentration by the Precipitation Reaction

Concentration of antibody in a serum can be determined by measuring the quantity of precipitate formed in an antigen–antiserum mixture. A known amount of viral antigen solution is added to varying quantities of antiserum and the mixtures are allowed to stand overnight in the cold. The precipitate is then collected in a refrigerated centrifuge, washed twice with saline, and the quantity of nitrogen in the sediment is determined by the micro-Kjeldahl method. The amount of antibody-nitrogen is calculated by subtracting the antigen-nitrogen from the total nitrogen in the precipitate. In those instances when the concentration of antigen in the test solution is not known, the amounts of precipitable antigen- and antibody-nitrogen can be calculated from the quantities of the total precipitable nitrogen, determined at two different antigen:antibody ratios in the proximity of the equivalence zone.[19, 20]

---

[34] F. M. Burnet, *Brit. J. Exp. Pathol.* **14**, 93 (1933).
[35] R. L. Libby, *J. Immunol.* **34**, 269 (1938).

iii. Application of Phage Agglutination and Precipitation Reaction

In addition to the titration of antibody in sera, the agglutination reaction can be used for detection of viral antigens, especially of those that do not react with neutralizing antibody. By means of this method it has been shown that the head membranes of hybrids, derived from crosses between T2 and T6, contain antigens of both parental phages.[16a] The precipitation reaction has been employed for determination of viral antigens present either in bacteria infected with isotopically labeled phage or in the virus-infected microorganisms grown in media containing radioactive amino acids.[36-38]

e. COMPLEMENT FIXATION REACTION

The complexes of viral antigens and their specific antibodies are capable of binding complement.[9, 39] The complement fixation reaction, therefore, can be employed for study of any of the viral constituents. This method has advantages over the agglutination tests, for it can be used with both impure and particulate materials. Several techniques are available to perform the complement fixation tests.[9, 39-42] The quantitative procedure of Mayer et al.,[40] adapted for phage work, is outlined below. For procedural details and theoretical discussion, the reader is referred to Chap. 17.B.

i. Procedure

The capacity of a phage to bind complement is determined as follows. All dilutions of antigen, antiserum, and guinea pig complement are made in buffered saline, containing 0.14 M NaCl, 0.005 M sodium Veronal buffer at pH 7.3, 0.5 mM MgCl$_2$, 0.15 mM CaCl$_2$, and 0.05% bovine serum albumin.[40] One milliliter portions of a anti-T6-serum dilution, having a neutralization constant K of 25 per minute, are added to a series of tubes containing 7 ml of ice-cold buffered saline and mixed with 1.0 ml of diluted guinea pig complement containing twenty 50%-hemolytic units. Then, 1.0-ml portions serial dilutions of T6 phage containing 10^9 to 10^{12} particles per milliliter are added to appropriate tubes and the mixtures are incubated either for 1 hour at 37° or for 18 hours at 4°. The

[36] O. Maaløe and G. S. Stent, Acta Pathol. Microbiol. Scand. 30, 149 (1952).
[37] O. Maaløe and N. Symonds, J. Bacteriol. 65, 177 (1953).
[38] G. Koch and A. D. Hershey, J. Mol. Biol. 1, 260 (1959).
[39] M. Rountree, Brit. J. Exp. Pathol. 32, 341 (1951).
[40] M. M. Mayer, A. G. Osler, O. G. Bier, and M. Heidelberger, J. Immunol. 59, 195 (1948).
[41] A. Peterkofsky, L. Levine, and R. K. Brown, J. Immunol. 76, 237 (1956).
[42] E. Wassermann and L. Levine, J. Immunol. 87, 290 (1961).

controls containing complement alone, complement and antiserum, as well as complement and antigen, are also prepared and incubated at the same time. Aliquots of the contents of each tube are then diluted 4-fold in chilled buffer, and 2-, 3-, and 4-ml samples of each dilution are added to a series of centrifugation tubes containing 1.0 ml of sensitized sheep red blood cells and buffer giving a total volume of 7.5 ml. The tubes are then incubated for 1 hour at 37° and immediately chilled. The non-hemolyzed cells are removed by centrifugation, and the percentage of hemolysis is determined by measuring the absorbance of the supernatant solution at 541 nm in a spectophotometer. In those instances when the sample of the diluted phage, complement, and antiserum mixture fails to lyse the erythrocytes, the hemolysis determination must be repeated using the undiluted mixture. From the data so obtained, the number of the hemolytic units of complement fixed is calculated using conversion factors calculated from the von Krogh equation[43] (see Chap. 17.B.2.b.iii). The quantity of complement fixed is then plotted against the amount of viral antigen used for fixation, and from this curve the minimum amount of phage necessary to cause the fixation of one unit of complement in the presence of given antiserum can be estimated. When the quantity of viral antigen is very small, a micro-complement fixation technique should be used[42] (see Chap. 17.B.3.a.ii).

ii. Application of Complement Fixation

Complement fixation tests have a wide application in virus research. Using such methods, it has been shown that viral antigens appear in phage-infected bacteria before the formation of infectious virus[39] and that there are no viral antigens in lysogenic bacteria grown in a medium in which they do not liberate phage.[27] It has also been demonstrated by the means of this technique that the head constituents of the T-even phages are serologically different from those of the tail,[9] and that an internal protein is present in the viral particle.[7] In addition, it has been found that antisera of animals immunized with ruptured T-even phages contain antibodies that fix complement in presence of the nucleic acids of these viruses, a fact indicating that the nucleic acids of T-even phages are immunologically active.[8] (See also Vol. II, Sections 12.D.1.b.i, c.ii, and d.) A study of the inhibition of the complement fixation reaction of nucleic acids by various sugars and nucleotides has revealed that the determinants of serological specificity of the viral nucleic acids are glucosides and gentiobiosides of hydroxymethylcytidylic acid.[44]

[43] M. M. Mayer, A. G. Osler, O. G. Bier, and M. Heidelberger, *J. Exp. Med.* **84**, 535 (1946).

[44] E. Townsend, W. T. Murakami, and H. Van Vunakis, *Fed. Proc., Fed. Amer. Soc. Exp. Biol.* **20**, 438 (1961).

2. ANTIBODY REACTIONS WITH CHEMICALLY MODIFIED BACTERIOPHAGES*

a. INTRODUCTION

The immunospecific inactivation of bacteriophages is among the most sensitive methods for the detection of very small amounts of antibodies and has for this reason been used extensively in immunological studies. However, this assay is limited to the detection of antibodies directed against bacteriophages. It is, therefore, of great importance to extend this sensitive assay to any desirable antigen. This is achieved by the chemical attachment to the bacteriophage of various antigens and haptens.

The procedure for coupling of antigens to bacteriophages is in principle the same as for coupling of antigens to proteins† (Vol. I, Chap. 1.E). However, the extent of conjugation to the phage is a crucial point in determining its capacity to be inactivated by antibodies. For this reason, optimal conditions for coupling should be found by varying the conditions of the coupling reaction.

The antigens chemically attached to bacteriophages include the following: nitro, iodo, and bromo derivatives of 4-hydroxyphenylacetyl,[1-3] nitrophenyl groups,[4-11] penicillin[12] and penicillin polymers,[13] prostaglandin,[14] steroids,[15] nucleosides,[16] oxazolone,[17] dansyl,[18] fluorescein,[18]

* Section 18.C.2 was contributed by Joseph Haimovich and Michael Sela.

† It is obvious that only procedures that do not lead to a complete loss in the viability of the phage may be used.

[1] O. Mäkelä, *Immunology* **10**, 81 (1966).
[2] S. Jormalainen and O. Mäkelä, *Eur. J. Immunol.* **1**, 471 (1971).
[3] V. Hatcher, and O. Mäkelä, *Immunochemistry* **9**, 1139 (1972).
[4] B. G. Carter, S. L. Yo, and A. H. Sehon, *Can. J. Biochem.* **46**, 261 (1968).
[5] C. L. Hornick, and F. Karush, *Isr. J. Med. Sci.* **5**, 163 (1969).
[6] S. Segal, A. Globerson, M. Feldman, J. Haimovich, and M. Sela, *J. Exp. Med.* **131**, 93 (1970).
[7] P. Barber and M. B. Rittenberg, *Immunochemistry* **6**, 163 (1969).
[8] O. N. Witte and L. I. Slobin, *J. Immunol.* **108**, 927 (1972).
[9] H. G. Bluestein and C. W. Pierce, *J. Immunol.* **11**, 130 (1973).
[10] L. K. Curtiss, and R. G. Krueger, *J. Immunol.* **110**, 167 (1973).
[11] H. Mossman and D. K. Hammer, *Z. Naturforsch.* **28c**, 83 (1973).
[12] J. Haimovich, M. Sela, J. M. Dewdney, and F. R. Batchelor, *Nature (London)* **214**, 1369 (1967).
[13] S. Shaltiel, R. Mizrahi, and M. Sela, *Proc. Roy. Soc. Ser. B* **179**, 411 (1971).
[14] F. Dray, E. Maron, S. A. Tillson, and M. Sela, *Anal. Biochem.* **50**, 399 (1972).
[15] J. M. Andrieu, S. Mamas, and F. Dray, *Eur. J. Immunol.* **4**, 417 (1974).
[16] B. Bonavida, S. Fuchs, and M. Sela, *J. Immunol. Methods* **1**, 155 (1972).
[17] S. Jormalainen, J. Aird, and O. Mäkelä, *Immunochemistry* **8**, 450 (1971).

plant hormones,[19, 20] inhibitors of acetylcholinesterase,[21] p-azobenzene-arsonate,[22, 23] picolinimidyl,[10] N-acetyl-p-aminophenyl lactoside,[24] biotin,[25] poly(amino acid) chains,[26, 27] as well as a variety of proteins and peptides.[28-36]

Detection of antibodies by inactivation of chemically modified bacteriophages and inhibition of the inactivation by haptens and proteins, facilitated the study of a wide variety of immunological phenomena, such as several aspects of the primary and secondary responses[6, 37-54] and tol-

[18] D. Blakeslee, D. F. Antczak, and D. T. Rowlands, *Immunochemistry* **10**, 61 (1973).

[19] S. Fuchs, J. Haimovich, and Y. Fuchs, *Eur. J. Biochem.* **18**, 384 (1971).

[20] Y. Fuchs, S. Mayak, and S. Fuchs, *Planta* **103**, 117 (1972).

[21] D. Gurari, and S. Fuchs, *Eur. J. Biochem.* **42**, 269 (1974).

[22] M. J. Becker, A. Conway-Jacobs, M. Wilchek, J. Haimovich, and M. Sela, *Immunochemistry* **7**, 741 (1970).

[23] M. J. Becker, H. Levin, and M. Sela, *Eur. J. Immunol.* **3**, 131 (1973).

[24] P. V. Gopalakrishnan and F. Karush, *J. Immunol.* **113**, 769 (1974).

[25] J. M. Becker and M. Wilchek, *Biochim. Biophys. Acta* **264**, 165 (1972).

[23] J. Haimovich and M. Sela, *J. Immunol.* **97**, 338 (1966).

[27] D. Gurari, H. Ungar-Waron, and M. Sela, *Eur. J. Immunol.* **3**, 196 (1973).

[28] J. Haimovich, E. Hurwitz, N. Novik, and M. Sela, *Biochim. Biophys. Acta* **207**, 115 (1970).

[29] E. Hurwitz, F. M. Dietrich, and M. Sela, *Eur. J. Biochem.* **17**, 273 (1970).

[30] O. Felsenfeld, *in* "Protides of the Biological Fluids" (T. Peeters, ed.), pp. 431–434. Pergamon, Oxford, 1971.

[31] S. Fuchs, M. Sela, and C. B. Anfinsen, *Arch. Biochem. Biophys.* **154**, 601 (1973).

[32] A. W. Steiner and F. M. Dietrich, *Z. Immunitaetsforsch. Allerg. Klin. Immunol.* **145**, 275 (1973).

[33] A. Maoz, S. Fuchs, and M. Sela, *Biochemistry* **12**, 4238 (1973).

[34] J. Eder and R. Arnon, *Immunochemistry* **10**, 535 (1973).

[35] J. Oger, B. G. W. Arnason, N. Pantazis, J. Lehrich, and M. Young, *Proc. Nat. Acad. Sci. U.S.* **71**, 1554 (1974).

[36] A. Aharonov, D. Gurari, and S. Fuchs, *Eur. J. Biochem.* **45**, 297 (1974).

[37] O. Mäkelä, E. Kostiainen, T. Koponen, and F. Ruoslahti, *in* "Nobel Symposium" (J. Killander, ed.), Vol. 3, pp. 505–515. Almqvist & Wiksell, Stockholm, 1967.

[38] S. Kontiainen and O. Mäkelä, *Int. Arch. Allergy Appl. Immunol.* **34**, 417 (1968).

[39] D. H. Plotkin, S. Kontiainen, A. B. Stavitsky, and O. Mäkelä, *Immunology* **15**, 799 (1968).

[40] A. M. Cross and O. Mäkelä, *Immunology* **15**, 389 (1968).

[41] O. Mäkelä and V. J. Pasanen, *Int. Arch. Allergy Appl. Immunol.* **35**, 468 (1969).

[42] S. Segal, A. Globerson, M. Feldman, J. Haimovich, and D. Givol, *Nature (London)* **223**, 1374 (1969).

[43] S. Segal, A. Globerson, and M. Feldman, *Cell. Immunol.* **2**, 205 (1971).

[44] S. Segal, A. Globerson, and M. Feldman, *Cell. Immunol.* **2**, 222 (1971).

[45] S. Kunin, G. M. Shearer, S. Segal, A. Globerson, and M. Feldman, *Cell. Immunol.* **2**, 229 (1971).

[46] S. Kontiainen, *Eur. J. Immunol.* **1**, 276 (1971).

[47] R. Tarrab, A. Sulica, J. Haimovich, and M. Sela, *Eur. J. Immunol.* **1**, 231 (1971).

erance,[55] antibody production by single cells[56] and in animals with a small number of lymphocytes,[57] the maturation of the immune response,[58-61] the biological importance of the bivalency of antibodies,[5, 24, 62] the size of the active site of antibodies of IgM and IgG classes,[63] the presence of antibodies in unimmunized animals,[2, 64] in allergic patients,[12] in newborn infants,[65] and in bronchial secretions of immunized dogs,[66] the genetics of the specificity of antibodies,[67] and the cross-reactions among haptens and antigens.[3, 14, 67-72] Conditions were established for the quantitative determination of several substances.[14, 15, 20, 29, 73, 74] Chemically modified bacteriophages were also used as potent immunogens *in vivo*[11] and in primary *in vitro* cultures[9] and for the detection of antigen receptors on lymphocytes.[75-77]

[48] A. Sulica, R. Tarrab, J. Haimovich, and M. Sela, *Eur. J. Immunol.* **1**, 236 (1971).

[49] M. Bustin, R. Tarrab, P. H. Strausbauch, A. Sulica, and M. Sela, *Eur. J. Immunol.* **2**, 288 (1972).

[50] P. H. Strausbauch, R. Tarrab, A. Sulica, and M. Sela, *J. Immunol.* **108**, 236 (1972).

[51] P. Del Guercio and E. Leuchars, *J. Immunol.* **109**, 951 (1972).

[52] I. Nakamura, S. Segal, A. Globerson, and M. Feldman, *Cell Immunol.* **4**, 351 (1972)

[53] S. Kunin, G. M. Shearer, A. Globerson, and M. Feldman, *Cell. Immunol.* **5**, 951 (1972).

[54] I. Nakamura, A. Ray, and O. Mäkelä, *J. Exp. Med.* **138**, 973 (1973).

[55] I. J. T. Seppala and O. Mäkelä, *Eur. J. Immunol.* **1**, 221 (1971).

[56] O. Mäkelä, *J. Exp. Med.* **126**, 159 (1967).

[57] J. Haimovich and L. Du Pasquier, *Proc. Nat. Acad. Sci. U.S.* **70**, 1898 (1973).

[58] J. Haimovich and M. Sela, *J. Immunol.* **103**, 45 (1969).

[59] H. Sarvas and O. Mäkelä, *Immunochemistry* **7**, 963 (1970).

[60] B. G. Carter, *Immunology* **19**, 429 (1970).

[61] L. Du Pasquier and J. Haimovich, *Eur. J. Immunol.* **4**, 580 (1974).

[62] C. L. Hornick and F. Karush, *Immunochemistry* **9**, 325 (1972).

[63] J. Haimovich, I. Schechter, and M. Sela, *Eur. J. Biochem.* **7**, 737 (1969).

[64] J. Haimovich, R. Tarrab, A. Sulica, and M. Sela, *J. Immunol.* **104**, 1033 (1970).

[65] S. Levin, Y. Altman, E. Nir, E. Hurwitz, and M. Sela, *Pediat. Res.* **7**, 675 (1973).

[66] G. A. Leslie and R. H. Waldman, *Experientia* **25**, 1096 (1969).

[67] T. Imanishi and O. Mäkelä, *Eur. J. Immunol.* **3**, 323 (1973).

[68] R. Arnon and E. Maron, *J. Mol. Biol.* **51**, 703 (1970).

[69] E. Maron, Y. Eshdat, and N. Sharon, *Biochim. Biophys. Acta* **278**, 243 (1972)

[70] B. Bonavida and S. Fuchs, *Immunochemistry* **9**, 443 (1972).

[71] A. Maoz, S. Fuchs, and M. Sela, *Biochemistry* **12**, 4246 (1973).

[72] M. Fainaru, A. C. Wilson, and R. Arnon, *J. Mol. Biol.* **84**, 635 (1974).

[73] J. Haimovich, E. Hurwitz, N. Novik, and M. Sela, *Biochim. Biophys. Acta* **207**, 125 (1970).

[74] E. Maron and B. Bonavida, *Biochim. Biophys. Acta* **229**, 273 (1971).

[75] F. Karush and C. L. Hornick, *in* "Cellular Recognition" (R. T. Smith and R. A. Good, eds.), pp. 281-285. Appleton-Century-Crofts, New York, 1969.

[76] A. Sulica, J. Haimovich, and M. Sela, *J. Immunol.* **106**, 721 (1971).

[77] S. Ben-Efraim, R. Teitelbaum, R. Ophir, R. Kleinman, and D. Weiss, *Isr. J. Med. Sci.* **10**, 972 (1974).

Bacteriophages were also modified by the specific attachment to the phage of Fab fragments of anti-phage antibodies. This immunological modification enabled the detection of anti-Fab antibodies[78] as well as antiallotypes of the particular Fab attached.[79] By coupling of antigens to the Fab it also served for the detection of antibodies against the antigens attached to the Fab.[80-81] Inactivation of immunologically modified bacteriophages is based on the fact that Fab is far less efficient than intact antibodies in inactivating phages, but the complex phage–Fab is efficiently inactivated by antibodies against determinants present on the Fab.[82-85]

b. HAPTEN-BACTERIOPHAGE CONJUGATES

i. General Procedure

Attachment of haptens to bacteriophages is performed by allowing purified bacteriophage preparations (Vol. I, Chap. 1.D.3) to react with the activated hapten at the appropriate conditions of temperature, pH, time of reaction, and concentrations of both activated hapten and bacteriophage. The reaction is terminated by diluting the reaction mixture 10- to 100-fold with 0.05 M phosphate buffer, pH 6.8, containing 20 μg/ml of gelatin (GPB)* and dialyzing against the same buffer† without gelatin. Large losses in viability of phage usually result from the coupling process. However, the high proportion of nonviable coupled phage does not interfere with the immunospecific inactivation of the survivors.[26] The surviving modified phage concentration is determined by plating‡ aliquots of serial 50-fold dilutions of the modified phage preparations to determine the number of plaque-forming units (PFU/ml). The different

[78] M. J. Taussig, *Immunology* 18, 323 (1970).

[79] E. Maron and S. Dray, *J. Immunol. Methods* 3, 347 (1973).

[80] H. E. Amos, D. W. Wilson, M. J. Taussig, and S. J. Carlton, *Clin. Exp. Immunol.* 8, 563 (1971).

[81] D. Gurari, B. Bonavida, M. J. Taussig, S. Fuchs, and M. Sela, *Eur. J. Biochem.* 26, 247 (1972).

[82] K. J. Lafferty, *Virology* 21, 76 (1963).

[83] J. W. Goodman and J. J. Donch, *Immunochemistry* 2, 351 (1965).

[84] G. W. Stemke and E. S. Lennox, *J. Immunol.* 98, 94 (1967).

[85] N. R. Klinman, C. A. Long, and F. Karush, *J. Immunol.* 99, 1128 (1967).

* This buffer is used as a diluent for phage, antisera, and inhibitors.

† Gel filtration may also be used for the separation of the modified phage from the unreacted hapten.

‡ The agar gel for preparation of the plates contains: 10 gm of Bacto tryptone, 12 gm of Bacto agar, 8 gm of NaCl, 2 gm of sodium citrate, and 3 gm of glucose dissolved into 1 liter of water. Soft agar for the top layer contains the same ingredients at the same concentrations except for the agar, which is at lower concentration, 7 gm/liter.

preparations of modified phages are tested for their capacity to be inactivated by the specific antiserum.

Hapten–bacteriophage preparations are kept at 4° in GPB. They are usually very stable and can be kept for years without a drop either in viability or in sensitivity to antibodies. In some instances there is a drop in the concentration of viable phage (up to 90% after a year), but even then, sensitivity to the inactivation by antibodies is not considerably changed.

ii. Penicilloyl-Bacteriophage T4 (Penicilloyl T4)[12]

Bacteriophage T4 solution (2 ml of 10^{11} PFU/ml) in sodium carbonate buffer, pH 9.5,* is added to penicillin G (200 mg) or to other penicillins of choice. The reaction mixture is allowed to stand at 37°. Samples are withdrawn after 10, 15, 20, and 25 hours and dialyzed against PB. One percent to 10% of the phage population survives the coupling process.

iii. 3-Iodo-4-hydroxy-5-nitrophenylacetyl-Bacteriophage T2(NIP-T2)[1]

Bacteriophage T2 (2×10^{10}/ml in 0.3 M sodium carbonate buffer, pH 9.5) is added to NIP-acetyl chloride (final concentration of 15 mg/ml). Reaction mixture is kept at room temperature with occasional shaking. Aliquots are withdrawn at 5, 10, 15, and 20 hours, diluted a hundredfold in GPB, and dialyzed against PB. Usually, the optimal reaction time is about 10 hours, at which time about 90% of the phage becomes inactive.

iv. 2,4-Dinitrophenyl-Bacteriophage T4 (DNP-T4)[4, 6]

Bacteriophage T4 (10^{11} PFU/ml) in 0.3 M sodium carbonate buffer, pH 9.5, is added to an equal volume of a solution of 2,4-dinitrobenzene sulfonate (100 mg/ml) in the same buffer. The reaction mixture is allowed to stand at 24° in the dark with occasional mixing for 5–30 hours. Aliquots removed at 5-hour intervals are dialyzed against PB. Usually, only 0.1 to 1% of the phage population survives the coupling process.

DNP-bacteriophage ΦX174 conjugate has been prepared, with only 50% loss of viability, by holding 2×10^{10} PFU overnight in 5% dinitrobenzene sulfonate in 0.2 M sodium carbonate buffer, pH 11.[5]

v. 3-Indoleacetyl-Bacteriophage T4 (IA-T4)[19]

Eighty milligrams of indoleacetic acid in 1 ml of dioxane are allowed to react with 60 mg of N,N'-dicyclohexyl carbodiimide for 30 minutes

---

* Bacteriophage solutions in buffers other than GPB are prepared by diluting the concentrated stock suspension (1 to 2×10^{13} PFU/ml) in the appropriate buffer.

with stirring. The mixture is centrifuged and aliquots of the supernatant (0.05–0.2 ml) are added dropwise to 1 ml of bacteriophage T4 solution (10^{12} PFU/ml in 0.1 M borate buffer, pH 8.5). The reaction is allowed to continue for 10 minutes at 4° with stirring, and is stopped by diluting the mixture a hundredfold in GPB. The diluted solution is dialyzed against PB. Similar procedures were employed for the preparation of gibberellyl-T4.[19]

c. POLYPEPTIDYL-BACTERIOPHAGES

i. General Procedure

Attachment of polypeptides to bacteriophages is performed in two ways: (1) direct polymerization of N-carboxy-α-amino acid anhydrides with bacteriophages as multifunctional initiators (Section 18.C.2.c.ii); (2) coupling of the polypeptides with the aid of bifunctional coupling agents (Sections 18.C.2.c.iii, 18.C.2.d.i–iii). The direct polymerization of N-carboxy-α-amino acid anhydrides on the bacteriophage protein is similar to the method for polymerization on proteins (Vol. I, Chap. 1.E.7).

ii. Poly-DL-alanyl-Bacteriophage T4 (Poly-DL-alanyl T4) by Polymerization of N-Carboxy-DL-alanine Anhydride on the Phage[26]

N-Carboxy-DL-alanine anhydride is dissolved in dioxane (20 mg/ml), and 0.1 ml of the solution is added to 1.9 ml of bacteriophage T4 solution (10^{12} PFU/ml in PB). The reaction mixture is allowed to stand at 0°. Aliquots of 0.1 ml are withdrawn after 5, 10, 15, and 20 minutes, diluted into 9.9 ml of GPB, and dialyzed against PB.* Usually, 1 to 10% of the phage population survives the polypeptidylation process.

iii. Poly-L-prolyl-Bacteriophage T4 (Poly-L-prolyl T4) Using 1,3-Difluoro-4,6-dinitrobenzene (DFDNB)[27]

A solution of 4.5 mg of DFDNB in 25 μl of acetone as bifunctional reagent, is added to a solution of 50 mg of poly-L-proline in 0.5 ml of 0.05 M sodium bicarbonate. After 20 minutes' reaction at 24°, T4 (1.5×10^{11} PFU in 0.5 ml of 0.1 M carbonate, pH 9.5) is added and the mixture is left for 18 hours at 24°. The conjugate is separated from the unreacted peptide by two successive centrifugations for 1 hour at 20,000 g, the pellet being resuspended in GPB.

---

* When tritiated N-carboxy-DL-alanine anhydride was allowed to react at a final concentration of 0.82 mg/ml, about 10,000 alanine residues were coupled per phage particle.

d. PROTEIN-BACTERIOPHAGE T4 CONJUGATES

i. *Tolylene 2,4-Diisocyanate (TDIC) Method*[28]

To 0.3 ml of bacteriophage T4 solution ($OD_{260nm}^{1cm} = 200$) is added 0.3 ml of several concentrations (10 to 50 mg/ml) of protein solution in PB; note that insulin is dissolved in 0.3 M sodium carbonate buffer, pH 9.5. To this mixture 0.1 ml of a solution of TDIC in dioxane (0.03% to 3% v/v) is added slowly with stirring. Smaller volumes of the same concentrations may be used. The reaction mixture is allowed to stand for 1 hour at 24°. At the end of the reaction, 5 ml of GPB are added and the reaction mixture is dialyzed against 6 liters of 0.05 M plain phosphate buffer, pH 6.8. Any precipitate is removed by centrifugation at low speed. The protein–bacteriophage conjugate is separated from the lighter un- reacted protein by two successive centrifugations for 1 hour at 20,000 g, the pellet being resuspended in GPB. The concentration of phage particles is determined by the absorbancy at 260 nm, and the concentration of viable phage is determined by plating serial 50-fold dilutions of the prepa- rations. From the above concentrations the percentage of the modified bacteriophage surviving the coupling process is calculated. Optimal con- ditions for coupling of several proteins are given in Table I.

ii. *Glutaraldehyde Method*[28]

To 0.1 ml of bacteriophage T4 solution ($OD_{260nm}^{1cm} = 200$) is added 0.1 ml of protein solution in PB (10 to 50 mg/ml). To this mixture, 0.025 ml of glutaraldehyde (0.05 to 0.2% v/v) is added; the reaction is left for 1 hour at 24°. The mixture is then diluted, dialyzed, centrifuged, and assayed as in the procedure for preparation of protein–bacteriophage conjugates with TDIC as the bifunctional reagent. The optimal condi- tions for coupling of RNase and lysozyme to bacteriophage T4 are given in Table I.

iii. *Bisdiazobenzidine (BDB) Method*[28]

To 0.1 ml of bacteriophage T4 solution ($OD_{260nm}^{1cm} = 200$) is added 0.1 ml of protein solution in PB (10 to 50 mg/ml). To this mixture 0.03- to 0.1-ml portions of active, bis-diazotized benzidine solution (Vol. I, Chap.1.E.6.h) diluted 1:15 in PB is added, the reaction mixture is left for 15 minutes at 24° and then diluted, dialyzed, centrifuged, and assayed as in the preparation of protein–bacteriophage conjugates in which TDIC is used as the bifunctional reagent. The best preparation of ribonuclease–T4 conjugate (highest sensitivity to inactivation by anti- RNase serum) was achieved with 10 mg of RNase per milliliter and 0.03 ml of BDB solution (Table I).

TABLE I

COUPLING OF PROTEINS TO BACTERIOPHAGE T4, AND INACTIVATION OF THE
SURVIVING PHAGE WITH SPECIFIC ANTISERA

Protein coupled to bacteriophage via bifunctional reagent	Protein (mg/ml)[a]	Bifunctional reagent (% v/v)[a]	Surviving phage (%)[b]	Antibody detected (ng/ml)[c]
Tolylene 2,4-diisocyanate				
RNase	7	0.008	1.1	2
BSA	11	0.2	0.05	2
RSA	17	0.6	0.05	1
Rabbit IgG	9	0.016	0.6	0.5
Lysozyme	21	0.0025	80.0	0.2
Insulin	17	0.2	0.1	ND[d]
(T,G)-A–L[e]	9	0.14	5.0	2.5
Glutaraldehyde				
RNase	4.5	0.01	7.4	2
Lysozyme	10	0.01	36.0	0.2
Bisdiazobenzidine				
RNase	4.3	See text	5.0	12

[a] Final concentration in the reaction mixture.

[b] The percentage of phage surviving the coupling process was calculated from the number of plaque-forming units and the optical density of the modified phage preparation.

[c] This is the lowest concentration of antibody detected from the dilution of serum (of known antibody content), which gives 50% inactivation of the protein–phage conjugate after reaction for 10 hours at 37°.

[d] ND, not determined. A guinea pig anti-insulin serum inactivated 50% of the insulin-T4 conjugate after 10 hours reaction at 37° at a final dilution of $1:10^7$. The concentration of antibodies in the serum could not be evaluated as antibodies could not be precipitated by the antigen.

[e] M. Sela, S. Fuchs, and R. Arnon, *Biochem. J.* **85**, 223 (1962).

e. IMMUNOLOGICALLY MODIFIED BACTERIOPHAGES: CONJUGATES OF
BACTERIOPHAGE T4 WITH DENATURED DNA-ANTI-T4 FAB'[81]

DNA is denatured by heating a solution (4 mg/ml) for 10 minutes in a boiling water bath and then cooling rapidly in ice. Fab' of anti-T4 is prepared by pepsin digestion. Denatured DNA (2.4 mg) is mixed with 5 mg of Fab' and 10 mg of 1-ethyl-3-(3-dimethylaminopropyl) carbodi-imide hydrochloride in a total volume of 1 ml of 0.1 M Tris buffer, pH 7.5. The mixture is dialyzed to remove excess coupling reagent, and 0.1 ml is added to 0.1 ml of T4 solution (10^9 PFU/ml). Reaction is terminated after 1 hour by adding 20 ml of PB. Five percent to 10% of the phage survive the coupling process.

f. Immunospecific Inactivation of Chemically Modified Bacteriophages, and Inhibition of Inactivation by Added Antigen

i. General Considerations

The inactivation of chemically modified bacteriophages by antibodies specific for the chemical substance attached to their protein coat is similar in its characteristics to the inactivation of unmodified phage (Section 18.C.1). The reaction follows first-order kinetics, although deviation from a first-order reaction has been observed in some instances. As with unmodified phage, this phenomenon may result from the dissociation of the phage–antibody complex during plating due to the low avidity of some antibodies reacting with the phage.[26] If the modified phages are allowed to react with antibodies and then plated by the decision technique,[86*] the deviation from first-order kinetics is considerably reduced.[26] The heterogeneity of the modified phage population, caused by the random coupling of the chemical substance attached, may also give rise to a reaction different from that which displays first-order characteristics. In addition, the high proportion of inactive phage in the modified phage preparation may limit the range at which a first-order reaction is achieved.[7]

Similar to the inactivation of unmodified phages,[87] the rate of inactivation may sometimes be increased by adding an antiserum against the type of specific antibody used for inactivation (for instance, when rabbit antiserum is used for inactivation, goat anti-rabbit globulin can be added at the end of the inactivation reaction and allowed to react for a few minutes prior to plating).

It should be emphasized that the rate of inactivation of the modified phage is not a direct measure of the amount of antibodies tested. Other parameters, such as affinity, the class of antibody, and the chemical nature and density of the antigenic determinant, play an important role in determining the efficiency of the antibodies to inactivate the phage.[58, 88]

Components other than antibodies present in the serum do not play a role in the inactivation of modified bacteriophages, as shown by the

[86] N. K. Jerne and P. Avegno, *J. Immunol.* **76**, 200 (1956).
* The decision technique of N. K. Jerne and P. Avegno [*J. Immunol.* **76**, 200 (1956)] consists in blocking phage reactivation during the plating period. An extra step is introduced in the test: the bacteria to be plated are mixed with phage, and a 10-minute period is allowed for infection of the bacteria. Then free phage are killed by application of a highly avid antiphage antiserum for 5 minutes, after which a sample is mixed with fluid agar and plated. [Editors]
[87] W. M. Krummel and J. W. Uhr, *J. Immunol.* **102**, 772 (1969).
[88] S. Koskimies, O. Mäkelä, and I. J. T. Seppala, *Scand. J. Immunol.* **1**, 33 (1972).

fact that isolated antibody preparations are as efficient as whole sera in this reaction.[58]

Specificity of the inactivation of the modified phages is proved by the inhibition of the inactivation with the free chemical substance identical to that attached to the phage (either hapten or protein). As undiluted sera may nonspecifically inactivate modified bacteriophages because of the presence of naturally occurring anti-bacteriophage antibodies, *each serum should be tested for anti-bacteriophage activity with unmodified phage.*

ii. Inactivation of Penicilloyl-Bacteriophage T4 by Anti-Penicilloyl Serum

To sterile test tubes (12 × 100 mm) are added 0.2 ml of penicilloyl-T4 solution (3 × 10³ PFU/ml) and 0.2-ml aliquots from serial 10-fold dilutions of anti-penicilloyl serum. (Smaller volumes of phage and antibody solutions may be used if necessary.) The mixtures are kept at 37° in a water bath for 1 to 5 hours. Soft agar (2.5 ml) and bacteria (3 × 10⁸ of *E. coli* B) are added to the reaction mixtures, which in turn are plated by the double agar layer method.[89] The plates are incubated for 8 to 20 hours at 37°, and the number of plaques are counted.

For determination of K (the first-order rate constant) of the serum, an inactivation experiment is performed as described above with 4 to 5 serum dilutions in the range previously found to cause 10 to 99% inactivation of the penicilloyl-T4 at the conditions employed. Plotting of the results (logarithm of surviving phage concentration as a function of the serum dilution) yields a straight line. K is calculated from the formula $K = 2.3D/t \times \log(P_0/P)$, where $P_0 =$ initial phage concentration, $P =$ phage concentration at time (t) of reaction, and $D =$ serum dilution. Figure 2 shows the results of a typical experiment.

iii. Inactivation of Poly-DL-alanyl-Bacteriophage T4 by an Antiserum with Polyalanyl Specificity

Poly-DL-alanyl T4 (1 ml of 10⁶ PFU/ml) and anti-polyalanyl serum (1 ml diluted 50-fold) are mixed (both solutions being prewarmed at 37° for 15 minutes). Aliquots of 0.1 ml are withdrawn at 2-minute intervals and diluted into 9.9 ml of GPB to stop the inactivation. From the diluted reaction mixtures, aliquots of 0.1 to 0.7 ml are plated as described above (direct plating).

For the decision method (see text footnote to Section f.i above), the aliquots to be plated are added to 0.2 ml of bacteria (10⁹/ml) and the tubes are shaken gently for 10 minutes at 37° A strong anti-T4 serum

[89] M. H. Adams, "Bacteriophages," pp. 450–451. Wiley (Interscience), New York, 1959.

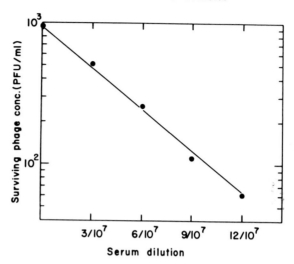

Fɪɢ. 2. Inactivation of penicilloyl-bacteriophage T4 by anti-penicilloyl serum. The reaction mixtures were incubated for 3 hours at 37°.

is then added (0.1 ml) in a final dilution found to inactivate 99.9% of the poly-ᴅʟ-alanyl T4 after 3 minutes of incubation. Reaction mixtures are shaken for an additional 4 to 5 minutes, top agar is poured into the tubes, and the whole mixture is plated. The results of such an experiment are summarized in Fig. 3.

iv. Inhibition of Inactivation of Penicilloyl-Bacteriophage T4

To a series of tubes containing 0.2 ml of anti-penicilloyl serum described in Fig. 2 (at a dilution of 3.6×10^{-6}), the inhibitor penicillin G or penicilloyl-ϵ-aminocaproic acid (0.2 ml) is added to a final concentration of 10^{-4} to 10^{-9} M. To a few tubes, buffer is added instead of inhibitor. The mixtures are kept at 37° for 30 minutes. Penicilloyl-T4 is added (0.2 ml containing about 600 PFU), and the mixtures are kept at 37° for an additional 3 hours and plated.

By preincubation of anti-penicilloyl antibodies with the inhibitor, the extent of inactivation of penicilloyl-T4, as compared to that obtained in the absence of inhibitor, is reduced and corresponds to an extent characteristic of a lower concentration of free antibody. For example, penicilloyl-T4 at an initial concentration of 10^3 PFU/ml was reduced to a concentration of 60 PFU/ml when allowed to react for 3 hours at 37° with anti-penicilloyl serum at a final dilution of $12:10^7$ (Fig. 2). By preincubating the antiserum at the same final dilution with penicillin G at a final concentration of 3×10^{-7} M, the amount of inactivation was reduced so that the concentration of viable phage dropped to only 200

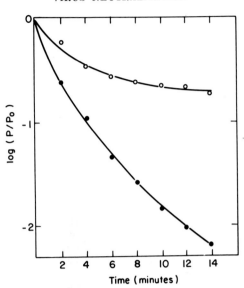

FIG. 3. Inactivation of poly-DL-alanyl-bacteriophage T4 by anti-poly-DL-alanyl RNase serum diluted 1:100 at 37°: ○, assays of survivors by direct plating; ●, assays of survivors by the "decision" technique. P = surviving phage concentration (PFU/ml). P_0 = initial phage concentration (PFU/ml). From J. Haimovich and M. Sela, *J. Immunol.* **97**, 338 (1966).

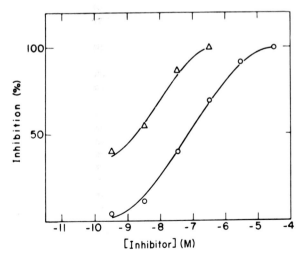

FIG. 4. Inhibition of the inactivation of penicilloyl-bacteriophage T4 by anti-penicilloyl serum with: ○, penicillin G; △, penicilloyl-ε-aminocaproic acid. For conditions, see text.

PFU/ml. This amount of inactivation corresponds to that obtained by only 60% of the initial concentration of antibody (see Fig. 2) and is therefore considered to be due to 40% inhibition of the antibodies by the inhibitor. Obviously, 100% inhibition results in no inactivation of the penicilloyl-T4 by the antiserum added.

An inhibition experiment performed as described above is summarized in Fig. 4.

For detection and quantitation of penicillin G, the same procedure is employed with 0.2 ml of the sample to be tested. By the extent of inhibition achieved and with the aid of the results summarized in Fig. 4 the amount of penicillin G in the sample tested is determined.

v. Inhibition of Inactivation of Protein–Phage Conjugates by Added Protein

Inhibition of the inactivation of protein–phage conjugates by free protein is performed in a similar manner except that protein and antibodies are allowed to react for longer times prior to the addition of phage (20 hours at 4° and an additional 2 hours at 37°).

World Health Organization Report on Nomenclature of Complement*

NOMENCLATURE OF COMPLEMENT*

The term "complement" is applied to a system of factors occurring in normal serum that are activated characteristically by antigen–antibody interaction and subsequently mediate a number of biologically significant consequences.

Study of the nature of complement has been concentrated to a large extent on analysis of the process of immune haemolysis,[1] and the nomenclature proposed for complement is based primarily on the haemolytic sequence. Nevertheless, it is recognized that not only may there be pathways of complement activity that diverge from the haemolytic pathway and require the participation of factors not required for immune haemolysis, but also parts of the complement system may be activated by mechanisms distinct from the sequential interactions occurring in immune haemolysis.

Complement, as it participates in immune haemolysis, comprises 9 components. It now appears established that these 9 factors are essentially similar, although not necessarily interchangeable, in the two species most studied—man and the guinea-pig—and it appear probable that this similarity extends to other mammalian species at least. For this reason it is now proposed that a uniform nomenclature be adopted for the various species that have been studied.

Several components of complement have been shown to have enzyme activity and it is to be anticipated that such activity will be described for more, and possibly for most, components. Eventually, therefore, a nomenclature may be envisaged for complement that follows the general

---

* Reprinted from *Bull. W.H.O.* **39**, 935–938 (1968).

* This memorandum was drafted as a result of a series of informal discussions arranged by the World Health Organization on the occasion of a number of international meetings. Those who participated in its drafting are denoted by an asterisk in the list of signatories . . .

[1] Immune haemolysis is the process whereby fresh normal serum (from any of a number of species) lyses red blood cells (usually from the sheep) treated with antibody to them (usually prepared in the rabbit).

biochemical conventions for the naming of enzymes. The notation proposed here should therefore be regarded as provisional until the necessary information becomes available.

THE COMPONENTS OF COMPLEMENT

A numerical notation is used for those complement components participating directly in the reaction of immune haemolysis. Hitherto the numbers have been preceded by the symbol C'. It is now suggested that this usage be changed and that the symbol C be used to denote complement components.

Although it would be desirable for the numerical symbols to parallel the reaction sequence—this being the procedure followed for all the more recently described components—it nevertheless appears unjustifiable to interfere with the well-established use of C1, C2 and C4 for particular components. In the order of their reaction the complement components should therefore be designated:

$$C1, C4, C2, C3, C5, C6, C7, C8, C9$$

The numbers (and letters) denoting complement components should not be subscript.

Other designations that have been used for complement components and some of their identifying properties are listed in Table 1.

First Component (C1)

The first component of human complement comprises 3 distinct protein subcomponents to which the provisional names C1q, C1r and C1s have been given. C1q was previously known as the 11S component or C'0.

Although the 3 subcomponents are separate molecules, they appear to function as a unit and to occur as a macromolecular complex *in vivo*. For these reasons it is recommended that the term C1 be used wherever possible, but that, where required, the existing nomenclature be retained for the present, although in general the use of lettered suffixes or subscripts for subcomponents should be given up.

INTERMEDIATE COMPLEXES

E is used for erythrocyte, S for a single site of initiation of complement fixation, and A for antibody in conjunction with C followed by those components which have interacted. The components enumerated after EAC denote a state of reactivity, not necessarily their physical presence.

In current usage the intermediate complex is often written with the lower-case letter "a" suffixed to components showing enzyme or other bio-

TABLE 1

NOMENCLATURE OF COMPLEMENT COMPONENTS

Recommended nomenclature for complement component	Previous designation	Approximate electrophoretic mobility (human C)	Approximate sedimentation coefficient (Svedberg units) (human C)
C1 C1q	11S component, C'0	$\gamma 2$	11
C1r		β	7
C1s	C'1-esterase (after activation)	$\alpha 2$	4
C4	β1E globulin	$\beta 1$	10
C2		$\beta 2$	6
C3	C'3c, C'3a, β1C globulin	$\beta 1$	10
C5	C'3b, C'3b, β1F globulin	$\beta 1$	8.7
C6	C'3e, C'3α	$\beta 2$	6
C7	C'3f, C'3β	$\beta 2$	6
C8	C'3a, C'3c	$\gamma 1$	8
C9	C'3d, C'3d	$\alpha 2$	5

logical activity when on that complex. For example, EAC'1a, 4, 2a, 3 represents the complex produced by the reaction of the first 4 components.

It is proposed that in future the intermediate complex should be written without suffixes, e.g., EAC1423 for the complex above. Alternatively, the example may be shortened to EAC1–3.

Where the activity of components is lost from the intermediate complex, the components concerned are deleted. Thus EAC43 represents the intermediate complex resulting from the loss of C1 and C2 activity from EAC1423.

The functional cell-membrane lesion at a site of complement fixation is denoted as S*.

Where the fragments of components fixed on the intermediate complex or the activation or inactivation of a particular reactive site are to be denoted, it is recommended that this be done in a separate description according to the conventions outlined below.

Complement Components Showing Altered Activity

At present, the suffix "a" is used to denote the acquisition by a component or group of components of an enzymatic or other biological activity. Thus C1a denotes the activated form of C1, which has esterase activity in relation to a number of amino-acid esters and destroys C4 and C2 in solution. The C1s subcomponent from C1a (which has been called C1-esterase) is itself enzymatically active and is therefore denoted C1sa. Similarly C(42)a denotes the activity described as C3-convertase, and C(567)a the chemotactic factor derived from C5, C6 and C7.

It is proposed to substitute for the suffix "a" a bar or rule placed over the affected component. Thus $\overline{C1}$ will replace C'1a, $\overline{C42}$ will replace C(42)a and $C\overline{567}$ will replace C(567)a.

Similarly, the loss by a complement component of a defined activity has been denoted by the suffix "i", and it is proposed that this usage be continued. However, it is highly probable that in many cases the inactivated compounds represent fragments produced by cleavage of the parent molecule. When sufficient information is available to designate the inactivated components as fragments (see below), this is to be preferred.

Fragments and Chains

It is anticipated that growing attention will be given to the molecular structure of individual components and that a consistent nomenclature will be helpful both for the fragments produced by peptide-bond breakage and for separated polypeptide chains.

It is proposed that fragments produced during the complement-fixation reaction by peptide-bond cleavage should be denoted in the general form Cn a, b, c . . . As examples, the fragments of C3 and C5 showing anaphylatoxin activity are designated C3a and C5a.

Where fragments are produced artificially by peptide-bond cleavage, the enzyme or other agent used may be placed after the fragment, e.g., C3a (trypsin) for the anaphylatoxin from C3 by trypsin. Where an artificial fragment is shown to be structurally identical with a fragment produced during complement fixation, the designation of the artificial treatment may be omitted.

The mechanism of the interaction of SA with the first four components, which yields the product SAC1423, could thus be written in terms of fragments and active enzymes:

$$C4 + C2 \rightleftarrows C4,2 \cdot \xrightarrow{\ \overline{C1}\ } C\overline{4,2a} \qquad\qquad C3 \xrightarrow{\ C\overline{4,2a}\ } C\overline{4,2a,3b} + C3a$$

TABLE 2

FACTORS[a] OTHER THAN COMPLEMENT COMPONENTS REACTING
IN THE COMPLEMENT SEQUENCE

Factor	Abbreviation or synonym in use	Approximate electrophoretic mobility	Relation to complement
C$\bar{1}$ inactivator	C1 esterase inhibitor	$\alpha2$	Inactivates C$\bar{1}$, both fixed and in free solution. Also inhibits kallikrein and PF/Dil.[b]
C3 inactivator (Conglutinogen Activating Factor)	KAF	$\beta1$	Reacts with fixed C3 making this reactive with conglutinin and reducing its haemolytic and immune adherence activity
C6 inactivator		$\beta2$	Inactivates fixed C6
Conglutinin	K	$\beta2$	Aggregates intermediate complexes containing fixed C3 which has been acted upon by KAF (C3 inactivator)
Immunoconglutinins	IK	γ	Autoantibodies to fixed C3 and C4
Plasmin	Fibrinolysin	$\beta1$	Acts upon C1s to activate it to C1-esterase and upon C3 in solution to yield a chemotactic fragment
Properdin		γ	In conjunction with naturally occurring antibodies, complement components and magnesium ions, plays a part in killing certain bacteria and neutralizing certain viruses

[a] These factors should be designated in full; if abbreviations are used, however, they should be explicitly described.

[b] Miles, A. A. & Wilhelm, D. L. (1955) *Brit. J. exp. Path.*, **36**, 71–81.

Note added by Editors: The alternative pathway of complement activation (Section 17.A.2) was not established in 1968. Likewise, the role of properdin was unknown.

Polypeptide chains would in an analogous way be designated α, β, chain Cn.

COMPLEMENT FACTORS NOT DIRECTLY INVOLVED IN THE HAEMOLYTIC SEQUENCE

A number of serum factors are known to react with the intermediate complex or with the products of complement fixation, although they play no essential role in immune haemolysis. They are enumerated in Table 2. It is not proposed that any systematic nomenclature be devised for them at the present time apart from the application, where appropriate, of the foregoing complement-component nomenclature.

GLOSSARY OF ABBREVIATIONS

E	Erythrocyte
S	Single site of complement activation
A	Antibody
C	Complement
C1, C2 . . . C9	Complement components
SAC1234 . . . n SAC 1–n	Intermediate complexes formed by the reaction of the first n complement components
Cn, a, b, c . . .	Fragments of complement components produced by peptide-bond cleavage
α, β, γ . . . chain Cn	Polypeptide chains of complement components
$C\bar{n}$	Complement component that has acquired enzymatic or other biological activity
Cni	Complement component that has lost a defined activity

* * *

* K. F. AUSTEN, Robert Bent Brigham Hospital, Harvard Medical School, Boston, Mass., USA

* E. L. BECKER, Walter Reed Army Institute of Research, Washington, D.C., USA

C. E. BIRO, Instituto Nacional de Cardiologia, Mexico City, Mexico

* T. BORSOS, National Institutes of Health, Bethesda, Md., USA

A. P. DALMASSO, Instituto de Biologia y Medicina Experimental, Buenos Aires, Argentina

W. DIAS DA SILVA, Universidade de Minas Gerais, Belo Horizonte, Brazil

H. ISLIKER, Institut de Biochimie, Université de Lausanne, Lausanne, Vaud, Switzerland

P. KLEIN, Institut für Medizinische Mikrobiologie der Johannes Gutenberg-Universität, Mainz, Federal Republic of Germany

* P. J. LACHMANN, Department of Pathology, University of Cambridge, Cambridge, England

M. A. LEON, Department of Pathology Research, St Luke's Hospital, Cleveland, O., USA

* I. H. LEPOW, Health Center, University of Connecticut, Hartford, Conn., USA

* M. M. MAYER, School of Medicine, Johns Hopkins University, Baltimore, Md., USA

* H. J. MÜLLER-EBERHARD, Scripps Clinic and Research Foundation, La Jolla, Calif., USA

* R. A. NELSON, University of California, San Diego, Calif., USA

U. NILSSON, Institute of Medical Microbiology, Lund, Sweden (present address: Hospital of the University of Pennsylvania, Philadelphia, Pa., USA)

I. NISHIOKA, National Cancer Research Institute, Tokyo, Japan

* H. J. RAPP, National Institutes of Health, Bethesda, Md., USA

* F. S. ROSEN, Children's Hospital, Harvard Medical School, Boston, Mass., USA

* Z. TRNKA, Immunology, World Health Organization, Geneva, Switzerland

P. A. WARD, Armed Forces Institute of Pathology, Washington, D.C., USA

A. C. WARDLAW, School of Hygiene, University of Toronto, Toronto, Canada

APPENDIX II

The International System of Units: SI Nomenclature*

Recommendations that all scientific and technical journals should adopt the system of units known as SI (Système International d'Unités) have come from the Royal Society Conference of Editors, Great Britain, The American Chemical Society, the Institute of Electrical and Electronic Engineers, the American Society for Testing and Materials, and others.

SI, which is an extension and refinement of the traditional metric system, was formally approved by the Conférence Générale des Poids et Mesures in 1960, and indorsed by the International Organization for Standardization.

BASIC UNITS AND MULTIPLIERS

There are only six basic units: metre (meter), m; kilogramme (kilogram), kg; second, s; ampere, A; degree Kelvin, $°K$; candela for luminous intensity, cd. None is pluralized. To these are added: amount of substance, mole (mol), defined as the amount of substance of a system which contains as many elementary units (atoms, molecules, ions, electrons, photons, et cetera) as there are carbon atoms in exactly 0.012 kg of the pure nuclide ^{12}C.

Multiples and fractions of the six basic units take the following forms:

Multiple	Prefix	Symbol	Fraction	Prefix	Symbol
10^{12}	tera	T	$(10^{-1}$	deci	d)
10^9	giga	G	$(10^{-2}$	centi	c)
10^6	mega	M	10^{-3}	milli	m
10^3	kilo	k	10^{-6}	micro	u
$(10^2$	hecto	h)	10^{-9}	nano	n
$(10$	deka	da)	10^{-12}	pico	p
			10^{-15}	femto	f
			10^{-18}	atto	a

* Appendix II was submitted by Merrill W. Chase.

Multiples of units are normally to be restricted to steps of a thousand, and fractions to steps of a thousandth. Expressions in parentheses are to be restricted to the early days of metrication where the centimeter has been the unit of length in certain biological measurements. Also the gram will be retained at present (as, μg, ng).

The attaching of a prefix constitutes in effect a new unit: $1\ km^2 = 1\ (km)^2$. Only a single prefix should be attached to basic units.

SUPPLEMENTARY UNITS

These units are dimensionless.

Physical quantity	Name of unit	Symbol for unit
plane angle	radian	rad
solid angle	steradian	sr

DERIVED SI UNITS WITH SPECIAL NAMES[a]

Physical quantity	Name of unit	Symbol	Definition
energy	joule[b]	J	$kg\ m^2/s^2 = N\ m = W\ s$
force	newton[c]	N	$kg\ m/s^2 = J/m$
power	watt	W	$kg\ m^2/s^3 = J/s$
electric charge[d]	coulomb	C	$A\ s$
electric potential difference[d]	volt	V	$kg\ m^2/s^3\ A = J/A\ s$
electric resistance[d]	ohm	Ω	$kg\ m^2/s^3\ A^2 = V/A$
electric conductance[d]	Siemen	S	$\Omega^{-1} = A/V$
electric capacitance[d]	farad	F	$A^2\ s^4/kg\ m^2 = A\ s/V$
magnetic flux	weber	Wb	$kg\ m^2/s^2\ A = V\ s$
inductance	henry	H	$kg\ m^2/s^2\ A^2 = V\ s/A$
magnetic flux density	tesla	T	$kg/s^2\ A = V\ s/m^2$
luminous flux	lumen	lm	$cd\ sr$
illumination	lux	lx	$cd\ sr/m^2$
frequency	hertz	Hz	cycle per second
customary temperature, t	degree Celsius	°C	$t/°C = T/°K - 273.15$

[a] New derived units can be added, such as the Siemen, the Pascal.

[b] The joule (newton × meter) is the unit of energy, while joule/sec (watt) is the unit of power. Accordingly, kilowatt hour, B.t.u., horsepower, and calories are superseded.

[c] The unit of force, the newton (kg m/s²), being independent of terrestrial gravitation, allows the removal of g in equations.

[d] SI electrical units replace electrostatic and electromagnetic units.

EXAMPLES OF OTHER DERIVED SI UNITS

Physical quantity	SI unit	Symbol for unit
area	square metre	m^2
volume	cubic metre	m^3
density	kilogramme per cubic metre	kg/m^3
velocity	metre per second	m/s
angular velocity	radian per second	rad/s
acceleration	metre per second squared	m/s^2
pressure	⎰newton per square metre ⎱Pascal	⎰N/m^2 ⎱Pa
kinematic viscosity, diffusion coefficient	square metre per second	m^2/s
dynamic viscosity	⎰newton second per square metre ⎱Pascal-second	⎰$N\ s/m^2$ ⎱Pa s
electric field strength	volt per metre	V/m
magnetic field strength	ampere per metre	A/m
luminance	candela per square metre	cd/m^2

UNITS TO BE ALLOWED IN CONJUNCTION WITH SI

Physical quantity	Name of unit	Symbol	Definition
length	parsec	pc	30.87×10^{15} m
area	barn	b	$10^{-28} m^2$
	hectare	ha	$10^4\ m^2$
volume	litre	l	$10^{-3}\ m^3 = dm^3$
pressure	bar	bar	$10^5\ N/m^2$
mass	tonne	t	$10^3\ kg = Mg$
kinematic viscosity, diffusion coefficient	stokes	St	$10^{-4} m^2/s$
dynamic viscosity	poise	P	$10^{-1}\ kg/m\ s$
magnetic flux density (magnetic induction)	gauss	G	10^{-4} T
radioactivity	curie	Ci	$3.7 \times 10^{10}/s$
energy	electronvolt	eV	1.6021×10^{-19} J

The common units of time (e.g., hour, year) will persist, and also, in appropriate contexts, the angular degree.

EXAMPLES OF UNITS *Contrary to SI*, WITH THEIR EQUIVALENTS[a]
Use of these terms is to be discouraged

Physical quantity	Unit	Equivalent
length	ångström	10^{-10} m
	inch	0.0254 m
	foot	0.3048 m
	yard	0.9144 m
	mile	1.60934 km
	nautical mile	1.85318 km
area	square inch	645.16 mm^2
	square foot	0.092903 m^2
	square yard	0.836127 m^2
	square mile	2.58999 km^2
volume	cubic inch	1.63871×10^{-5} m^3
	cubic foot	0.0283168 m^3
	Imperial gallon	0.004546092 m^3
	U.S. gallon	0.003785412 m^3
mass	pound	0.45359237 kg
density	pound/cubic inch	2.76799×10^4 kg/m^3
	pound/cubic foot	16.0185 kg/m^3
force	dyne	10^{-5} N
	poundal	0.138255 N
	pound-force	4.44822 N
	kilogramme-force	9.80665 N
pressure	atmosphere	101.325 kN/m^2
	torr	133.322 N/m^2
	pound (f)/sq. in.	6894.76 N/m^2
energy	erg	10^{-7} J
	calorie (I.T.)	4.1868 J
	calorie (15°C)	4.1855 J
	calorie (thermochemical)	4.184 J
	B.t.u.	1055.06 J
	foot poundal	0.0421401 J
	foot pound (f)	1.35582 J
power	horse power	745.700 W
temperature	degree Rankine	5/9 °K
	degree Fahrenheit	$t/°F = 9/5T/°C + 32$

[a] Fuller lists are to be found in the National Physical Laboratory's "Changing to the Metric System" (Anderton and Brigg) H.M.S.O., London, 1966, and "Units, Symbols and Abbreviations. A Guide for Biological and Medical Editors and Authors," (G. Ellis, ed.), The Royal Society of Medicine, London, 1972.

Author Index

Numbers in parentheses are footnote reference numbers and indicate that an author's work is referred to although his name is not cited in the text.

A

Aaronson, S. A., 317(28, 29), 321, 369, 373, 374(242, 266)
Abeyounis, C. J., 61, 65(f), 66
Accolla, R. S., 353
Ackermann, W. W., 333
Ada, G. L., 91
Adams, M. H., 276, 316(16), 321, 376, 377, 378(3, 16), 380(3), 395
Adebahr, M .E., 16
Adler, F. L., 41
Aebi, H., 349
Ager, J. A. M., 121
Agnello, V., 191, 194(34), 198, 269
Aguilu, L. A., 7
Aharonov, A., 387
Aiken, B. S., 132
Ainslie, R. B., 141
Aird, J., 386
Aitken, R. M., 62
Akeroyd, J. H., 4, 73
Albert, D. M., 374
Albrecht, F., 318(58), 322, 330
Allain, D. S., 121
Allen, F. H., Jr., 16
Allen, K., 293, 294(2)
Allison, W. S., 359(73), 361
Almeida, J., 340, 341, 342(102)
Alouf, J. E., 287, 288
Alper, C. A., 130, 258, 259, 350
Alsever, J. B., 141
Altman, Y., 388
Altmann, G., 116, 117, 118(3)
Amano, T., 318(64, 68, 69, 70, 71, 72), 322, 323, 335, 344, 351(68), 356, 368
Amiraian, K., 319(89), 323, 359(59), 361
Amos, H. E., 389
Anderson, B., 13
Anderson, R. L., 372
Andres, G. A., 326
Andrewes, C. H., 378
Andrieu, J. M., 386, 388(15)

Anfinsen, C. B., 317(43, 44, 45, 46, 47), 322, 331, 335(50), 344, 351, 352, 355, 387
Angeletti, P. U., 317(35), 322
Antczak, D. F., 387
Aoki, T., 99
Appella, E., 359(21), 360, 364, 365
Armstrong, S. H., Jr., 21
Arnason, B. G. W., 387
Arnheim, N., Jr., 368, 369
Arnon, R., 315, 318(67), 319(90, 92), 323, 335, 336, 340, 342, 344, 349, 351(65, 66), 356, 359(74, 81, 82), 361, 368, 369, 387, 388, 393
Aronson, T., 212
Arquilla, E. R., 31, 45
Arroyave, C. M., 131, 217, 270
Asahi, M., 319(95), 323
Askonas, B. A., 34
Aston, W. P., 183, 185(5), 251, 252(32)
Attardi, G., 373, 381(5)
Atwood, K. C., 20
Austen, K. F., 133, 179, 210, 245, 250, 251, 254, 255, 269, 270, 336
Austin, C. M., 91
Avegno, P., 394
Avery, O. T., 88
Avrameas, S., 222, 251, 326, 359(26), 360
Aye, M. T., 374

B

Babinet, C., 317(26), 321
Bach, M. L., 366
Badin, J., 68
Baechtel, S., 319(101), 324
Bailey, A., 15
Bailey, L. H., 22(a), 23
Baker, J. R., 102
Baltimore, D., 373, 374(264)
Bandhauer, K., 109
Bandhaur, K., 104, 109(37)
Barber, P., 386, 394(7)

Subject Index

Page numbers in italic type refer to figures, tables, or reaction schemes.

A

AbH$_{50}$, unit of hemolytic antibody, 152

ABO blood groups, 11, 13, 20, 24, 25;
  see also Blood group cellular antigens; Blood group substances; Blood typing (human)
  Ii specificity concealed in A substances, 13
  lectins to determine groups, 20
  soluble secretor substances precipitated by sieva lectin, 24, 25

Acatalasemia (Swiss type), defective enzyme in, 349

α-Acceptors, 353

ω-Acceptors, 353, 354

ACD (acid–citrate–dextrose) solution, 33, 138, 141, 142; see also Alsever's solution
  NIH formula A, 138, 141; NIH formula B, 17, 141; other formulations, 141
  stabilization period for RBC, 142

N-Acetyl-p-aminophenyl lactoside (LAC), coupling to bacteriophage, 387

Acetylcholinesterase, stabilization by Ab, 348

β-N-Acetylgalactosamine, 371

Acetyl(tri)-glucosamine, lysozyme inhibitor, 356

N-Acetyl-β-hexosaminodase, 371
  deficiency in human diseases, 371
  molecular forms, 371

N-Acetyl lactosamine, 371

Acetyl lysine methyl ester, esterolysis by urokinase, 245

N-Acetyl-L-phenylalanine ethyl ester, hydrolysis by C1s̄, 201

N-Acetyl-L-tyrosine ethyl ester (ATE), substrate for C1̄, C1s̄, 184, 185, 190, 201, 204, 249, 370

N-Acetyl-L-tyrosine methyl ester, hydrolysis by C1s̄, 201

Adenosine diphosphate (ADP), regulatory molecule for glutamic dehydrogenase, 330

Adenosine triphosphatase (ATPase), 320, 335, 365
  antigenic sites, 335
  inhibition by Ab, 320
  isozymic forms, 365

Adenosine triphosphate (ATP), substrate for creatine kinase, 331

5'-Adenylic acid deaminase, 320, 330
  inhibition by Ab, 320
  protection by substrate, 330

Adjuvants in immunization, 55, 268, 270
  alumina, 268
  Freund's adjuvant, 55, 270

ADP, see Adenosine diphosphate

Affinity (antibodies), 67; see Antibodies; Avidity

Affinity chromatography, 19, 221, 222, 267
  C1q binding to Sepharose-IgG, 195
  C8 purified by insolubilized anti-IgG, 221, 222

Agar, 77, 133
  activation of alternative C-pathway, 133
  cross-reaction with blood group substances, 77

Agglutination, see also Agglutination of bacteria; Antiglobulin mixed reactions; Bentonite flocculation test; Hemagglutination, direct; Hemagglutination, passive; Latex fixation test; Lectins; Mixed agglutination
  bacteria, 76–90
  erythrocytes
    direct, 1–20, 67–75
    indirect by anti-globulin Ab, 10–12, 36, 49–66
    passive hemagglutination, 26–66
  human blood groups: by antisera, 1–20, by lectins, 19–26, 68
  lattice hypothesis, 21, 57
  "pattern" (IgM vs IgG), 39, 44
  phage, 377, 383

Bacterial immobilization, 91ff
　anti-H antibody production by Ab and
　　Ab-producing cells, 91ff
　end-point counts, 92, 93
　maintenance of motile cultures, 83, 91
　procedure, 92: counting chamber, 92
Bacterial species, 26–30, 36, 37, 76, 77,
　　80–86, 88–90, 113, 136, 275–282,
　　284–287, 292, 316, 317, 319, 331, 332,
　　349, 353, 366, 367, 381, 382; *see also*
　　Spores (bacterial)
　bacilli: *B. anthracis*, 84, 86; *B. botu-*
　　linus, 312, 313; *B. cereus*, 82,
　　320, 367; *B. licheniformis*, 320; *B.*
　　palustris, 319; *B. subtilis*, 318, 320,
　　351
　Bordetella pertussis, 76, *85, 86*
　Brucellae, 76, 77, 80, *85*
　Citrobacter, *86*
　clostridia: *C. histolyticum*, 319, *C.*
　　oedematiens, 319, *C. tetani*, 284,
　　319; *C. welchii* (*perfringens*), 292,
　　317, 319, 332
　Corynebacterium diphtheriae, 36, 37,
　　275–282
　Diplococcus pneumoniae, 26–30, 76, 77,
　　81, 85, 88, 90, 136
　Escherichia coli, 27, 29, 30, 84, 86, 113,
　　316, 317, 319, 349, 353, 366, 367, 381,
　　382
　gonococci, 71
　Klebsiella (polysaccharides), 30
　mycobacteria, 27, 82, 84–86, 317, 319:
　　atypical, 82, 84–86; *M. bovis*, 319;
　　M. phlei, 317; *M. tuberculosis*, 27
　Pasteurella (*Francisella*) *tularensis*, 77,
　　85, 86
　Proteus: OX-19, 90; spp., 80
　Pseudomonas aeruginosa ("PC-9 anti-
　　gen"), 29
　salmonellae, 77, 80, 83, 85, 86, 90; *S.*
　　typhi O antigen, 28, 30, 80, 83, 84,
　　89, 90
　Serratia marcescens (P-15 antigen), 29
　shigellae, 76
　staphylococci, 76, 81, 83, *85*, 317, 331
　streptococci (hemolytic), 76, 285–289
Bacterial spores, *see* Spores, bacterial
Bacteriophage, 376, 377, 380–385, 390, *see*
　　also Bacteriophage–antibody inter-

actions; Bacteriophage, chemically
　modified; Viruses, animal; Viruses,
　types of; Vol. I, Chapter 1.D.3
antigens, *see also* Vol. I, Chapter 1.D.3
　internal: proteins, nucleic acids, 376,
　　377
　surface: membranes, tails, sheaths,
　　375, 377
　anti-phage antibodies (preparation),
　　376, 377
　f2 phages, 377
　homogeneity, 380
　hybrids, 381, 384: head membranes
　　with parental antigens, 384
　mutants, 382
　ϕX-174, 377, 390
　proflavin: prevention of phage multi-
　　plication, 382
　radiolabeling, 384
　ruptured phages as antigens, 40, 165,
　　376, 385
　T-even phages, 376, 377, 384, 390
　　head and tail: antigen differences,
　　　385
　　nucleic acids as antigens, 385
　　solubilized T2 on tanned RBC, 40
　　T2/T6 hybrids, 384
　　T6: denatured DNA in cross reac-
　　　tions with T2, T4, 165
　　T6 antiserum, 384
　UV light to inactivate, 382
　viral antigens prior to infectivity, 385
Bacteriophage–antibody interactions,
　　375–386, 394, 395, 397; *see also*
　　Bacteriophage; Viruses, animal;
　　Viruses, types of; Vol. I, Chapter
　　1.D.3
　antibody reactions
　　agglutination, 377, 383: detection of
　　　antigens not involved in neutral-
　　　ization, 384
　　complement fixation tests, 384, 385
　　neutralization (tail, sheath antigens),
　　　375–382, 386: neutralization con-
　　　stant, 378, 379, *380*
　　precipitation (quantitative), 382–384
　antigenicity, 376
　antigens detected within host bacteria,
　　375, 380

Complement-related proteins, Factor D
(*continued*)
  assay: tryptic conversion to $\bar{D}$,
    + CoF + Factor B, then sheep
    RBC + serum, 255
  procedure, 255
  resistance to DFP, 254
  Factor $\bar{D}$ (C3-proactivator-convertase
    or C3PA*ase*; GBG*ase*), 130, 133,
    242, 254, 256, 258
    guinea pig $\bar{D}$, 256–258
      assay: ZX (zymosan-properdin),
        decay to C3b: ZX^d + Factor
        B +C3 + Factor $\bar{D}$, assess C3
        inactivation, 258
      procedure, 256, 257; purity, 258
    human $\bar{D}$ (serine esterase)
      assay: CoF + Factor B + Factor
        $\bar{D}$, then sheep RBC + serum, 256
      inactivation by DFP, 254
      procedure, 256
      tryptic conversion D → $\bar{D}$, 254
  Factor E (properdin), 130, 133, 256
  properdin (P), 130, 132, 133, 253, 254
    assay: inactivated serum + P +
      factor B: C3 conversion in IEA;
      solid-phase radioimmunoassay, 254
    characteristics, 253
    procedure, 253, 254; purity, 254
Concanavalin A (jack bean), pan-
  hemagglutinin for human RBC, 20,
  21
Conductivity measurements, 206, 225
Conglutinin, 129, 213, 252
Conglutinogen-activating factor (KAF;
  C3b-In), 130, 133, 136, 250, 252
Conjugation methods (protein–protein,
  protein–cell surface, protein–bac-
  teriophage), 41, 47, 48, 326, 390, 392
  BDB: 41, 47, 48, 392; CrCl$_3$: 48;
    DCCI: 390; DFDNB: 48; ECDI:
    48; glutaraldehyde, 326, 392;
    TDIC, 392
Coombs tests, *see* Antiglobulin consump-
  tion test; Antiglobulin reactions
  with erythrocytes; Mixed agglutina-
  tion; Mixed antiglobulin reactions;
  Mixed hemadsorption
Conformational changes, 131, 330–337,
  348–356

during cleavage of complement components, 131
effect of Ab on enzymes, 330, 331, 335–
  337, 348–350, 354
Corynebacterium diphtheriae, 36, 37,
  275–282
  bacteriophage as toxin, 275–282
  toxoid, 36, 37
Coulter counter for RBC standardization, 5, 7: use with partially agglutinated RBC, 7, 8
Craigie U-tubes (bacterial motility), 83,
  91
C-reactive protein (latex agglutination
  test), 120
Creatine-ATP phosphotransferase, inhibition by Ab, 317
Creatine hydrate, 331
Creatine kinase, 330, 331
  failure of protection by substrate, 330
  protection: 2 substrates, 331
Crotalaria aegyptica, Crotolaria falcata:
  sources of anti-A lectins, 22
Crotalus terrificus, lecithinase, 317
CVF (cobra venom factor), *see* Complement-related proteins
Cyclic cytidylic acid, *see* Cytidylic acid
Cyclic uridylic acid, *see* Uridylic acid
Cytidylic acid (cytidine phosphate) as
  enzyme substrate, 327–329, 339, 340,
  344–346
  cyclic form, 339, 344, *345, 346*
  methyl ester, 339
Cytisus sessifolia, source of anti-H lectin,
  23
Cytochrome *c,* evolutionary development, 369
Cytotoxicity, 244; *see also* Immune
  hemolysis
  amnion cells protected *vs* Ab by
    C$\bar{1}$-INH, 244
  staphylotoxin, 290

D

Dansyl chloride (5-dimethylamino-
  naphthalene sulfonyl chloride),
  haptenation of bacteriophage, 386
Danysz phenomenon, 340–342
DCCI, *see* Dicyclohexyl carbodiimide